Education and Communication in Veterinary Clinical Practice

Education and Communication in Veterinary Clinical Practice

Guest Editor

Paul Mills

MDPI

Basel • Beijing • Wuhan • Barcelona • Belgrade • Novi Sad • Cluj • Manchester

Guest Editor
Paul Mills
School of Veterinary Science
The University of Queensland
Gatton
Australia

Editorial Office
MDPI AG
Grosspeteranlage 5
4052 Basel, Switzerland

This is a reprint of the Special Issue, published open access by the journal *Animals* (ISSN 2076-2615), freely accessible at: https://www.mdpi.com/journal/animals/special_issues/7CR95Y3SG3.

For citation purposes, cite each article independently as indicated on the article page online and as indicated below:

Lastname, A.A.; Lastname, B.B. Article Title. *Journal Name* **Year**, *Volume Number*, Page Range.

ISBN 978-3-7258-4933-8 (Hbk)
ISBN 978-3-7258-4934-5 (PDF)
https://doi.org/10.3390/books978-3-7258-4934-5

Contents

About the Editor

Paul Mills

Paul Mills is a veterinary pharmacologist and a veterinary educator. He has led nationally funded projects on veterinary education and received institutional and national teaching excellence awards. He served a term on the Editorial Board for the *Journal of Veterinary Medical Education* and was the inaugural Australian member for the Committee for International Veterinary Medical Education (CIVME). Prof Mills holds several qualifications for education, including a Graduate Certificate in Higher Education and an MPhil in Veterinary Education, and is a Principal Fellow of the Higher-Education Academy.

animals

MDPI

Editorial

Education and Communication in Veterinary Clinical Practice

Paul C. Mills

School of Veterinary Science, The University of Queensland, Gatton Campus, Gatton, QLD 4343, Australia; p.mills@uq.edu.au

Effective communication is a hallmark of successful veterinary clinical practice. Communication underpins professionalism, establishes effective teamwork, and is essential to veterinary–client relationships. Teaching or developing effective communication is an increasingly important component of the 'hidden' curriculum for veterinary educators, introduced and reinforced throughout the teaching program. Effective communication is also a focus for prospective employers when considering a new graduate. Successful communication must also consider the rapidly changing modalities of how people communicate and, importantly, how important communication will be toward resilience in a highly stressful profession.

The 'intervention' of COVID-19 rapidly taught everyone that traditional approaches to communication were not always feasible or safe. A paradigm shift occurred for many higher education providers, particularly during the peak stages of the pandemic, when face-to-face (F-2-F) teaching was either not permitted or impractical. Indeed, the emergency response teaching [1] largely consisted of rapid, large-scale online adaptation of teaching and assessment strategies [2]. eLearning became the new paradigm as teachers and educators attempted to maintain student learning within pandemic restrictions that varied by country and region. Blended learning and flipped classrooms have been reported to be educationally sound [3–6], so it was pleasing to include examples in this Special Issue where veterinary educators have also used these approaches successfully. Using flipped classrooms and/or blended learning to successfully teach cardiac auscultation and anatomical structure are examples of teaching that would normally only be considered effective in an F-2-F setting. An important outcome of using flipped classrooms is that students are more likely to engage in deep learning strategies due to a reduction in cognitive load [7,8].

It was interesting that several articles in this Special Issue focused on enhancing interpersonal and interprofessional communication skills. Returning to the impact of COVID-19, it was highlighted that human physicians tend to consider veterinarians as having a superior knowledge and understanding of zoonoses [9,10]. This superior comprehension and ability to diagnose [11] places veterinarians in a unique position at the human–animal interface [12], elevating the importance of interprofessional communication.

An important underlying theme of this Special Issue is that successful and safe graduate transition to veterinary clinical practice is associated with communication competency development [13,14]. It was therefore pleasing to see veterinary educators describing their success in using blended learning approaches to improve communication and establish personal relationships between veterinarians and the pet owners, which has been reported to improve the quality and outcomes of medical treatments [15,16]. This Special Issue takes this further by teaching students to self-assess their communication skills, adding an important cognitive alignment to the increasingly popular use of self-directed learning (SDL).

The importance of effective communication exceeds many barriers that could normally be expected to restrict learning. What the papers included in this Special Issue have in common is veterinary educators adopting and adapting aspects of learning theory to enhance the outcomes in veterinary science students by focusing on communication at multiple levels of the curriculum.

Conflicts of Interest: The author declares no conflict of interest.

List of Contributions:

1. Singh, A.A.; Shapter, F.M.; Bernard, A.; Whitworth, D.J.; Holt, M.G.; Waller, P.S.; Bond, S.L. Applying Iterative Student Feedback across Flipped Classroom and Flexible Teaching Approaches: Impact on Veterinary Students' Learning Experience. *Animals* **2024**, *14*, 2335; https://doi.org/10.3390/ani14162335.
2. Arnecke, A.L.; Schwarz, S.; Lübke-Becker, A.; Jensen, K.C.; Herre, C.; Bahramsoltani, M. Risk Communication on Zoonoses and Antimicrobial Resistance—How Do Exotic Pet Owners Perceive the Communication of Their Veterinarians? *Animals* **2024**, *14*, 2035; https://doi.org/10.3390/ani14142035.
3. Wood, A.; Shapter, F.M.; Stewart, A.J. Assessment of a Teaching Module for Cardiac Auscultation of Horses by Veterinary Students. *Animals* **2024**, *14*, 1341; https://doi.org/10.3390/ani14091341.
4. Heise, S.A.C.; Tipold, A.; Rohn, K.; Kleinsorgen, C. Measuring Veterinarian Professions' Readiness for Interprofessional Learning in a Pre- and Post-Intervention Study. *Animals* **2024**, *14*, 229; https://doi.org/10.3390/ani14020229.
5. van Gelderen, I.; Taylor, R. Developing Communication Competency in the Veterinary Curriculum. *Animals* **2023**, *13*, 3668; https://doi.org/10.3390/ani13233668.
6. MacMartin, C.; Wheat, H.; Coe, J.B. Conversation Analysis of Clients' Active Resistance to Veterinarians' Proposals for Long-Term Dietary Change in Companion Animal Practice in Ontario, Canada. *Animals* **2023**, *13*, 2150; https://doi.org/10.3390/ani13132150.
7. Gómez, O.; García-Manzanares, M.; Chicharro, D.; Juárez, M.; Llamazares-Martín, C.; Soriano, E.; Terrado, J. Application of Blended Learning to Veterinary Gross Anatomy Practical Sessions: Students' Perceptions of Their Learning Experience and Academic Outcomes. *Animals* **2023**, *13*, 1666; https://doi.org/10.3390/ani13101666.
8. Blázquez-Llorca, L.; Morales de Paz, L.; Martín-Orti, R.; Santos-Álvarez, I.; Fernández-Valle, M.E.; Castejón, D.; García-Real, M.I.; Salgüero-Fernández, R.; Pérez-Lloret, P.; Moreno, N.; et al. The Application of 3D Anatomy for Teaching Veterinary Clinical Neurology. *Animals* **2023**, *13*, 1601; https://doi.org/10.3390/ani13101601.
9. Kneissl, S.M.; Tichy, A.; Mitlacher, S.F. Flipped Classroom to Facilitate Deeper Learning in Veterinary Undergraduate Students: An Educational Change Pilot Study Limited to the Imaging Module Bones. *Animals* **2023**, *13*, 1540; https://doi.org/10.3390/ani13091540.
10. Bahramsoltani, M.; Bröer, S.; Langforth, S.; Eule, C.; Prior, A.; Vogt, L.; Li, T.-T.; Schirone, R.; Pohl, A.; Jensen, K.C. Outcome of Communication Training in Veterinary Studies: Influence on the Perception of the Relevance of Veterinary Competencies and Self-Assessment of Communication Skills. *Animals* **2023**, *13*, 1516; https://doi.org/10.3390/ani13091516.
11. Heise, S.A.C.; Wissing, S.; Nerschbach, V.; Preussing, E.; Tipold, A.; Kleinsorgen, C. Evaluation of an Interprofessional Blended Learning Course Focusing on Communication within Veterinary Teams. *Animals* **2024**, *14*, 729; https://doi.org/10.3390/ani14050729.

References

1. Mercer-Mapstone, L.; Dvorakova, S.L.; Matthews, K.E.; Abbot, S.; Cheng, B.; Felten, P.; Knorr, K.; Marquis, E.; Shammas, R.; Swaim, K. A systematic literature review of students as partners in higher education. *Int. J. Stud. Partn.* **2017**, *1*, 15–37. [CrossRef]
2. Hodges, C.; Moore, S.; Lockee, B.; Trust, T.; Bond, A. The Difference between Emergency Remote Teaching and Online Learning. 2020. Available online: https://er.educause.edu/articles/2020/3/the-difference-between-emergency-remote-teaching-and-online-learning (accessed on 21 August 2024).
3. Goyal, M.; Krishnamurthi, R.; Yadav, D. *E-Learning Methodologies—Fundamentals, Technologies and Applications*; Institution of Engineering and Technology: London, UK, 2021.
4. Reidsema, C.; Kavanagh, L.; Hadgraft, R.; Smith, N. *The Flipped Classroom: Practice and Practices in Higher Education*, 1st ed.; Springer: Singapore, 2017.
5. Abeysekera, L.; Dawson, P. Motivation and cognitive load in the flipped classroom: Definition, rationale and a call for research. *High. Educ. Res. Dev.* **2015**, *34*, 1–14. [CrossRef]
6. O'Flaherty, J.; Phillips, C. The use of flipped classrooms in higher education: A scoping review. *Internet High. Educ.* **2015**, *25*, 85–95. [CrossRef]
7. Sweller, J.; Ayres, P.; Kalyuga, S. *Cognitive Load Theory*; Springer Science+Business Media: New York, NY, USA, 2011.
8. Sweller, J.; Chandler, P. Why some material is difficult to learn. *Cogn. Instr.* **1994**, *12*, 185–233. [CrossRef]
9. Grant, S.; Olsen, C.W. Preventing zoonotic diseases in immunocompromised persons: The role of physicians and veterinarians. *Emerg. Infect. Dis.* **1999**, *5*, 159–163. [CrossRef] [PubMed]

10. Hill, W.A.; Petty, G.C.; Erwin, P.C.; Souza, M.J. A survey of Tennessee veterinarian and physician attitudes, knowledge, and practices regarding zoonoses prevention among animal owners with HIV infection or AIDS. *J. Am. Vet. Med. Assoc.* **2012**, *240*, 1432–1440. [CrossRef] [PubMed]
11. Garcia-Sanchez, P.; Romero-Trancón, D.; Sainz, T.; Calvo, C.; Iglesias, I.; Perez-Hernando, B.; Hurtado-Gallego, J.; Sánchez, R.; Alcolea, S.; Moya, L.; et al. The role of veterinarians in zoonosis prevention: Advising families of immunocompromised children with pets. *One Health* **2024**, *18*, 100662. [CrossRef] [PubMed]
12. de Melo, R.T.; Rossi, D.A.; Monteiro, G.P.; Fernandez, H. Veterinarians and One Health in the Fight Against Zoonoses Such as COVID-19. *Front. Vet. Sci.* **2020**, *7*, 576262. [CrossRef] [PubMed]
13. Cake, M.A.; Bell, M.A.; Williams, J.C.; Brown, F.J.L.; Dozier, M.; Rhind, S.M.; Baillie, S. Which professional (non-technical) competencies are most important to the success of graduate veterinarians? A Best Evidence Medical Education (BEME) systematic review: BEME Guide No. 38. *Med. Teach.* **2016**, *38*, 550–563. [CrossRef] [PubMed]
14. Hodgson, J.L.; Pelzer, J.M. (Eds.) *Veterinary Medical Education: A Practical Guide*; Wiley Blackwell: Hoboken, NJ, USA, 2017.
15. Hamood, W.J.; Chur-Hansen, A.; McArthur, M.L. A qualitative study to explore communication skills in veterinary medical education. *Int. J. Med. Educ.* **2014**, *5*, 193–198. [CrossRef] [PubMed]
16. Pun, J.K.H. An integrated review of the role of communication in veterinary clinical practice. *BMC Vet. Res.* **2020**, *16*, 394. [CrossRef] [PubMed]

animals

MDPI

Article

Outcome of Communication Training in Veterinary Studies: Influence on the Perception of the Relevance of Veterinary Competencies and Self-Assessment of Communication Skills

Mahtab Bahramsoltani [1,*], Sonja Bröer [2], Susann Langforth [3], Corinna Eule [4], Alina Prior [1], Lena Vogt [5], Ting-Ting Li [3], Rebecca Schirone [1], Alina Pohl [6] and Katharina Charlotte Jensen [7]

1 Institute of Veterinary Anatomy, School of Veterinary Medicine, Freie Universität Berlin, Koserstraße 20, 14195 Berlin, Germany
2 Institute of Pharmacology and Toxicology, School of Veterinary Medicine, Freie Universität Berlin, Koserstraße 20, 14195 Berlin, Germany
3 Institute of Food Safety and Food Hygiene, School of Veterinary Medicine, Freie Universität Berlin, Königsweg 67, 14163 Berlin, Germany
4 Centre for Veterinary Clinical Services, Veterinary Hospital, School of Veterinary Medicine, Freie Universität Berlin, Oertzenweg 19b, 14163 Berlin, Germany
5 Veterinary Skills Net, School of Veterinary Medicine, Freie Universität Berlin, Oertzenweg 19b, 14163 Berlin, Germany
6 Clinic of Animal Reproduction, School of Veterinary Medicine, Freie Universität Berlin, Königsweg 65, 14163 Berlin, Germany
7 Institute for Veterinary Epidemiology and Biostatistics, School of Veterinary Medicine, Freie Universität Berlin, Königsweg 67, 14163 Berlin, Germany
* Correspondence: mahtab.bahramsoltani@fu-berlin.de

Simple Summary: Communication is of great importance in all veterinary fields. An e-learning course in the second year and a practical course based on role plays in the third year were set up in the veterinary studies program at Freie Universität Berlin. This study investigated the effects of the communication courses on the assessment of the skills that veterinarians need in their professional work and on the students' self-perception of their own communication skills. Students conducted the survey before and after the e-learning course as well as before and after the practical course. Additionally, veterinarians were surveyed regarding which professional skills seem relevant from their point of view. The results show that students who have just completed the practical course rated communicative competencies for veterinary professional success higher than the other groups. These students also rated their own communication skills higher than all other students. This indicates that the practical course in combination with the e-learning course they had attended in their second year helped them to improve their self-assessment of communication skills, which is something they will benefit from in their professional lives.

Abstract: Since communication skills contribute significantly to professional success among veterinarians, there is a particular focus on developing communication classes in veterinary curricula. At Freie Universität Berlin, an e-learning course covering the basics of communication and a practical communication course based on role plays with and without simulation persons have been established. The outcome of these communication courses on the assessment of the relevance of several veterinary competencies and on the self-assessment of communication skills using the SE-12 questionnaire was investigated. For this purpose, students were surveyed before and after the e-learning course as well as before and after the practical course. Veterinarians were also surveyed on the relevance of veterinary competencies. The relevance of communicative competencies for professional success was rated significantly higher by the students after completing the practical course than by the other students and the veterinarians. Self-assessment of communication skills showed little increase after the e-learning course, but a significant increase after the practical course. Thus, an effective outcome of the communication classes was observed mainly after the practical course. However, the effect of the e-learning course cannot be ruled out since the students participating in the practical course have also completed the e-learning course beforehand.

Keywords: veterinary studies; communication trainings; communication skills; veterinary competencies; self-assessment; e-learning; simulation training

1. Introduction

The majority of veterinary students desire to work in general (46%) or specialist (12%) clinical practices [1]. Usually, students decide to study veterinary medicine because they want to work with animals, have had exposure to companion animals or livestock, have veterinary professionals as role models, and/or have a fondness or talent for the natural sciences [2]. Special competencies such as interpersonal and business skills do not typically play a role in the decision-making process to become a veterinarian or to attend pre-veterinary courses [3]. However, the students might realize during the course of their degree program that communication is one of the most important skills for a medical practitioner [4]. Adequate and successful communication in the medical setting significantly contributes to better compliance and adherence to treatment plans and, consequently, treatment success, a good doctor–patient relationship, as well as the healthcare professional's well-being [5]. In Germany, the importance of communication skills in medical professions has been acknowledged by implementing communication training as a core subject into the Medical Studies Masterplan to allow students to be prepared for efficient patient-physician communication in their clinical practice [5,6]. Similarly, communication skills are listed by the European Association of Establishments for Veterinary Education (EAEVE) as "Day One Skills" for veterinarians [7]. These skills include effective communication with different audiences such as animal owners, employees, colleagues, business partners, and the public. In addition, veterinarians should be able to actively listen and communicate comprehensibly adapted relevant information to the target audience [8]. Indeed, communication skills are regarded as being among the most important key competencies for veterinarians and define subsequent success in veterinary practice [9]. However, interaction and communication with pet owners are a particular challenge for veterinarians [10,11], and a perceived lack of communication skills leads to the experience of cognitive dissonance and stress, which can lead to mental disorders [11]. Conversely, it has been shown that learning and training communication skills lead to a lower stress experience and are associated with higher professional success for veterinarians [9,10]. Nevertheless, education in communication is not yet a mandatory part of veterinary teaching in Germany; no competencies are anchored in the ordinance for the licensing of veterinarians (TAppV) [12]. The urgent need to include communication in TAppV and in the German veterinary curriculum has been demonstrated by Gruber et al. (2021) [13].

At the School of Veterinary Medicine at Freie Universität Berlin, different modules for teaching communication skills have been integrated into compulsory modules over the last five years: The theoretical foundations of communication, such as the 4-sides model [14], transactional analysis [15], strategies of conversation [16], and the Calgary-Cambridge observation guide [17], are taught in the second semester (first year) in the form of a mandatory e-learning course [18]. A newer addition is a practical communication course, in which communication and conversation skills are trained within small groups in various scenarios from the veterinary profession in role plays with and without trained simulation persons (actors or actresses). This training takes place for students in the fifth semester (third year).

The aim of this study was to determine the impact of these communication courses on the students' awareness of the relevance of communicative competencies in the veterinary profession and their self-assessment of their own communication skills.

2. Participants, Materials and Methods

2.1. Participants

For this study, different groups of veterinary students at Freie Universität Berlin on the one hand and veterinarians in Germany on the other hand were surveyed. The online surveys were conducted between November and December 2022 via the online survey application LimeSurvey Version 3.28.21®. All individuals were informed of the purpose of the study, that their participation in the study was voluntary, and that their data would be collected anonymously. All participants gave their informed consent for inclusion before they participated in the study.

The first group consisted of students enrolled in the first semester (first year). These students represented the participants who had not yet participated in any communication course as part of their studies. The second group of students were third-semester students (second year). These students had taken the mandatory e-learning course on the basics of communication (see below for description) in the previous semester. The survey of these two groups of students took place during the dissection courses in the first and third semesters, respectively, in which all students in the semester participated. The students were informed about the content and objectives of the study at the beginning of the respective course and were then given the QR code to take part in the survey. The third group was represented by the students in the fifth semester (third year). These students were surveyed at the beginning and at the end of the mandatory practical communication course (see below for description). The last group were veterinarians. The questionnaire for this group was distributed to various groups on social media.

2.2. Communication Courses

2.2.1. E-Learning Course on the Basics of Communication

The e-learning course, which has been mandatory for students of the second semester since 2019, was created with the authoring tool tet.folio Version 2019 [19] and made available via the learning management system Blackboard Learn Version 9.1 Q4 2019® [20], which is used at Freie Universität Berlin.

The beginning of the e-learning course is designed to raise awareness of the topic. In several videos, students see bad practice examples, e.g., an exam situation, a veterinary consultation interview, as well as statements from pet owners about the quality of veterinary consultations. In addition, students have the task of searching for good and bad ratings of veterinarians online, in which pet owners address the communication skills of veterinarians.

The first communication model introduced is Schulz von Thun's 4-sides model [14]. Students will use a variety of videos to identify potential communication faults at the factual level and learn the method of paraphrasing as part of active listening [21]. Next, the appeal level is addressed, which consists of the aspect of a message for which the sender tries to influence the receiver [14]. To understand the effects of appeals, students are asked to indicate the extent to which they would like to comply with appeals, which are expressed in different ways. Subsequently, the students have the opportunity to see how their fellow students responded. Following it, the students are then invited to indicate how an appeal should be phrased for them to like or dislike following it. The unit concludes with several videos of situations involving veterinary consultations, whereby students are asked to identify positive and negative aspects of the formulation of each appeal. To understand self-disclosure in communication situations, students learn about methods that people use on the one hand to impress ("impression techniques"), or on the other hand to hide unpleasant aspects of themselves ("facade techniques") [14]. In this unit, students also practice recognizing the nature of self-disclosure using different video examples. The meaning of the relationship level is introduced with a self-reflection exercise. The students are first presented with the statement of a pet owner as a text and are asked to assess the pet owner's age, gender, occupation, appearance, and socioeconomic status. Afterwards, they can view the corresponding assessments of their fellow students. In the next steps, they listen to the same statement first in an audio file and then in a video. When assessing the same parameters again, the students recognize possible changes in their assessments. This exercise serves to realize how much the assessment of people is determined by the projection of one's own unpleasant behaviors and the transfer of previous experiences with other people [14]. The unit ends with lessons on the phenomena of "projection" and "transfer" [14] as well as on the meaning and value of empathy in communication. The learning objectives in this module are to recognize the impact of structure, conciseness, and comprehensible language on the factual level, to get to know convincing strategies on the appeal level, to perceive behaviors on the level of self-disclosure as "impression and facade techniques" and to manage them, as well as to become aware of the role of "projection" and "transfer" on the relationship level [14].

The second module of the e-learning course is about transactional analysis [15]. The first unit focuses on the different ego states, i.e., parent ego state, adult ego state, and child ego state [15], which are introduced in animation videos. Following each video, the students are presented with various statements from the field of veterinary study and profession that they are to assign to the respective ego state. At the end of the unit, the students have the task of responding to a statement by a veterinarian as a pet owner from different ego states. The second unit on transactional analysis deals with the different types of transactions (complementary, crossed, and ulterior [15]), which are also introduced in animation videos. In the associated exercises, students are asked to match statements in such a way that complementary or crossed transactions are created and then to determine from which ego state the respective statements originate. Additionally, they are to identify the ulterior messages in various statements as well as specify from which ego state these ulterior messages originate and to which ego state they are addressed. Moreover, several dialogues are presented where students are asked to indicate the type of transaction using respective arrows. The unit on transactional analysis ends with an application example from veterinary practice. The learning objectives in this module are to identify verbal and non-verbal elements in communication that indicate the different ego states, as well as to recognize complementary, crossed, and ulterior transactions and to apply strategies to avoid crossed and ulterior transactions [15].

The third module is focused on the methods of conversation. The first unit introduces the five stages of conversation [16]. Afterwards, the students have the task of assigning sentences to the individual stages of the conversation in different conversational situations, i.e., in a study group, in a team, or in a veterinary consultation. In the second unit, the students get to know the Calgary-Cambridge observation guide (CCOG) [17]. The subsequent exercises are focused on the phases of the veterinary consultation as defined in the CCOG, i.e., preparation, initiation, gathering information, explanation and planning, and closure [17]. For the phase "preparation", students have to decide whether different aspects and activities belong to this phase or not. For the phase "initiation", the exercise consists of students evaluating different ways in which the veterinarian welcomes pet owners presented in videos. Since asking questions is of particular significance in the phase "gathering information", the tasks for this phase refer to the different types of questions and in which situation each type of question is appropriate. The phase "explanation and planning" is addressed in a task in which students assess whether different aspects and actions contribute to the success of this phase. In addition, the principles of participatory decision-making are introduced [22,23]. "Closure", as the last phase, is presented with two different video representations of the end of a veterinary consultation. The students' task is to identify positive aspects of a successful closing phase in the videos. The learning objectives in this module are to learn about an optimal structure for the veterinary consultation by the CCOG, recognize what belongs to a good preparation of the consultation, which behaviors contribute to an appreciative welcome of the pet owner, formulate open and closed questions appropriately, bring about participatory decision-making, as well as to shape the closure of the consultation to mutual satisfaction [17,22,23].

The e-learning course ends with a knowledge test in the form of a multiple-choice quiz that students complete as a self-test.

2.2.2. Practical Communication Course

The practical communication course has been mandatory for fifth-semester students since 2022. The course is based on a flipped classroom concept [24] and includes e-learning units for preparation as well as four lessons, 90 min each. In each lesson, a case is worked on that deals with communicating in a situation of the veterinary profession. In two cases, the task consists of anamnesis (cat with conjunctivitis, mastitis case on a dairy farm), the third case is about breaking bad news (equine asthma), and the last case focuses on a conflict situation (improper use of an electric prod by an animal transporter at the abattoir). In the lessons on anamnesis, the learning objectives are to apply the CCOG to take a structured anamnesis, to create a trusting atmosphere for conversation, and to ask targeted questions to obtain relevant information [17]. The learning objectives of the lesson on breaking bad news are to explain the pet's disease in accordance with the pet owner's prior knowledge, to communicate the treatment options in a precise and understandable way, and to bring about participatory decision-making with the pet owner [25]. In the lesson on conflict situations, the learning objectives are to adequately assess the conflict situation [26], understand the perspective of the animal transporter and thus the cause of his misbehavior, and apply verbal and non-verbal strategies for de-escalation [27] in order to make the animal transporter realize that his behavior was not appropriate. The cases were developed in cooperation with the team "Special Teaching Formats" of the Charité-Universitätsmedizin Berlin, who also conducted the training of the simulation persons as well as a workshop to qualify the lecturers for the delivery of the lessons [28,29].

For all cases, the e-learning material for preparation includes information on medical and legal background knowledge. Additionally, students receive e-learning material for each case that addresses the respective communicative competencies. In preparation for the anamnesis, an animated video was used to refresh their knowledge of the CCOG [17]. For the equine asthma case, the six-step protocol for delivering bad news (SPIKES) [25] was introduced with a poster. To prepare for communicating in the conflict situation, students were provided with an animated video on Glasl's escalation stages [26] and a poster on verbal and non-verbal de-escalation strategies [27], with a special focus on the change of perspective. Also included in the e-learning material for all cases are the rules for giving and receiving feedback [30].

The lessons (concept and schedule adapted from [28]) take place in groups of about 20 students each. Each lesson starts with the lecturer explaining the conversation setting and focus to the students, as well as the learning objectives. In the next step, the students' prior knowledge acquired in the e-learning phase is activated by giving them cards with keywords related to the case, which they have to explain. Students who wish to perform the role play are then identified. In the two cases for the anamnesis as well as for the conflict situation, a simulation person takes on the role of the animal owner or animal transporter, so that only one student is selected for the role of the veterinarian. In the role play involving breaking bad news, all roles are taken on by students: the veterinarian, animal owner, and stable owner. The remaining students are observers during the following role play and are given specific observational tasks focusing on the following aspects: conversation structure, problem exploration, relationship building, empathy/understanding the other person's perspective, and arranging the end of the conversation. Then the setting for the role play is prepared, with dummies serving as animals. In cases where a simulation person is involved, this person joins the lesson at the beginning of the role play. During the role play, the lecturer switches to the role of an observer. The role play can only be interrupted and stopped by the students participating in the role play with a previously agreed time-out sign, in order to receive tips if they do not know how to proceed. After the role play, the observers and the simulation person write down and structure their feedback. When everyone has finished, the student who played the veterinarian is given the opportunity to express his or her own perception of the conversation situation. Subsequently, he or she receives 360° feedback, starting with the simulation person or the fellow students involved in the role play, followed by the observing students, and finally by the lecturer. After the joint discussion of the case and possible clarifications of open questions, the lesson ends with the lecturer revisiting the learning objectives and formulating the corresponding take-home messages.

2.3. Questionnaires

At the beginning of the online survey, before taking the questionnaires, third-year students who were surveyed at the end of the practical communication course were asked to indicate whether they participated in the role plays as a veterinarian, animal owner, or solely as an observer. The veterinarians were asked to indicate the number of years they have worked as a veterinarian (<2 years, 2–5 years, 6–10 years, >10 years).

A self-developed questionnaire (questionnaire 1) was used to obtain an assessment of which competencies the respondents perceived as relevant to the veterinary profession. Within this questionnaire, participants were asked to select exactly five from a list of potential veterinary competencies (defined by the authors) that they consider most relevant to professional career success (Table 1). This questionnaire was used with both students and veterinarians.

Table 1. Questionnaire 1: Respondents were asked to select five competencies from the list of 15 that they consider most relevant to a successful career for veterinarians (translation of the original German statements).

For veterinarians to be successful in their careers, it is important that they …
… can argue convincingly.
… are good at mental arithmetic.
… can resolve conflicts.
… can use medical terminology correctly.
… are good with people.
… can ask targeted questions.
… can take the perspective of the other person.
… are good listeners.
… are tidy.
… have manual skills.
… are good with animals.
… always have the specialist knowledge at hand.
… are always up to date with the latest knowledge.
… can structure.
… have technical skills.

Another questionnaire (questionnaire 2) was used to assess students' self-efficacy regarding their own communication skills (Table 2). For this purpose, the SE-12 questionnaire, which was developed for assessing clinical communication competencies for healthcare professionals [31], was used. The questionnaire was translated into German and adapted to veterinary medicine by replacing "patient" with "patient owners" (a common term for owners of companion and farm animals in Germany) in all cases. The participants rated the statements on a 10-point Likert scale from 1 (very uncertain) to 10 (very certain); alternatively, the statement could also be rated as "not relevant" [31].

2.4. Statistical Analysis

Data was exported in Microsoft Excel 2019®. The data of the people who clicked on the link but did not answer any questions were deleted (n = 29). As the students in the third year were invited to participate before and after the practical communication course, we planned to merge the answers by an individual code of five letters, consisting of the third letter of the month of birth of their mother, the third letter of their month of birth, the second letter of their mother's first name, the second letter of their first name, and the second letter of their birthplace. However, 91 answers could not be matched to a corresponding code. Moreover, a few codes did not explicitly match another code. Due to concerns about data loss, we did not match the answers and regarded them as independent in the following.

Table 2. Questionnaire 2: SE-12 questionnaire for the self-assessment of self-efficacy regarding communication skills [31], adapted to veterinary medicine by replacing "patient" with "patient owners". Respondents indicated their assessment on a 10-point Likert scale ranging from 1 (very uncertain) to 10 (very certain) or they indicated "not relevant".

How certain are you that you are able to successfully . . .
. . . identify the issues the patient owners wish to address during the conversation?
. . . make an agenda/plan for the conversation with the patient owners?
. . . urge the patient owners to expand on his or her problems/worries?
. . . listen attentively without interrupting or changing of focus?
. . . encourage the patient owners to express thoughts and feelings?
. . . structure the conversation with the patient owners?
. . . demonstrate appropriate nonverbal behavior (eye contact, facial expression, placement, posture, and voicing)?
. . . show empathy and acknowledge the patient owners' views and feelings?
. . . clarify what the patient owners know in order to communicate the right amount of information?
. . . check patient owners' understanding of the information given?
. . . make a plan based on shared decisions between you and the patient owners?
. . . close the conversation by assuring, that the patient owners' questions have been answered?

The analyses were conducted with IBM SPSS Statistics Version 27®. The assessment of the competencies (questionnaire 1) was displayed in cross tables stratified by group. For each competency, Pearson's chi-square tests were calculated. For the self-assessment of communication skills (questionnaire 2), descriptive analyses were carried out, again stratified by group. As the scores were not always distributed normally, Kruskal–Wallis tests were calculated. For the pairwise comparison of the groups, p-values were adjusted for multiple testing (Bonferroni correction). The significance level was set at 5%. The results are presented as bar charts for questionnaire 1 and boxplots for questionnaire 2 using Microsoft Excel 2019®.

3. Results

3.1. Number of Participants

A total of 618 participants were included in the analysis of questionnaire 1. They were distributed as follows. From the first-year students, 144 students participated out of a total of 192 students, and from the second-year students, 101 students participated out of a total of 181 students. Out of the total of 149 third-year students, 106 completed the questionnaire before the practical communication course and 97 at the end of the course. Among the 97 third-year students surveyed at the end of the course, 24 students (25%) reported being involved in the role plays as veterinarians, 14 students (14%) confirmed being involved as animal owners, and the remaining 59 students (61%) reported being observers only. From the group of veterinarians, 160 people participated in this survey. Of these, 12 participants (8%) had <2 years of work experience, 38 individuals (24%) had 2–5 years, 32 individuals (20%) had 6–10 years, and 77 individuals (48%) had >10 years; one person did not specify his or her work experience.

Questionnaire 2 was used to survey students only and was completed by a total of 419 students. These were 121 first-year students and 93 second-year students. Of the third-year students, 108 students participated in the survey before the practical communication course and 97 at the end of the course.

3.2. Assessment of the Relevance of Competencies

Both veterinary students (first-year, second-year, and third-year before and after the practical communication course) and veterinarians were asked to select from a list of

15 competencies, which they considered to be the five most relevant for a successful career of veterinarians. Since there were no significant differences by role (veterinarian, pet owner, or observer) among the group of third-year students surveyed after the practical communication course, these students were included as one group in the analyses. Similarly, there was no significant relationship between the length of professional experience and the assessment of the relevance of the competencies among the veterinarians (except for "being tidy"). Therefore, the group of veterinarians was not divided according to professional experience in the further analysis.

Regarding the top five competencies, there were almost no differences between the surveyed groups. For all groups surveyed, the top five included the competencies of being good with people, being good with animals, asking targeted questions, and being a good listener. For the second-year and third-year students, the competencies of taking the perspective of the other person and resolving conflicts were also included. Among the top five were the competency of being up to date with the latest knowledge for the first-year students and the competency of structuring for the veterinarians. However, there were differences between the groups regarding individual competencies.

Figure 1 shows the percentage of people in each group who selected or did not select each competency for all 15 listed competencies. Table 3 displays the results of the chi-square test. For four competencies, there was no significant difference between the group of respondents and the assessment of the relevance of the competency. Two of these competencies, i.e., being good with people and the competency of asking targeted questions, were given high relevance by all groups. The competency of always having specialist knowledge at hand was considered relevant by around 20–36% in all groups. The least relevance was attributed to the competency of being good at mental arithmetic, as only nine respondents chose this competency. Due to the sparse data, no calculations were carried out for the competency of being good at mental arithmetic.

Table 3. Differences concerning the relevance of competencies in the veterinary profession between different groups of veterinary students and veterinarians (chi-square test; n = 618; degrees of freedom = 4).

Competency	Chi-Square	*p*-Value
Arguing convincingly	52.9	<0.001
Resolving conflicts	54.4	<0.001
Using medical terminology	25.3	<0.001
Being good with people	6.6	0.158
Asking targeted questions	8.2	0.084
Taking the perspective of the other person	27.6	<0.001
Being good listener	25.7	<0.001
Being tidy	10.5	0.033
Having manual skills	41.1	<0.001
Being good with animals	36.2	<0.001
Having the specialist knowledge at hand	11.1	0.260
Being up to date with the latest knowledge	19.6	<0.001
Structuring	52.0	<0.001
Having technical skills	21.0	<0.001

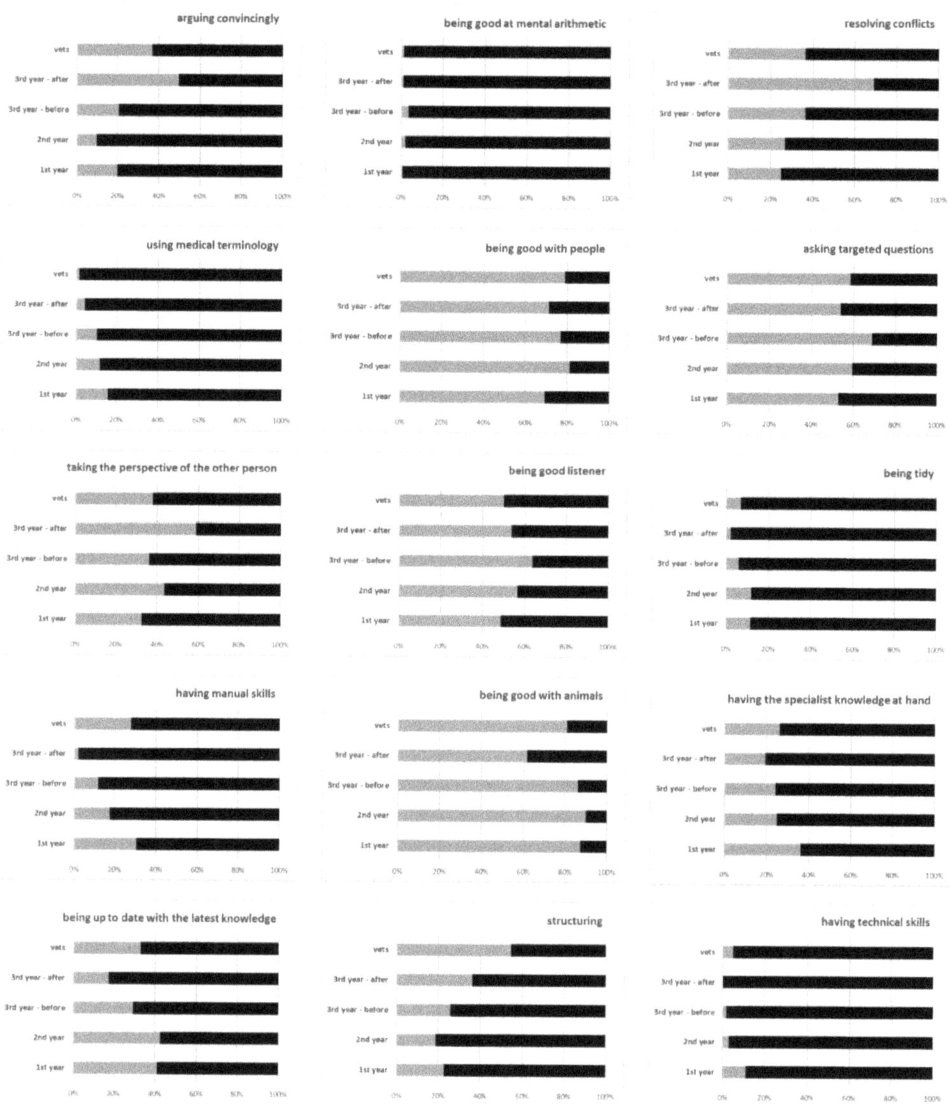

Figure 1. Assessment of the different competencies as relevant (grey = selected, black = not selected) for a successful veterinary career by first-year students (1st year, n = 144), second-year students (2nd year, n = 101), third-year students before (3rd year—before, n = 106) and after (3rd year—after, n = 97) the practical communication course, and veterinarians (vets, n = 160).

For the assessment of the other competencies, significant differences existed between the groups. The relevance of being good with animals was rated as relevant by 81–91% of all groups except the third-year students after the course (62%). The relevance of being a good listener was rated highest by third-year students before the course (64%), followed by second-year students (56%), third-year students after the course (54%), veterinarians (50%), and first-year students (50%). The relevance of arguing convincingly and the relevance of resolving conflicts were rated significantly higher by third-year students after the course (50% and 69%) than by the other groups (10–37% and 25–36%). Interestingly, the veterinarians rated these two competencies higher than the other groups of students. Moreover, the relevance of taking the perspective of the other person was rated highest by third-year students after the course (59%), followed by second-year students (44%). The relevance of structuring was rated highest by veterinarians (54%) and was less often chosen by students (19–36%). The relevance of being up to date with the latest knowledge was rated highly by second-year students (43%) and first-year students (41%), but less often by veterinarians (33%), third-year students before the course (29%), and third-year students after the course (18%). The relevance of having manual skills and the relevance of having technical skills were rated highest by first-year students (31% and 11%), followed by veterinarians (28% and 5%), but were less often chosen by the other groups of students. The relevance of using medical terminology declined within veterinary education: 16% of first-year students but only 1% of veterinarians chose this competency. The relevance of being tidy was chosen more often by first- and second-year students (12%) and fewer by the other groups (2–7%).

3.3. *Self-Assessment of Communication Skills*

For an overall analysis of students' self-assessment of communication skills, a total score summed across items was calculated for each participant (Figure 2). Generally, the students assessed themselves quite favorably, with a median score of 7.3. However, the score differed significantly between the groups of students (chi-square (3) = 18.5, $p < 0.001$, n = 419). The pairwise comparison illustrated that the third-year students' self-assessment of communication skills after the practical communication course was significantly higher than that of the first-year students ($p = 0.004$), the third-year students before the practical course ($p = 0.001$), and slightly higher compared to the second-year students ($p = 0.055$). The other comparisons showed no significant differences.

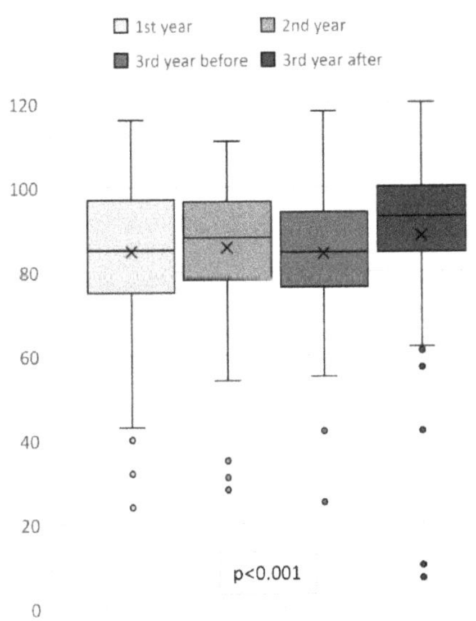

Figure 2. Self-assessment of communication skills by first-year students (1st year, n = 121), second-year students (2nd year, n = 93), and third-year students before (3rd year before, n = 108) and after (3rd year after, n = 97) the practical communication course using the SE-12 questionnaire [31] adapted to veterinary medicine, total score calculated from the sum of the results of the 12 items; cross: mean, whiskers: 10th and 90th percentile.

However, the results differed between the individual items of the questionnaire (Figure 3). Generally, the students assessed themselves worse concerning the planning of the conversation (median = 7, mean = 6.4) and structuring of the consultation (median = 7; mean = 6.5) and better concerning showing empathy (median = 8; mean = 7.9), active listening (median = 8, mean = 7.8), and encouraging the patient owners to express their thoughts and feelings (median = 8, mean = 7.8). For six out of twelve items, the Kruskal–Wallis test revealed differences between the groups concerning the self-assessment of the respective communication skill (Table 4).

Table 4. Comparison of the self-assessment of communication skills between different groups of students (1st = first year students, n = 121; 2nd = second-year students, n = 93; 3rd(b) = third year students before the practical communication course, n = 108; 3rd(a) = third year students after the practical communication course, n = 97).

Communication Skill	Kruskal–Wallis Test		Post Hoc Tests (Adjusted *p*-Values)					
	Chi-Square	*p*-Value	1st to 2nd	1st to 3rd(b)	1st to 3rd(a)	2nd to 3rd(b)	2nd to 3rd(a)	3rd(b) to 3rd(a)
Identify the issues the patient owners wish to address	11.6	0.009	1.0	1.0	0.037	1.0	0.405	0.023
Make an agenda/plan for the conversation	22.3	<0.001	1.0	1.0	0.001	1.0	0.099	<0.001
Urge the patient owners to expand problems	3.4	0.332	Not performed					
Listen without changing of focus	0.7	0.863	Not performed					
Encourage to express thoughts and feelings	1.9	0.599	Not performed					
Structure the conversation	27.3	<0.001	1.0	1.0	<0.001	1.0	0.007	<0.001
Demonstrate appropriate nonverbal behavior	7.0	0.073	Not performed					
Show empathy	2.2	0.529	Not performed					
Clarify the patient owners' knowledge	17.0	<0.001	1.0	1.0	0.008	1.0	0.226	0.001
Check patient owners' understanding	16.3	<0.001	1.0	1.0	0.001	1.0	0.046	0.049
Make a plan based on shared decisions	16.6	<0.001	1.0	1.0	0.099	1.0	0.109	0.001
Close the conversation	6.8	0.078	Not performed					

The first skill was structuring the conversation with the patient owners. For this skill, the third-year students rated themselves significantly higher than the other groups. Also concerning the second skill regarding checking the patient owners' understanding of the information given, the third-year students after the practical communication course rated their abilities higher than the other groups of students. Concerning the next three skills (identify the issues the patient owners wish to address during the conversation, make an agenda/plan for the conversation with the patient owners, and clarify what the patient owners know in order to communicate the right amount of information), the self-assessment was significantly higher among third-year students after the practical course than among first-year students and third-year students before the course. However, third-year students after the course did not rate themselves significantly higher than second-year students concerning these three skills. The sixth skill was to make a plan based on shared decisions with the patient owners. Self-assessment in this skill was only significantly higher among third-year students after the practical course compared to third-year students before the course, but not compared to the other two groups.

Regarding the other skills, i.e., urging the patient owners to expand on their problems/worries, listening attentively without interrupting or changing of focus, encouraging the patient owners to express thoughts and feelings, demonstrating appropriate nonverbal behavior, showing empathy and acknowledging the patient owners' views and feelings, and closing the conversation by assuring, that the patient owners' questions have been answered, the groups' self-assessment of the respective communication skill did not show any significant differences.

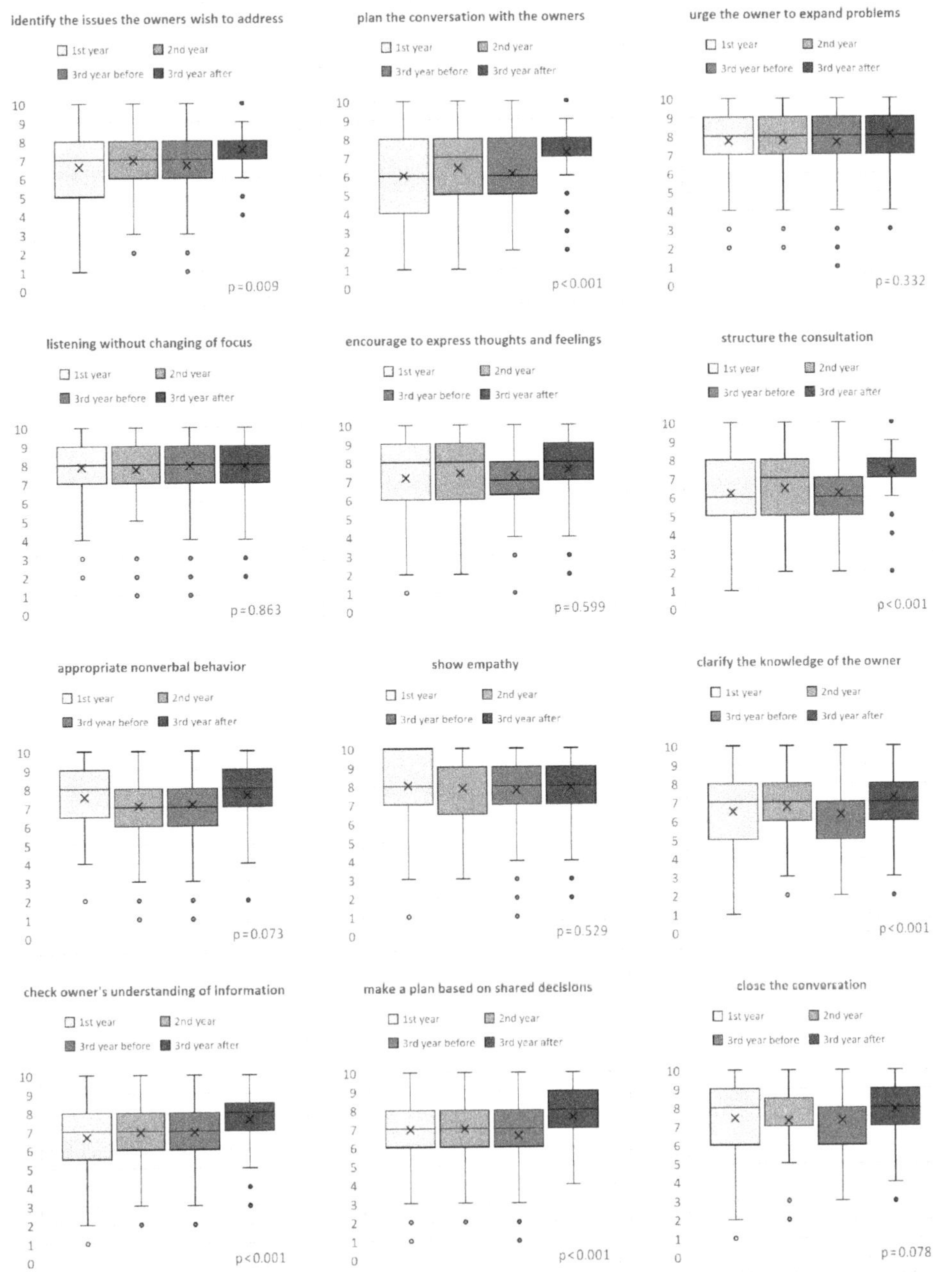

Figure 3. Self-assessment of communication skills by first-year students (1st year, n = 121), second-year students (2nd year, n = 93), and third-year students before (3rd year before, n = 108) and after (3rd year after, n = 97) the practical communication course using the SE-12 questionnaire [23] adapted to veterinary medicine, results for each of the communication skills defined in SE-12; cross: mean, whiskers: 10th and 90th percentile.

4. Discussion

As evidenced by numerous studies, it is undisputed that communication skills are among the key competencies of veterinarians [4,7,32,33]. For this reason, all veterinary schools in Germany are working to establish and expand curricula for teaching communication skills, even though communication teaching is not yet required as per the TAppV [18]. Thus, an e-learning course to teach the basics of communication for first-year students and a practical communication course for third-year students were introduced as mandatory courses at the veterinary school of Freie Universität Berlin in 2019 and 2022, respectively. This study examined the possible effects of the skills taught in these communication courses on perceptions of the relevance of different competencies in the veterinary profession and on self-assessments of communication skills.

With the first questionnaire, students and veterinarians were asked to select from a list of 15 competencies the five they considered most relevant to a successful veterinary career. The list included competencies from the area of methodological and self-competencies that the authors, as veterinarians, considered potentially relevant. The question was whether the students who completed the communication courses (e-learning and practical course) gave a higher relevance to the competencies related to communication and to what extent the students' assessment approached those of the veterinarians, assuming that veterinary professional activity sensitizes veterinarians to the relevance of communicative competencies.

Two competencies that were rated as very relevant by all groups were "being good with people" and "being able to ask targeted questions". Studies that surveyed veterinarians also found that they perceived having high empathy and compassion for people as highly relevant competencies for veterinarians [34,35]. Moreover, this assessment increased with work experience [34]. Although the differences were not significant, the competency of being good with people was rated higher by second- and third-year students than by first-year students who had not yet had communication classes. Therefore, the experiences in the communication courses may have increased the awareness of this aspect. Observations of veterinary consultations show the high value of targeted questions, both open-ended and closed-ended, for obtaining information [36]. This fact was apparently recognized by the students surveyed separately from communication classes. The assessment of the competencies of "arguing convincingly", "resolving conflicts", and "taking the perspective of the other person" differed significantly in the surveyed groups. These competencies were assessed as more relevant by the third-year students after the practical communication course than by the other surveyed groups. Veterinarians are constantly faced with the challenge of convincing pet owners of the strategies for treating their animals and the associated costs with plausible arguments [37,38]. The fact that the relevance of "arguing convincingly" was rated higher by the third-year students after the practical communication course could be due to the focus of the role play dealing with equine asthma in the course. In this role play, the task was to convince the animal owner and the stable owner of the necessary changes in the husbandry of the horse. During a focus group survey of veterinarians who were new to the profession, the skill of resolving conflicts was defined as one of the most important skills [39]. The management of a conflict situation was the focus of the role play on the improper use of the electric prod at the abattoir, demonstrating to the students the necessity of this skill for professional activity. This could be the reason why the competency "resolving conflicts" was rated the highest by the students after the practical communication course. Especially in difficult consultation situations in veterinary practice, the competency to take the perspective of the other person and thus develop empathy and compassion contributes to results that are satisfactory for both sides [40]. This became particularly comprehensible to the students in the role play on the improper use of the electric prod at the abattoir and could thus have led to the students attributing a very high relevance to this competency after the practical communication course. For effective communication, it is also important that veterinarians are good listeners [35,41]. The students who had completed the e-learning course on the basics of communication but had not yet participated in the practical communication course attributed a higher relevance to the competency "being a good listener" than the students after the practical course. In the e-learning course, the technique of active listening [21] was introduced and deepened in related exercises. Even though listening was part of the communication in the practical course, this aspect was not directly addressed again. Therefore, it can be assumed that other newly introduced communication techniques were more prominent for third-year students after the practical course. The competency of structuring is of particular significance in veterinary consultation [17]. For this purpose, the CCOG [17] was already introduced to the students in the e-learning course, refreshed in the e-learning preparation material for the practical communication course, and practically applied in the two role plays on anamnesis. Amongst the students surveyed, the relevance of this competency was rated highest among third-year students after the practical communication course, followed by third-year students before the practical course. However, the relevance of structuring was rated lowest by second-year students, thus lower than by first-year students. Therefore, it can be suggested that it was only with repetition, and even more so through practical application of the CCOG [17], that the relevance of structuring became apparent. Since the relevance of the competency of structuring was rated highest by the surveyed veterinarians, there is a tendency for the students to approximate the assessment of the veterinarians during their studies.

The competency of "being good with animals" is not only considered extremely relevant by pet owners but is also rated very highly by veterinarians [35]. Similarly, among the competencies not related to communication, the relevance of "being good with animals" was rated highest overall in this study. However, the rating of relevance was significantly lower among third-year students after the practical communication course. Furthermore, after having completed the practical communication course, the third-year students were the only group surveyed who ranked being good with animals lower than being good with people. This could be related to the intensive work on communication skills in the course, which may have made the students aware of the importance of appreciative interaction with people as a prerequisite for a successful veterinary consultation. The competencies of "having the specialist knowledge at hand" and "being up to date with the latest knowledge" were predominantly given greater relevance by the students in the first years of study. The stronger focus of these students on specialist knowledge could result from the observation that students usually find it easier to acquire specialist knowledge than to deal with aspects of personal identity development [42,43]. This may have been counteracted by the practical communication course, as the third-year students after this course indicated the least relevance to these specialist knowledge-related competencies. The relevance of manual and technical skills was rated rather low overall but was rated highest by first-year students and decreased continuously until the rating of third-year students after the practical communication course, which was the lowest. Veterinarians' ratings of the relevance of these competencies were lower than those of first-year students but higher than those of the other student groups surveyed. In another study, in which veterinary students and veterinarians were asked to indicate the importance of different skills for veterinary practice, technical and surgical skills were ranked higher by students than by veterinarians [44]. In the study presented here, this was only the case when comparing the results of first-year students and veterinarians. During the communication classes, manual and technical skills became decreasingly relevant. The competencies of "being tidy" and "using medical terminology" were rated as having very little relevance by all groups surveyed. The use of medical terminology was still attributed to the highest relevance by the students of the first year; in the following years, this competency was continuously attributed to a lower relevance. Since the importance of this competency was rated lowest by the veterinarians, the assessment showed a convergence with the veterinarians' rating over the course of the study. This could be an effect of the communication courses, as it has been shown that teaching communication clarifies that explaining medical terminology in language that pet owners can understand is of much higher significance [45]. The competency of being good at mental arithmetic was attributed the least relevance for the professional success of veterinarians by all groups surveyed.

Overall, after completing the practical communication course, students placed a higher significance on the relevance of competencies in the area of communication than the other student groups and veterinarians surveyed. At the same time, it was also these students who predominantly assigned the lowest significance to non-communicative competencies compared to the other groups surveyed. Although a similar effect was not observed among students who had already taken the e-learning course on the basics of communication, it cannot be ruled out whether the prior awareness of the relevance of communication skills through the e-learning course contributed to the practical course having this effect. This is because all the students who had participated in the practical course had also completed the e-learning course beforehand. It is not surprising that the assessment of the relevance of communication skills was higher among students after the practical communication course than among veterinarians, as recent studies indicate insufficient communication skills among veterinarians and strongly recommend integrating the teaching of communication skills into the veterinary curriculum [4]. Since such a curriculum, and thus an obligatory teaching of communication skills, does not yet exist in Germany [18], it can be assumed that the majority of the veterinarians who participated in the survey had no communication training. However, based on their professional experience, veterinarians have an implicit understanding of communicative competencies [33]. This could explain why they still rated the relevance of communicative competencies higher than the students who had not yet completed the practical communication course.

Another aspect investigated was whether the experiences in the communication courses (e-learning and practical course) could influence students' self-assessment of their communication skills. For this purpose, the SE-12 questionnaire, which was developed for measuring self-efficacy with regard to clinical communication skills in healthcare professionals [31], was adapted to veterinary medicine and used for the student survey. The analysis of the overall SE-12 scale showed no significant increase in self-evaluation of communication skills for the second-year students as well as the third-year students before the practical communication course. These students had taken the e-learning course on the basics of communication in the second semester of their first year of study. In two other studies, which also used the SE-12 questionnaire to assess the effects of online courses on communication, similar results were obtained [46,47]. The first of these studies examined the effect of an educational intervention on person-centered communication based predominantly on e-learning [48] for nursing assistants in home care [46]. They found no significant differences between outcomes measured before and after the intervention [46]. In the other study, a blended learning course for teaching patient communication to general practice residents was developed and evaluated at three different time points [47]. The first time of the survey was before the course, the second time after the e-learning section, and the third time after the practical training sessions [47]. This study also showed no significant increase in self-assessment of communication skills after the e-learning section [47]. However, the fact that the e-learning course did not have a significant effect on the self-assessment of communication skills in the study presented could also be because the students were not surveyed directly after the course, but more than three months (second-year students) or more than a year later (third-year students before the practical course). For instance, one study showed that among healthcare professionals, the significant increase in self-assessment of communication skills measured immediately after communication training decreased slightly but statistically significantly when the survey was repeated after six months [49]. This would also explain why the self-assessment of the third-year students before the practical communication course was lower on average than that of the second-year students. Third-year students after the practical communication course showed significantly higher self-assessments of communication skills than first-year students and third-year students before the practical course. This result is consistent with the findings of the study in which blended learning was used to teach communication skills; there too, a significant increase in self-assessment of communication skills was found only after practical training [47]. However, in a study in which communication skills were assessed following three different types of communication training (e-learning only, practical course only, and e-learning and practical course), it was found that while the combination of e-learning and practical course produced the best results, e-learning only had a higher effect than practical training only [50]. Therefore, also in the self-assessment of communication skills, it cannot be ruled out that the knowledge acquired in advance in the e-learning course could have had an influence on the significantly higher self-assessment of the students after the practical course.

The significantly higher self-assessment of communication skills among third-year students after the practical communication course in the total score was only confirmed for the results of six items of the SE-12 questionnaire. Third-year students' self-assessment after the practical course regarding skills in structuring the consultation and checking owners' understanding of the information was significantly higher than in all other student groups surveyed. Self-assessment in the skills of identifying the issues the owners wish to address, planning the conversation with the owners, and clarifying the knowledge of the owner were significantly higher among third-year students after the practical communication course than before the course, as well as among first-year students. For the skill of making a plan based on shared decisions, third-year students' self-assessment was significantly higher after than before the practical course. All these skills were explicitly addressed in the practical communication course. Planning the conversation, structuring the consultation, and identifying the owner's issues are elements of the CCOG [17] taught in the e-learning course and applied in the practical course during the anamnesis role plays. Clarifying the owner's knowledge, checking the owner's understanding, and making a plan based on shared decisions are elements of the SPIKES model [25] applied in the practical course during the equine asthma role play. No significant differences between student groups were found for the self-assessment in the skills of urging the owner to expand problems, listening without changing focus, encouraging the owner to express thoughts and feelings, showing appropriate nonverbal behavior, showing empathy, and closing the conversation. What is notable is that these skills are more about the relationship level. As studies with medical students have shown, little prior experience with consultations and thus few existing cognitive schemas lead to working memory resources being directed primarily toward cognitive processes and thus fewer resources being available for processing emotions [51]. Therefore, the lack of significant effects in the self-assessment of these skills after the practical communication course could be explained by the assumption that the working memory resources available to the students were predominantly bound by the cognitive processes required to implement the structural objectives in the role play, leaving them with few resources to perceive and attend to the emotional and relational aspects. With a stronger routine in the structural processes of conversation, students would have the space to focus more on the emotional aspects and subsequently feel more competent with these communication skills as well. For this purpose, it is necessary to expand the communication curriculum with further mainly practical courses.

Some limitations must be considered when interpreting the results. While the first-year, second-year, and third-year students were different cohorts of students, the same students were surveyed before and after the practical communication course. Therefore, the comparison of the cross-sectional and longitudinal data must be done carefully. On the one hand, the third-year students might have been focused on the relevance of communicative competencies by the survey before the practical communication course; on the other hand, knowing the questionnaire might have had an influence on the way they answered the questions after the practical course. This may have resulted in the attribution of the higher relevance of communicative competencies and the significantly higher self-assessment of communication skills. To test whether the repeated survey had an impact on the results, the survey should be delivered again to current first-year students at the same time in future years. It has been shown that self-assessment of communication skills yields favorable results immediately after communication training rather than several months later [49]. Therefore, the effects of the practical communication course might be overestimated since the survey was conducted immediately after the course, whereas the survey after the e-learning course on the basics of communication was conducted several months after completing the course. To take this fact into account, a follow-up survey of the students should be conducted six months after the practical course. In addition, when assessing the outcome of the e-learning course, it must be considered that although it was checked whether the pages had been worked on by the students, it was not possible to check how intense the attention and concentration and therefore the engagement with the content, was during this work. Moreover, the value of self-assessment as an instrument for measuring the outcome of communication courses must be critically viewed, because the assessment of communication skills by the students themselves may indeed turn out to be better than the assessment by the simulation person involved in the communication [52]. Consequently, it should be examined whether the effects of the practical communication course can also be replicated using third-party assessments or by examining communication skills, e.g., in an objectively structured clinical examination [53]. Finally, assessing veterinary communication skills using the SE-12 questionnaire [31] is limited to communication skills aimed at an interaction with pet owners that is comparable to the direct interaction between physician and patient. However, with the animal as the patient, the communication challenges for veterinarians go far beyond this and can range from being the pet's advocate to being a service provider for the pet's owner. Veterinarians do not only treat the animals and potentially deal with euthanasia, but also have to assess and discuss the financial situation and the compliance and skills of the owner to follow their treatment plans [37,38,54,55].

5. Conclusions

Teaching communication skills in the e-learning course and in the practical course resulted in different effects on students' perceptions of competencies relevant to veterinary careers. The relevance of communicative competencies was rated significantly higher by the students after completion of the practical communication course than by the surveyed veterinarians as well as by the students who had not completed any communication course or only the e-learning course. Students who were surveyed after the practical communication course also scored significantly higher on the self-assessment of their communication skills than students who did not take communication courses or who only completed the e-learning course. However, since all students who participated in the practical communication course also completed the e-learning course beforehand, the significant effects on recognizing the relevance of communicative competencies and the positive influence on self-assessment of communication skills cannot be attributed exclusively to learning in the practical course. It remains to be investigated whether these outcomes of the communication courses can also be confirmed in a longitudinal study as well as through third-party assessments or in objectively structured examinations.

Supplementary Materials: The following supporting information can be downloaded at: https://www.mdpi.com/article/10.3390/ani13091516/s1, Table S1: raw data.

Author Contributions: Conceptualization, M.B.; formal analysis, K.C.J.; investigation, T.-T.L., A.P. (Alina Prior), R.S. and L.V.; methodology, M.B., S.B., C.E., K.C.J., S.L., T.-T.L., A.P. (Alina Pohl), A.P. (Alina Prior), R.S. and L.V.; project administration and supervision, M.B.; visualization, M.B. and K.C.J.; writing—original draft, M.B., S.B., C.E., K.C.J. and S.L.; writing—review and editing, M.B. and S.B. All authors have read and agreed to the published version of the manuscript.

Funding: This research received no external funding.

Institutional Review Board Statement: The study was conducted according to the guidelines of the Declaration of Helsinki and approved by the Ethics Committee of Freie Universität Berlin (ZEA-Nr. 2022-025, 13 December 2022).

Informed Consent Statement: Informed consent was obtained from all subjects involved in the study.

Data Availability Statement: Data are contained within the article or supplementary material. The data presented in this study are available in the supplementary material.

Acknowledgments: The authors would like to express their sincere thanks to Victoria Ángeles Castrillejo Mojado and Sebastian Haase for their creative and excellent support in the development and technical implementation of the e-learning course, as well as to Susanne Lück and Peter Eberz for delivering the workshop for the lecturers, the professional support during the role development, and the training of the simulation persons. Special thanks also go to the students and veterinarians for their participation in the survey. The publication of this article was funded by Freie Universität Berlin.

Conflicts of Interest: The authors declare no conflict of interest.

References

1. Fraser, D.R.; McGregor, D.D.; Grohn, Y.T. Career paths of alumni of the Cornell Leadership Program for veterinary students. *Vet. Rec.* **2008**, *163*, 750–756. [PubMed]
2. Tomlin, J.L.; Brodbelt, D.C.; May, S.A. Influences on the decision to study veterinary medicine: Variation with sex and background. *Vet. Rec.* **2010**, *166*, 744–748. [CrossRef] [PubMed]
3. Lowrie, P.M. Tying art and science to reality for recruiting minorities to veterinary medicine. *J. Vet. Med. Educ.* **2009**, *36*, 382–387. [CrossRef] [PubMed]
4. Pun, J.K.H. An integrated review of the role of communication in veterinary clinical practice. *BMC Vet. Res.* **2020**, *16*, 394. [CrossRef]
5. Gebhardt, C.; Mehnert-Theuerkauf, A.; Hartung, T.; Zimmermann, A.; Glaesmer, H.; Götze, H. COMSKIL: A communication skills training program for medical students. *GMS J. Med. Educ.* **2021**, *38*, Doc83. [CrossRef]
6. Wulf, H. Masterplan Medizinstudium 2020. *Anästhesiol. Intensiv. Notf. Schmerzther.* **2017**, *52*, 313. [CrossRef]
7. EAEVE. List of Subjects and Day One Competences: (As Approved by ECCVT on 17 January 2019). Available online: https://www.eaeve.org/fileadmin/downloads/eccvt/List_of_subjects_and_Day_One_Competences_approved_on_17_January_2019.pdf (accessed on 25 February 2023).
8. European System of Evaluation of Veterinary Training. Manual of Standard Operating Procedure. Available online: https://www.eaeve.org/fileadmin/downloads/SOP/ESEVT_SOP_May_2016_amended_Annex_8_approved_by_ExCom_on_29_May_2019.pdf (accessed on 25 February 2023).
9. Bernigau, D.; Dilly, M. Fachgruppe im Fokus: DVG Forum. *Dtsch. Veterinärmedizinische Ges.* **2019**, *16*, 41–43.
10. Emmett, L.; Aden, J.; Bunina, A.; Klaps, A.; Stetina, B.U. Feminization and Stress in the Veterinary Profession: A Systematic Diagnostic Approach and Associated Management. *Behav. Sci.* **2019**, *9*, 114. [CrossRef]
11. Stetina, B.U.; Krouzecky, C. Reviewing a Decade of Change for Veterinarians: Past, Present and Gaps in Researching Stress, Coping and Mental Health Risks. *Animals* **2022**, *12*, 3199. [CrossRef]
12. Verordnung zur Approbation von Tierärztinnen und Tierärzten. (TAppV). Available online: https://www.gesetze-im-internet.de/tappv/ (accessed on 25 February 2023).
13. Gruber, C.; Dilly, M.; Bahramsoltani, M.; Kleinsorgen, C.; Engelskirchen, S.; Ramspott, S.; Ehlers, J.P. Communication as teaching content of veterinary studies—A joint position paper from the DVG specialist group "communication and didactics" and the GMA veterinary medicine committee. *GMS J. Med. Educ.* **2021**, *38*, Doc84. [CrossRef]
14. Schulz von Thun, F. *Miteinander Reden 1: Störungen und Klärungen. Allgemeine Psychologie der Kommunikation*, 1st ed.; Rowohlt E-Book: Reinbek, Germany, 2013; ISBN 9783644446410.
15. Berne, E. Strukturanalyse und Transaktionsanalyse. In *Spiele der Erwachsenen: Psychologie der Menschlichen Beziehungen*, 21st ed.; Berne, E., Ed.; Rowohlt Verlag GmbH: Hamburg, Germany, 2002; pp. 29–46. ISBN 3499613506.
16. Beebe, S.A.; Beebe, S.J.; Redmond, M.V. *Interpersonal Communication: Relating to Others*, 6th ed.; Allyn & Bacon: Boston, MA, USA, 2011; ISBN 9780205674534.
17. Gray, C.; Moffett, J. A Guide to the Veterinary Consultation Based on the Calgary-Cambridge Observation Guide. In *Handbook of Veterinary Communication Skills*; Gray, C., Moffett, J., Eds.; Wiley: Oxford, UK, 2013; pp. 27–36. ISBN 9781118699706.
18. Pohl, A.; Klass, L.G.; Kleinsorgen, C.; Bernigau, D.; Pfeiffer-Morhenn, B.; Arnhold, S.; Dilly, M.; Beitz-Radzio, C.; Wissing, S.; Vogt, L.; et al. Integration and potential of teaching communication skills in the study of veterinary medicine in Germany. *GMS J. Med. Educ.* **2021**, *38*, Doc53. [CrossRef] [PubMed]
19. Freie Universität Berlin. tet.folio. Available online: https://tetfolio.tu-berlin.de/ (accessed on 25 February 2023).
20. Blackboard. Germany. Available online: https://www.blackboard.com/de-de (accessed on 25 February 2023).
21. Weger, H.; Castle Bell, G.; Minei, E.M.; Robinson, M.C. The Relative Effectiveness of Active Listening in Initial Interactions. *Int. J. Listening* **2014**, *28*, 13–31. [CrossRef]
22. Charles, C.; Gafni, A.; Whelan, T. Decision-making in the physician-patient encounter: Revisiting the shared treatment decision-making model. *Soc. Sci. Med.* **1999**, *49*, 651–661. [CrossRef] [PubMed]

23. Elwyn, G.; Edwards, A.; Kinnersley, P.; Grol, R. Shared decision making and the concept of equipoise: The competences of involving patients in healthcare choices. *Br. J. Gen. Pract.* **2000**, *50*, 892–899. [PubMed]
24. Milman, N.B. The Flipped Classroom Strategy: What it is and how can it best be used? In *Distance Learning: ... for Educators, Trainers, and Leaders*; Simonson, M., Ed.; Information Age Publishing: Charlotte, NC, USA, 2014; pp. 9–11. ISBN 9781623969974.
25. Baile, W.F.; Buckman, R.; Lenzi, R.; Glober, G.; Beale, E.A.; Kudelka, A.P. SPIKES-A six-step protocol for delivering bad news: Application to the patient with cancer. *Oncologist* **2000**, *5*, 302–311. [CrossRef] [PubMed]
26. Glasl, F. The Process of Conflict Escalation and Roles of Third Parties. In *Conflict Management and Industrial Relations*; Bomers, G.B.J., Peterson, R.B., Eds.; Springer: Dordrecht, The Netherlands, 2013; pp. 119–140, ISBN 978-94-017-1134-0.
27. Price, O.; Baker, J. Key components of de-escalation techniques: A thematic synthesis. *Int. J. Ment. Health Nurs.* **2012**, *21*, 310–319. [CrossRef]
28. Kienle, R.; Freytag, J.; Lück, S.; Eberz, P.; Langenbeck, S.; Sehy, V.; Hitzblech, T. Communication skills training in undergraduate medical education at Charité—Universitätsmedizin Berlin. *GMS J. Med. Educ.* **2021**, *38*, Doc56. [CrossRef]
29. Lück, S.; Kienle, R.; Langenbeck, S.; Sehy, V.; Freytag, J. Motivierende Gesprächsführung mit Simulationspatient_innen lehren und prüfen. *Z. Klin. Psychol. Psychother.* **2021**, *50*, 159–167. [CrossRef]
30. Adkoli, B.V.; Parija, S.C. Feedback: How to Give and Take? In *Effective Medical Communication;* Parija, S., Adkoli, B., Eds.; Springer: Singapore, 2020; pp. 27–36. ISBN 978-981-15-3408-9.
31. Axboe, M.K.; Christensen, K.S.; Kofoed, P.-E.; Ammentorp, J. Development and validation of a self-efficacy questionnaire (SE-12) measuring the clinical communication skills of health care professionals. *BMC Med. Educ.* **2016**, *16*, 272. [CrossRef]
32. Abood, S.K. Effectively communicating with your clients. *Top. Companion Anim. Med.* **2008**, *23*, 143–147. [CrossRef]
33. Gaida, S.; Härtl, A.; Tipold, A.; Dilly, M. Communication identity in veterinary medicine: A grounded theory approach. *Vet. Rec. Open* **2018**, *5*, e000310. [CrossRef] [PubMed]
34. Colombo, E.S.; Crippa, F.; Calderari, T.; Prato-Previde, E. Empathy toward animals and people: The role of gender and length of service in a sample of Italian veterinarians. *J. Vet. Behav.* **2017**, *17*, 32–37. [CrossRef]
35. Mellanby, R.J.; Rhind, S.M.; Bell, C.; Shaw, D.J.; Gifford, J.; Fennell, D.; Manser, C.; Spratt, D.P.; Wright, M.J.H.; Zago, S.; et al. Perceptions of clients and veterinarians on what attributes constitute 'a good vet'. *Vet. Rec.* **2011**, *168*, 616. [CrossRef] [PubMed]
36. McArthur, M.L.; Fitzgerald, J.R. Companion animal veterinarians' use of clinical communication skills. *Aust. Vet. J.* **2013**, *91*, 374–380. [CrossRef] [PubMed]
37. Lam, T.J.G.M.; Jansen, J.; van den Borne, B.H.P.; Renes, R.J.; Hogeveen, H. What veterinarians need to know about communication to optimise their role as advisors on udder health in dairy herds. *N. Z. Vet. J.* **2011**, *59*, 8–15. [CrossRef]
38. Lavigne, S.H.; Louis, S.; Rankin, S.C.; Zaoutis, T.E.; Szymczak, J.E. How companion animal veterinarians in the United States perceive financial constraints on antibiotic decision-making. *Vet. Rec.* **2021**, *188*, e62. [CrossRef]
39. Reinhard, A.R.; Hains, K.D.; Hains, B.J.; Strand, E.B. Are They Ready? Trials, Tribulations, and Professional Skills Vital for New Veterinary Graduate Success. *Front. Vet. Sci.* **2021**, *8*, 785844. [CrossRef]
40. Morrisey, J.K.; Voiland, B. Difficult interactions with veterinary clients: Working in the challenge zone. *Vet. Clin. N. Am. Small Anim. Pract.* **2007**, *37*, 65–77. [CrossRef]
41. Hare, D. Good communication skills key to success. *Can. Vet. J.* **2003**, *44*, 621–622.
42. Armitage-Chan, E.; May, S.A. Developing a Professional Studies Curriculum to Support Veterinary Professional Identity Formation. *J. Vet. Med. Educ.* **2018**, *45*, 489–501. [CrossRef]
43. Matthew, S.M.; Taylor, R.M.; Ellis, R.A. Relationships between students' experiences of learning in an undergraduate internship programme and new graduates' experiences of professional practice. *High Educ.* **2012**, *64*, 529–542. [CrossRef]
44. Haldane, S.; Hinchcliff, K.; Mansell, P.; Baik, C. Expectations of Graduate Communication Skills in Professional Veterinary Practice. *J. Vet. Med. Educ.* **2017**, *44*, 268–279. [CrossRef] [PubMed]
45. Hafen, M.; Rush, B.R.; Nelson, S.C. Utilizing filmed authentic student-client interactions as a communication teaching tool. *J. Vet. Med. Educ.* **2009**, *36*, 429–435. [CrossRef] [PubMed]
46. Gustafsson, T.; Sundler, A.J.; Hedén, L.; Lindberg, E.; Maurin Söderholm, H. Communication in home care-A feasibility study of an educational intervention in self-efficacy and job satisfaction. *Nurs. Open* **2023**, *10*, 1375–1382. [CrossRef] [PubMed]
47. Houwen, J.; de Bont, O.A.; Lucassen, P.L.; Rosmalen, J.G.; Stappers, H.W.; olde Hartman, T.C.; van Dulmen, S. Development of a blended communication training program for managing medically unexplained symptoms in primary care using the intervention mapping approach. *Patient Educ. Couns.* **2022**, *105*, 1305–1316. [CrossRef] [PubMed]
48. Gustafsson, T.; Sundler, A.J.; Lindberg, E.; Karlsson, P.; Söderholm, H.M. Process evaluation of the ACTION programme: A strategy for implementing person-centred communication in home care. *BMC Nurs.* **2021**, *20*, 56. [CrossRef]
49. Wolderslund, M.; Kofoed, P.-E.; Ammentorp, J. The effectiveness of a person-centred communication skills training programme for the health care professionals of a large hospital in Denmark. *Patient Educ. Couns.* **2021**, *104*, 1423–1430. [CrossRef]
50. Gartmeier, M.; Bauer, J.; Fischer, M.R.; Hoppe-Seyler, T.; Karsten, G.; Kiessling, C.; Möller, G.E.; Wiesbeck, A.; Prenzel, M. Fostering professional communication skills of future physicians and teachers: Effects of e-learning with video cases and role-play. *Instr. Sci.* **2015**, *43*, 443–462. [CrossRef]
51. Son, D.; Shimizu, I.; Ishikawa, H.; Aomatsu, M.; Leppink, J. Communication skills training and the conceptual structure of empathy among medical students. *Perspect. Med. Educ.* **2018**, *7*, 264–271. [CrossRef]

52. Graf, J.; Loda, T.; Zipfel, S.; Wosnik, A.; Mohr, D.; Herrmann-Werner, A. Communication skills of medical students: Survey of self- and external perception in a longitudinally based trend study. *BMC Med. Educ.* **2020**, *20*, 149. [CrossRef]
53. Hecker, K.G.; Adams, C.L.; Coe, J.B. Assessment of first-year veterinary students' communication skills using an objective structured clinical examination: The importance of context. *J. Vet. Med. Educ.* **2012**, *39*, 304–310. [CrossRef] [PubMed]
54. Kleen, J.L.; Rehage, J. Kommunikationskompetenz in der tierärztlichen Praxis. *Tierärztliche Prax. Ausg. G Großtiere Nutztiere* **2008**, *36*, 293–297. [CrossRef]
55. Shaw, J.R.; Adams, C.L.; Bonnett, B.N. What can veterinarians learn from studies of physician-patient communication about veterinarian-client-patient communication? *J. Am. Vet. Med. Assoc.* **2004**, *224*, 676–684. [CrossRef] [PubMed]

animals

MDPI

Article

Applying Iterative Student Feedback across Flipped Classroom and Flexible Teaching Approaches: Impact on Veterinary Students' Learning Experience

Arti A. Singh [1,2], Frances M. Shapter [1], Anne Bernard [3], Deanne J. Whitworth [1], Marnie G. Holt [2], Philip S. Waller [4] and Stephanie L. Bond [1,*]

1 School of Veterinary Science, Faculty of Science, The University of Queensland, Gatton, QLD 4343, Australia; a.singh1@uq.edu.au (A.A.S.); f.shapter@uq.edu.au (F.M.S.); d.whitworth@uq.edu.au (D.J.W.)
2 Faculty of Science, The University of Queensland, Brisbane, QLD 4072, Australia; m.holt2@uq.edu.au
3 QCIF Bioinformatics, Institute for Molecular Bioscience, The University of Queensland, Brisbane, QLD 4072, Australia; a.bernard@qcif.edu.au
4 eLearning Innovations and Partnerships in Science and Engineering (eLIPSE), The University of Queensland, Brisbane, QLD 4072, Australia; p.waller@uq.edu.au
* Correspondence: steph.bond@uq.edu.au

Simple Summary: Iterative feedback from students using a research-supported, flipped classroom delivery within a foundational veterinary gastrointestinal anatomy and physiology course suggested a strong preference for change from flipped to flexible delivery. Integration of broader course feedback enhanced the student experience in the subsequent flexible delivery iteration. Feedback requested the following: that online teaching materials be made available earlier in the semester rather than progressively; the re-introduction of face-to-face lectures; and full-length lecture videos with a more conversational presentation style in addition to already provided shorter, modularized videos. Once the enhanced flexible learning approach was employed, a substantially improved student experience was reported, with enhanced work/study/life balance, reduced stress levels, and more efficient time use when studying. Our results highlight the importance of considering student perceptions and the student experience when designing and implementing educational interventions. This teaching method offers veterinary educators an innovative and efficient starting point for designing foundational coursework.

Abstract: No single teaching strategy supports all learning styles in veterinary science students. To facilitate more convenient and flexible teaching, learning, and revision, an innovative online digital learning platform—VetCloud—was developed to provide access to modularized programme content across courses to promote active, integrated learning. This study aimed to understand student perceptions regarding the enhancement of the student learning experience in a foundational course in gastrointestinal anatomy and physiology at The University of Queensland across two learning cycles, via applying iterative student feedback in transitioning a flipped classroom approach using VetCloud for the delivery of lecture content in 2022 to a flexible learning approach in 2023. By 2023, the use of VetCloud in the flexible learning approach improved students' work/study/life balance, reduced their stress levels, and enabled a more efficient use of their time when studying, compared to the flipped classroom approach in 2022. Surveying student perceptions was integral to maximizing their learning experience. Data clearly demonstrates that students will mix-and-match how they interact with available options provided via flexible delivery on an individualized basis. This teaching method offers veterinary educators an innovative and efficient approach to veterinary student education in anatomy and physiology while enhancing student well-being.

Keywords: blended learning; flipped classroom; veterinary medicine; veterinary science; anatomy; physiology

1. Introduction

Higher education has undergone a sector-wide shift in recent years, away from largely face-to-face classroom-based instruction led by the 'teacher as expert' towards flexible, multi-modal instruction and an increased recognition and engagement of 'students as partners' [1] in the teaching and learning process. While emergency response teaching [2] at the time of the COVID-19 pandemic necessitated a rapid, large-scale online adaptation of teaching and assessment strategies [3], the advantages and benefits of eLearning approaches [4–7] such as blended learning and the flipped classroom in higher education have been highlighted across disciplines, including anatomy and physiology, medicine, veterinary science, and other health professions [8–19].

In the context of veterinary education, the use of blended learning and flipped classroom approaches has been reported to benefit the student learning experience in classroom settings [12–14], practical laboratory settings [15], and clinical and professional skills contexts [16–18]. Benefits to teaching staff have also been reported [12], including increased satisfaction in their teaching. Veterinary science students face the challenge of comprehending vast anatomical, physiological, and pathological variations between and across different animal species within a finite curriculum limited by programme length. Challenges associated with implementing the flipped classroom approach in veterinary education [12] include student-related barriers such as resistance to change and a perceived increase in an already heavy student workload, lack of engagement, and lack of time; staff-related barriers such as an increase in workload and lack of time for preparation of eLearning resources; and institutional barriers such as the availability of technology and resources, logistics, training, and institutional support.

The Bachelor of Veterinary Science (Honours) degree (BVSc(Hons)) at The University of Queensland (Australia) is a five-year undergraduate programme based at the University's regional campus in Gatton, Queensland. The first four years of the degree involve a combination of lectures, tutorials, practical classes, and placements. Content is delivered and managed through the University's online learning management system (LMS), Blackboard™ (by Anthology, Boca Raton, FL, USA). LMS course sites for previously completed courses are available to BVSc(Hons) students as they progress through their degree. The final year of the degree consists of internal and external clinical placements. The BVSc(Hons) students are a diverse cohort, ranging in age from 17 to 50+ years and with a variety of living arrangements, work demands, caring responsibilities, and financial constraints that may affect their ability to participate in on-campus or synchronous online classes in their pre-clinical years.

In an effort to facilitate more convenient and flexible teaching, learning, and revision for BVSc(Hons) students across their degree, VetCloud—an innovative online digital learning platform—was conceived and developed as a cross-faculty collaboration, providing students with access to modularized programme content across courses to enhance search capability and promote active, integrated learning. In VetCloud-using courses, lectures are designed using a scaffolding approach, where content is broken down into modules based on single knowledge topics, each with clearly defined learning outcomes. Lecture content for these courses is presented on VetCloud both as a complete full-length recording and as short modular videos (3–12 min), accompanied by downloadable learning resources including lecture slides, notes, slides with an accompanying transcript, and extension resources. Active learning strategies are incorporated to maximize student engagement via the use of self-assessment quiz questions associated with each module provided on VetCloud. This enables students to learn at their own pace, consolidating knowledge and understanding, and easily locate material on VetCloud for revision of 'assumed knowledge' in later years of the programme. Iterative student feedback has informed enhancements to learning materials provided on VetCloud each active learning cycle, culminating in quantifiably improved student impact.

Gathering and responding to student feedback has been central to the iterative development of VetCloud to date. An important source of student feedback has been partnerships between VetCloud-using courses and the Student-Led Observation for Course Improvement (SLOCI) [20] Team within the Faculty of Science in 2022 and 2023. The Science SLOCI Team is a student-led team of current undergraduate students enrolled in programmes from across the Faculty of Science at The University of Queensland who work to gather information regarding current student perceptions of courses or projects on behalf of teaching staff. Based on the 'students as partners' philosophy [1], SLOCI aims to deliver the student voice to teaching staff in more targeted ways than institutional end-of-semester teaching evaluations allow, through a combination of tailored activities such as online surveys, focus group interviews, and class observations.

VETS1003: Digestion, Metabolism and Nutrition is a foundational one-semester gastrointestinal anatomy and physiology course for BVSc(Hons) students. Conducted in semester 2 each year, VETS1003 is taken by first-year BVSc(Hons) students in the second semester of their degree programme. VetCloud has been used in VETS1003 in two learning cycles to date: semester 2, 2022 and semester 2, 2023. The aim of this study was to enhance the student learning experience in VETS1003 via iterative feedback, based on the two learning cycles of first-year BVSc(Hons) student feedback obtained from online surveys facilitated through partnerships with the Faculty of Science SLOCI Team (i.e., from feedback obtained from the 2022 and 2023 cohorts of VETS1003 students).

2. Materials and Methods

VetCloud was used to deploy the anatomy and physiology lecture content during weeks 1–9 of the 13-week teaching semester in the first-year course VETS1003: Digestion, Metabolism and Nutrition in semester 2, 2022 (n = 145 students) and 2023 (n = 133 students).

2.1. Active Learning Cycle 1: VetCloud Used in a Flipped Classroom Approach

In semester 2, 2022, VETS1003 learning resources were provided to students via a flipped classroom approach on VetCloud, with progressive weekly release of lecture content just prior to timetabled 'lecture' timeslots (3 h per week) in weeks 1–9. Content was subsequently discussed during hybrid tutorials held concurrently face-to-face and online via Zoom^{TM} (San Jose, CA, USA), and then applied in practical classes. The 'complete lecture recording videos' provided in 2022 were not recordings of live lectures; they consisted of the relevant pre-recorded short topic videos joined together to cover all the topics relevant to each lecture within a single longer video.

2.2. Active Learning Cycle 2: VetCloud Used in a Flexible Learning Approach

In semester 2, 2023, all content for the anatomy and physiology modules of VETS1003 was provided on VetCloud from week 1 of the semester. In addition to VetCloud learning resources, face-to-face lectures (3 h per week) were offered in weeks 1–7 of the 13-week teaching semester. In 2023, the 'complete lecture recording videos' available in 2022 that consisted of the relevant short topic videos joined together were provided to students from the beginning of the semester (i.e., before the face-to-face lectures took place) and were replaced with a recording of each 2023 face-to-face lecture within one week of each lecture being delivered during the semester. Content was subsequently discussed during weekly face-to-face tutorials, then applied in practical classes.

2.3. Student Surveys

This study was approved by the Human Ethics Committee of The University of Queensland (project number 2019/HE001666). The SLOCI Team conducted online voluntary, anonymous surveys of VETS1003 students during week 8 of semester 2 in 2022 (Supplementary File S1) and weeks 6–9 of semester 2 in 2023 (Supplementary File S2) via the Microsoft Forms platform. VETS1003 students were informed about the surveys and invited to participate in them via weekly announcements made on the VETS1003 LMS course sites and sent via email. Implied consent was obtained from all students involved in the study by their voluntary choice to respond to a survey, and students were advised that survey responses would remain anonymous to VETS1003 teaching team members. Students were given the incentive of winning one of a limited number of AUD 20 Coles-Myer retail gift cards for their survey participation. Both the 2022 and 2023 surveys included two additional, voluntary open-response questions, through which students who wished to participate in the gift card draw could provide their names and contact email addresses. If provided, student names and contact details were used only for gift card draws.

The 2022 online survey (Supplementary File S1) consisted of 33 questions, including 11 Likert scale rating questions, 14 multiple-choice questions that all allowed for one response each, and eight open-response questions. Survey questions were refined for the 2023 online survey (Supplementary File S2) to obtain more nuanced information about how students interacted with VetCloud; the 2023 survey consisted of 32 questions, including nine Likert scale rating questions, seven multiple-choice questions that allowed for only one response each, six multiple-choice questions that allowed for multiple responses, and ten open-response questions.

2.4. Statistical Methods

Descriptive statistics were reported using frequencies and proportions for categorical data. Likert scales were considered in two ways: categorical, with five categories (1, 2, 3, 4, and 5), and ordinal (scale from 1 to 5), which were described using medians and inter-quartile ranges (IQR). Comparison of categorical variables between learning cycles (2023 vs. 2022) was performed using a chi-square test. Comparison of the ordinal Likert scales between the learning cycles was performed using a Mann–Whitney test. In figures, data from the 2022 learning cycle are presented in blue and those for 2023 are displayed in red. All analyses were performed using the R statistical software [21], and p-values were two-tailed with $p < 0.05$ considered statistically significant.

3. Results

VETS1003 student perceptions of VetCloud were compared between the implementation of a flipped classroom approach in 2022 ($n = 47$ students survey responses, 32% response rate) and a flexible learning approach in 2023 ($n = 46$ student survey responses, 35% response rate).

3.1. Students' Lecture Delivery Format Preferences during the Flipped Classroom and Flexible Learning Approaches

Due to COVID-19 and resultant staffing changes in 2021, the previous two VETS1003 student cohorts (2020 and 2021) had been provided with lecture recordings through the LMS when face-to-face lectures were not possible. In 2022, student preferences were assessed regarding a return to face-to-face lectures, recordings of previously delivered live lectures, or a flipped classroom approach with the VetCloud platform (Figure 1). Given the clear student preference for a return to the live lecture (Figure 1) when they were permitted to select only one favored lecture delivery format, live lectures were incorporated in 2023 and the survey questions were adjusted accordingly (Figure 2).

There was a clear student preference for a multi-modal delivery of content in 2023, with the majority of students ($n = 33/46$, 72%) selecting multiple formats (Figure 2) now that they were allowed to do so. Thirteen students (28%) selected only one lecture format, of which pre-recorded full-length (50 min) lecture videos were the most popular ($n = 7$ students, 15%). Overall, 31 of the 46 students (67%) reported a liking for pre-recorded full-length (50 min) lecture videos, 30 students (65%) a liking for short topic videos, and 24 students (52%) a liking for face-to-face lectures.

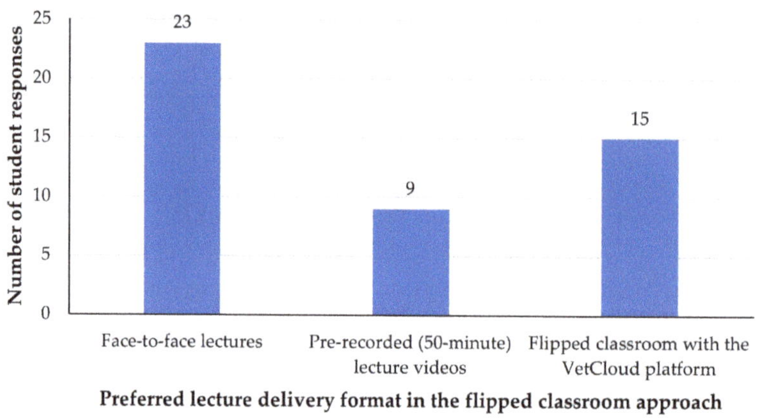

Figure 1. VETS1003 students' (n = 47) preferred lecture delivery formats during the flipped classroom approach employed in 2022. Face-to-face lectures and pre-recorded (50 min) lecture videos were not offered in 2022, and students were permitted to select only one of the three answer options.

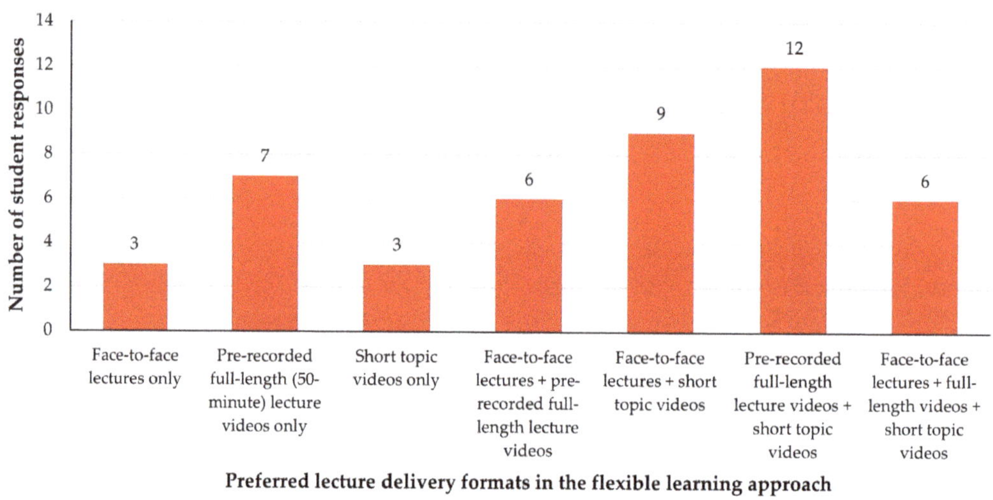

Figure 2. VETS1003 students' (n = 46) preferred lecture delivery formats during the flexible learning approach employed in 2023. Students were permitted to select as many of the three answer options as they wished.

3.2. Timeline of Student Engagement with Resources on VetCloud during the Flipped Classroom and Flexible Learning Approaches

In 2022, 28% of students (n = 13/47) engaged with the learning resources on VetCloud for weekly 'lectures' prior to the scheduled self-directed learning 'lecture time', while 25% (n = 12) interacted with the resources during the 'lecture time' (Figure 3). Almost half of the students (n = 22, 47%) engaged with the learning resources after the scheduled 'lecture time' (Figure 3).

In 2023, when face-to-face VETS1003 lectures were held, the learning resources on VetCloud were available to students from the beginning of the semester and multiple responses to the equivalent survey question were allowed. The 46 responding students provided 59 responses (Figure 3). Eleven students (24%) selected multiple answer options, including two (4%) who selected all three times, with 35 students (76%) indicating that they only engaged with VetCloud resources at one time (Figure 4). Nine students (20%) engaged with the resources on VetCloud before the face-to-face lectures, 12 students (26%) engaged with them during the lectures, and 38 (83%) engaged with them afterwards (Figure 4). Of the 38 students (83%) who engaged with the resources after the face-to-face lectures, 28 (61% of the total 46 survey respondents) engaged with the resources only after the lectures, three students (7%) engaged with them both before and after the lectures, and five students (11%) engaged with them both during and after the lectures (Figure 4).

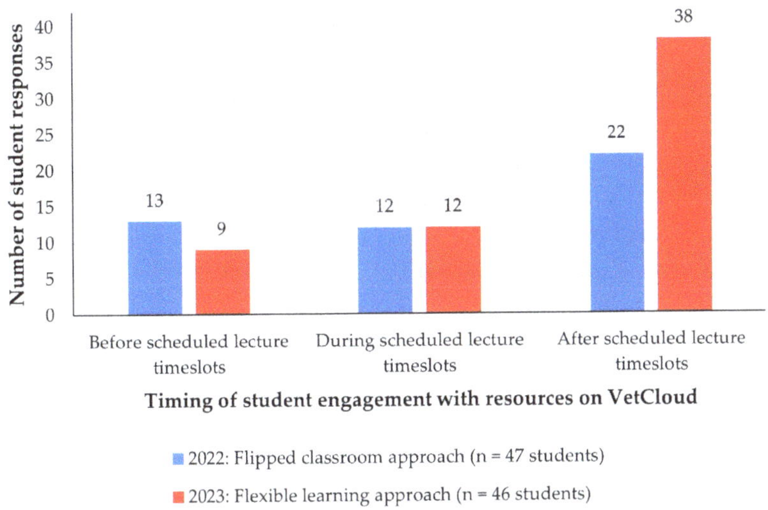

Figure 3. Timing of VETS1003 students' engagement with resources on VetCloud in relation to scheduled 'lecture' timeslots during the flipped classroom approach employed in 2022 and the scheduled face-to-face lectures during the flexible learning approach employed in 2023. Students in 2022 were permitted to select only one of the three answer options, while students in 2023 were permitted to select as many of the three answer options as they wished.

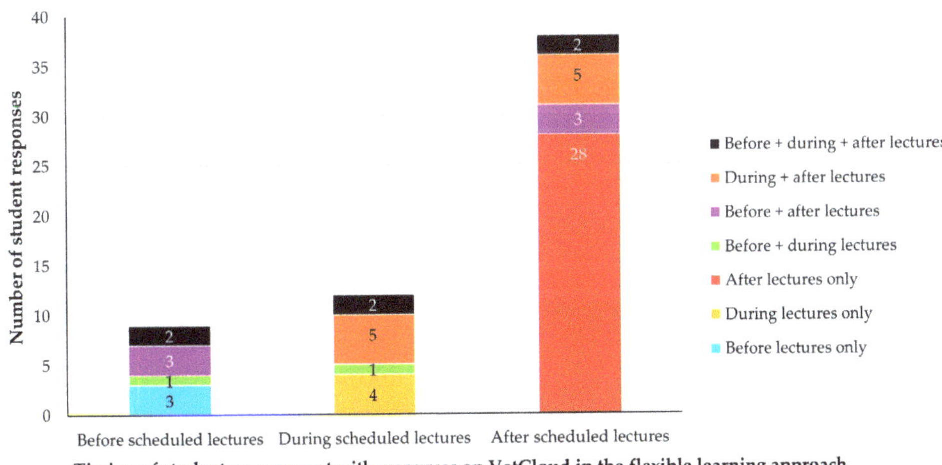

Figure 4. Timing of VETS1003 students' ($n = 46$) engagement with resources on VetCloud in relation to the scheduled face-to-face lectures during the flexible learning approach employed in 2023, showing the specific combinations of timing options they selected.

A chi-square test was performed to compare the timing of engagement with resources on VetCloud between the two learning cycles. For the purpose of the analysis, all responses by 2023 students were considered (n = 59 responses). No significant relationship was found (p = 0.16).

3.3. Students' Tutorial Attendance and Engagement during the Flipped Classroom Approach

In 2022, when face-to-face lectures were not held for VETS1003 and tutorials were held in-person and synchronously online via Zoom™, students were asked about their tutorial attendance and mode of engagement. They were first asked to respond to the Likert scale rating question *'How often do you attend the tutorial sessions, either in person or over Zoom?'*. After this, they were asked to respond to the multiple-choice question *'How do you generally engage with the weekly tutorial?'* by selecting one answer option (Figure 5). Students who selected the *'I do not engage with tutorials'* answer option were then directed to an open-response question that asked them to explain why this was the case.

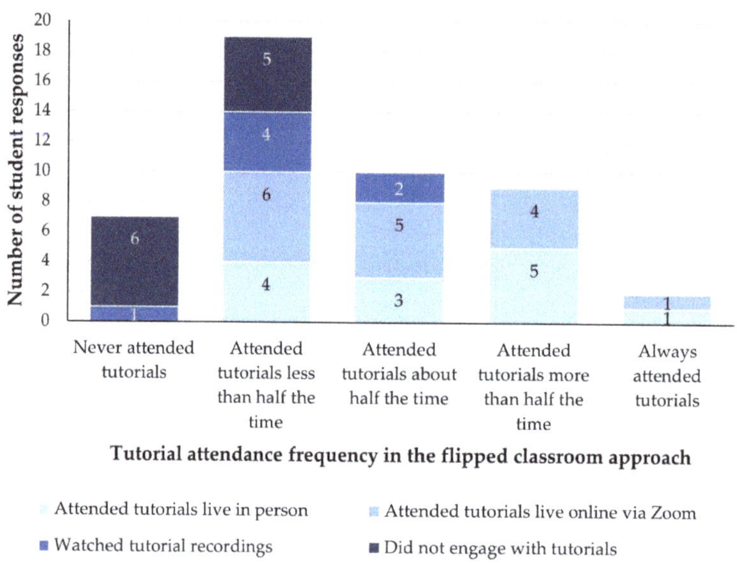

Figure 5. The reported frequency of tutorial attendance and mode of tutorial engagement of VETS1003 students (n = 47) during the flipped classroom approach employed in 2022.

The majority of students (n = 26/47, 55%) indicated that they attended tutorials less than half of the time or did not attend them at all (Figure 5). Ten students (21%) attended approximately half of the tutorial sessions, nine students (19%) attended more than half of the tutorial sessions, and two students (4%) indicated that they always attended the tutorials (Figure 5).

Of the 19 students who indicated that they attended less than half of the tutorials, six (13% of the responding 47 students) typically did so online via Zoom and four (9%) in person (Figure 5). Another four (9%) of these students indicated that they typically watched video recordings of the tutorials, as did one (2%) of the seven students who never attended tutorials. The remaining five students (11%) who attended less than half the tutorials and six students (13%) who never attended tutorials reiterated that they did not typically engage with tutorials at all (Figure 5).

3.4. Time Spent Engaging with Resources on VetCloud during the Flipped Classroom and Flexible Learning Approaches

In 2022, all 47 responding students reportedly engaged with the lecture content for an average of at least two hours each week, with just over half the students (n = 24, 51%) indicating that they spent at least five hours engaging with lecture content each week (Figure 6).

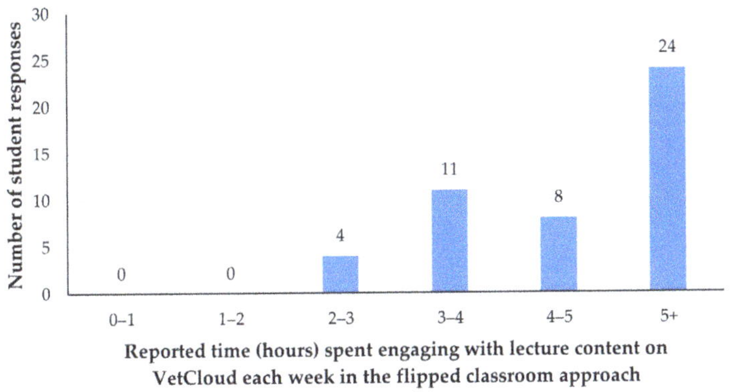

Figure 6. The average amount of time VETS1003 students (n = 47) reportedly engaged with lecture content/resources on VetCloud each week during the flipped classroom approach employed in 2022.

The broader multiple-choice question '*On average, how many hours do you engage with the lecture content a week?*' from the 2022 survey was replaced in the 2023 survey with two different multiple-choice questions aimed at teasing out more nuanced information about when and how students were spending time engaging with VETS1003 resources on VetCloud for **each** lecture. In 2023, students were first asked '*On average, for how many hours do you engage with the content for* ***each*** *lecture on VetCloud in the week that it is timetabled?*' and then '*On average, for how many hours do you engage with the content for* ***each*** *lecture on VetCloud in total, including revision for assessments?*' (Figure 7).

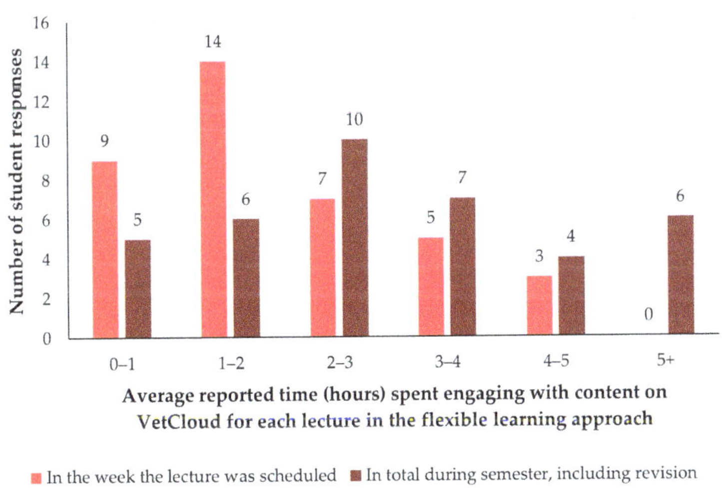

Figure 7. The average amount of time VETS1003 students (n = 38) reportedly spent engaging with content/resources on VetCloud for each lecture during the flexible learning approach employed in 2023, in the week each lecture was scheduled and in total during the semester including for revision.

Of the 46 survey respondents in 2023, eight selected a larger number of hours per lecture in the week that it was timetabled rather than in total during the semester; the responses to these two questions from these eight students have not been included in our analysis, and thus 38 responses for each of these two questions are reported and analysed here instead of 46 responses each. These 38 students spent a reported average of five hours or less engaging with content for each lecture in the week it was scheduled (Figure 7), most commonly (n = 14/38, 37%) spending 1–2 h on each lecture. In terms of total time spent engaging with content for each lecture during the semester including for revision, students most commonly (n = 10/38, 26%) indicated that they spent an average of 2–3 h engaging with the content for each lecture, followed closely by students (n = 7/38, 18%) who spent 3–4 h (Figure 7).

Eleven students (29% of 38) indicated that they engaged with lecture content/resources on VetCloud only in the week when each lecture was scheduled (Figure 8). The majority of the 38 students (n = 27, 71%) indicated that they did engage with lecture content/resources on VetCloud after the week when each lecture was scheduled; the largest proportion (n = 6, 16%) engaged with it for 1–2 h per lecture in the week each lecture was scheduled out of a total of 2–3 h per lecture over the semester, followed by four students (~11%) who engaged with it for 1–2 h per lecture in each scheduled lecture week out of a total of 3–4 h per lecture over the semester (Figure 8). Most students (n = 18/38, 47%) indicated that they spent an additional 1 h per lecture for revision over the semester (Figure 8).

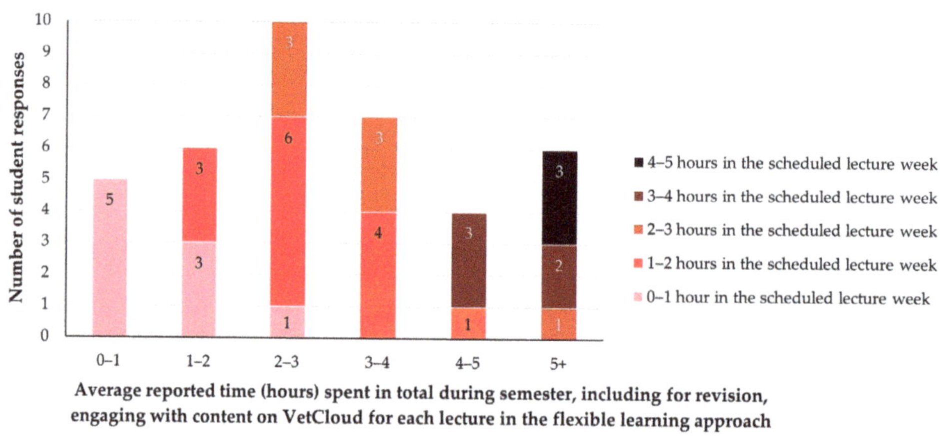

Figure 8. The average amount of time VETS1003 students (n = 38) reportedly spent engaging with content/resources on VetCloud for each lecture during the flexible learning approach employed in 2023, showing the number of hours each student spent during the week each lecture was scheduled out of the total number of hours they spent during the semester.

3.5. Student Opinions of Whether Sufficient Learning Materials Were Provided on VetCloud to Support Their Learning as Part of the Flipped Classroom and Flexible Learning Approaches

In 2022, students were asked the multiple-choice question '*Do you feel that the flipped classroom approach has provided sufficient learning materials to give you confidence that you understand the content, as outlined by the learning outcomes for each module?*' and were directed to select one answer option (Figure 9).

In 2023, after the flexible learning approach, with the online content available from the beginning of the semester, the multiple-choice question from the 2022 survey was replaced with a more clearly worded question that asked students to rate on a Likert scale of 1–5 how much they agreed with the statement '*VetCloud provides access to sufficient learning materials to support my learning in VETS1003*'.

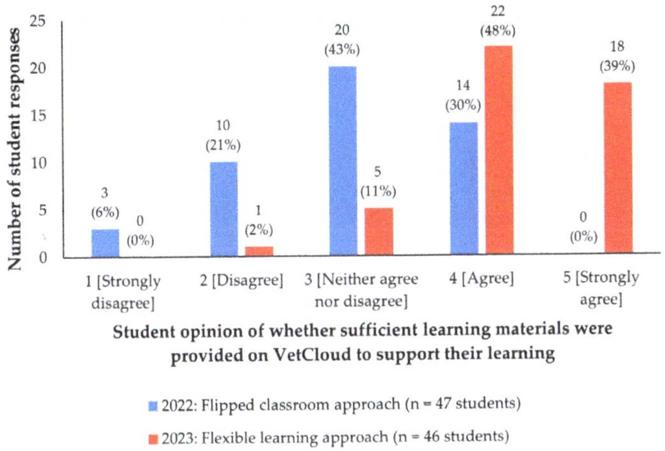

Figure 9. VETS1003 students' opinions of whether sufficient learning materials were provided on VetCloud to support their learning as part of the flipped classroom approach employed in 2022 ($n = 47$) and the flexible learning approach employed in 2023 ($n = 46$).

A chi-square test was performed to assess the relationship between student opinion and the learning cycle, and a significant difference was found ($p < 0.001$). In 2023, the majority (87%) of students agreed (48%) or strongly agreed (39%; Figure 9), compared to only 30% who agreed in 2022. The calculated median Likert rating value for the 2023 cohort was 4 (IQR 4–5), compared to the 2022 cohort's calculated median rating value of 3 (IQR 2–4; Figure 10). A Mann–Whitney test was performed to assess the difference between the two learning cycles and the result was significant ($p < 0.001$).

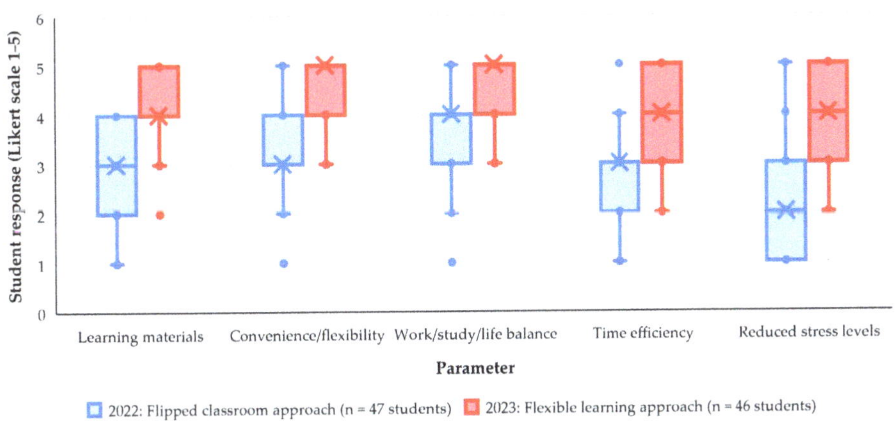

Figure 10. VETS1003 students' evaluations of VetCloud's impact on their learning experience; that is, whether it provided sufficient learning materials to support their learning, provided convenience and flexibility in their learning, supported their work/study/life balance, enabled them to use their time more efficiently when learning, and helped to reduce their stress levels as part of the flipped classroom approach employed in 2022 ($n = 47$) and the flexible learning approach employed in 2023 ($n = 46$). (× = median; lines = quartiles, median, and minimum and maximum values; dots = Likert scale answer values, including outliers).

3.6. Student Evaluations of Whether Having Access to VetCloud as Part of Flipped Classroom and Flexible Learning Approaches Provided Greater Convenience and Flexibility in Their Learning

In 2022, students were asked to rate how they found the flipped classroom approach using the VetCloud platform for providing convenience and flexibility in their learning in comparison to traditional course delivery (didactic lectures; Figure 11). In 2023 (flexible learning approach), students were asked *'On a scale of 1–5, how do you rate the VetCloud platform for providing convenience and flexibility in your learning, in comparison to traditional course delivery (didactic lectures delivered at set times)?'* (Figure 11).

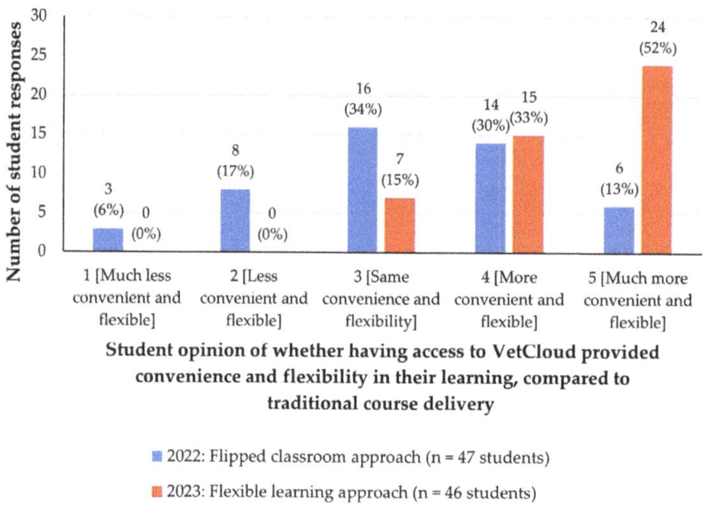

Figure 11. VETS1003 students' opinions of whether having access to VetCloud provided convenience and flexibility in their learning in comparison to traditional course delivery during the flipped classroom approach employed in 2022 (n = 47) and the flexible learning approach employed in 2023 (n = 46).

In 2022, when a flipped classroom approach was employed with online resources provided progressively over the semester in a 'just-in-time' manner, students provided a spread of responses across all five Likert scale levels, with the greatest proportion of them selecting a rating of 3 (same convenience and flexibility; n = 16, 34%; Figure 11) or 4 (more convenient and flexible; n = 14, 30%), with a calculated median rating value of 3 and IQR 3–4 (Figure 10). In 2023, all students selected a rating of 3–5 (calculated median rating 5 and IQR 4–5), with more than half of the students (n = 24, 52%) reporting that having access to VetCloud resources provided more convenience and flexibility in their learning, in comparison to traditional course delivery (Figures 10 and 11). A chi-square test was performed on the categorical data to assess the relationship between students' rating and learning cycle, and a significant increase in ratings was found for 2023 ($p < 0.001$), with 85% of students selecting a rating of 4 or 5 in 2023, compared to 43% in 2022. Similarly, a Mann–Whitney test was performed on the Likert scale data, which provided a similar interpretation ($p < 0.001$).

3.7. VetCloud's Facilitation of Students' Work/Study/Life Balance during the Flipped Classroom and Flexible Learning Approaches

Students were also asked to rate the VetCloud platform in terms of how well it supported their work/study/life balance. In 2022, they provided a spread of responses across all five Likert scale levels (Figure 12), with 81% rating VetCloud at 3–5 (neutral–excellent; Figure 11). In 2023, all 46 survey respondents rated VetCloud at 3–5 (neutral–excellent; Figure 12). Both a chi-square test on the categorical data and a Mann–Whitney test on the

Likert scale data presented evidence for a significant increase in ratings from 2022 to 2023 ($p < 0.001$ for both). The calculated median Likert scale rating was 5 (IQR 4–5) in 2023, whereas it had been 4 (IQR 3–4) in 2022. Figure 10 shows the increase in the calculated median ratings between the 2022 (4, IQR 3–4) and 2023 (5, IQR 4–5) cohorts.

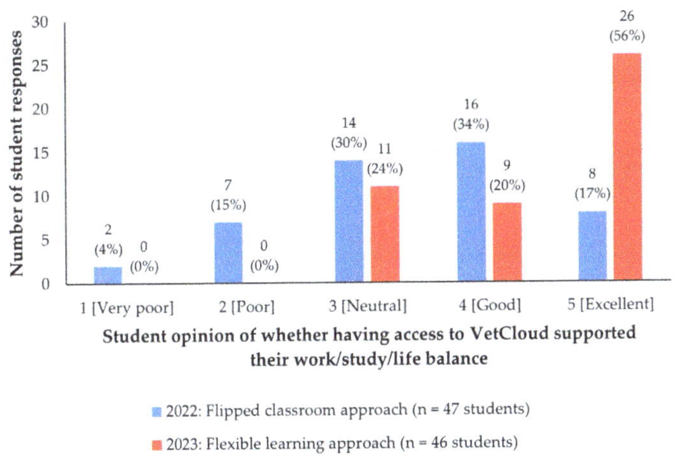

Figure 12. VETS1003 students' opinions of whether having access to VetCloud supported their work/study/life balance as part of the flipped classroom approach employed in 2022 (n = 47) and the flexible learning approach employed in 2023 (n = 46).

3.8. VetCloud's Facilitation of Efficient Time Use in the Flipped Classroom and Flexible Learning Approaches

In 2022, with the progressive release of the online content and no recordings of live lectures provided, students were asked '*Do you feel that you are using your time more efficiently learning in this format, compared to didactic teaching (traditional lectures)?*'. Cumulatively, 85% of students were neutral to being strongly in disagreement with this statement (Figure 13).

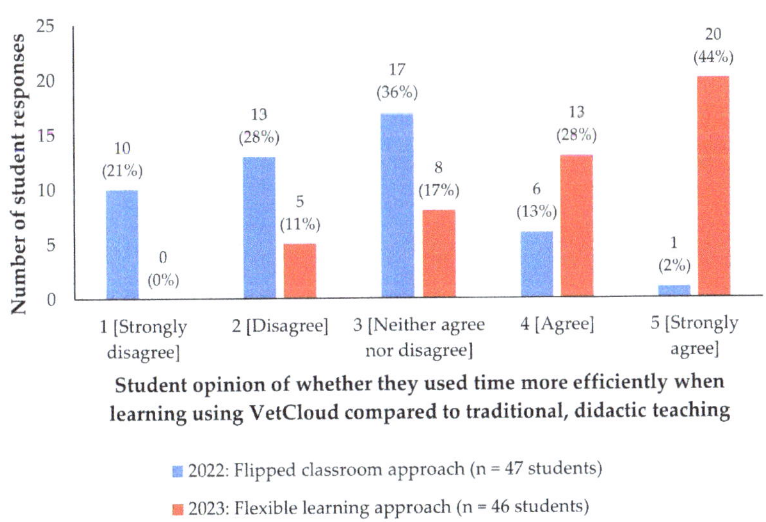

Figure 13. VETS1003 students' opinions of whether they used their time more efficiently when learning using VetCloud compared to traditional, didactic teaching as part of the flipped classroom approach employed in 2022 (n = 47) and the flexible learning approach employed in 2023 (n = 46).

In 2023, when the online content was available from the beginning of the semester, the multiple-choice question from the 2022 survey was replaced with a more clearly worded question that asked students to rate how much they agreed with the statement *'I use my time more efficiently when learning using VetCloud, compared to didactic teaching (traditional lectures)'*. This time, most students (Figure 13) either strongly agreed (n = 20/46, 44%) or agreed (n = 13, 28%) with the given statement. The calculated median rating value for this 2023 survey question was 4 (IQR 3–5)—a marked increase from the equivalent 2022 median rating value of 3 (IQR 2–3; Figure 10). Both a chi-square test on the categorical data and a Mann–Whitney test on the Likert scale data presented evidence for a significant increase in rating from 2022 to 2023 ($p < 0.001$).

3.9. Student Stress Levels during the Flipped Classroom and Flexible Learning Approaches

In the 2022 survey, students were asked *'Do you feel the flipped classroom approach using VetCloud has reduced your stress levels while learning the content throughout the semester?'*. Most students (n = 42/47, 89%) were neutral, disagreed, or strongly disagreed (Figure 14).

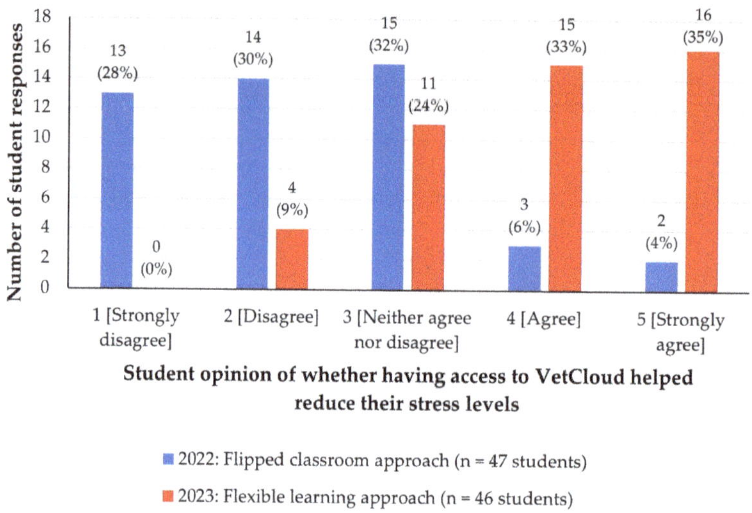

Figure 14. VETS1003 students' opinions of whether having access to VetCloud as part of the flipped classroom approach employed in 2022 (n = 47) and the flexible learning approach employed in 2023 (n = 46) helped to reduce their stress levels during the semester.

In 2023, the multiple-choice question from the 2022 survey was replaced with a question that asked students to rate how much they agreed with the statement *'Having access to VetCloud as a learning resource has reduced/is reducing my stress levels during the semester, including in the lead up to assessments'*. This time, with all the VETS1003 anatomy and physiology content provided on VetCloud from the beginning of the semester as part of the flexible learning approach, there was a positive trend, with most students either strongly agreeing (n = 16/46, 35%) or agreeing (n = 15, 33%) with the given statement (Figure 14). The calculated median rating value for this 2023 survey question was 4 (IQR 3–5) compared to 2 (IQR 1–3) in 2022 (Figure 10). Both a chi-square test on the categorical data and a Mann–Whitney test on the Likert scale data presented evidence for a significant increase in rating from 2022 to 2023 ($p < 0.001$).

3.10. Students' General Opinions of the Flipped Classroom and Flexible Learning Approaches

In the 2022 survey, students were asked three final open-response questions to gauge their general opinions about the flipped classroom approach. They were first asked *'What did you like/dislike about the VetCloud learning platform? Are there any improvements that you would suggest?'* (n = 40/47 responses, 85%) and finally *'Do you have any further comments, or feedback on the course thus far?'* (n = 28 responses, 60%). Across these three questions, students indicated that they appreciated several of the resources provided on VetCloud (e.g., self-assessment quizzes, short topic videos) and generally found the platform itself easy to navigate and use. However, students commonly felt that the use of VetCloud in the flipped classroom approach could be improved. Students did not like the restricted release of online content/resources on Thursdays before being expected to engage with it on Friday mornings (8–11 a.m.) in preparation for attending tutorials (12–1 p.m.) and practical classes (1–5 p.m.) on Friday afternoons. They found the same-day engagement/delivery of lecture content, tutorials, and practicals too overwhelming and fast-paced, and reiterated that it did not provide them enough time to 'digest' the information.

In 2022, students felt that there was too much lecture content and found the time allocated for engaging with it on Friday mornings unrealistic and stressful: *'the course is so content heavy that it is difficult to get the lectures done in the 3 hours before the prac on the Friday. And if I do get the lectures done, I don't have a good idea of the content going into the prac that day.'* Several students felt that the delivery of content in the short topic videos was too fast, which made the concepts covered more difficult to understand: *'I think VETS1003 is very detailed and complicated and therefore it requires more time and slower paced, in depth lectures.'* Students requested slower, more in-depth explanations of complicated concepts in videos delivered in a more conversational style, and earlier release of online content/resources on VetCloud before scheduled classes. Several students also expressed a preference for having—and requested the addition of—face-to-face lectures for VETS1003, to allow for more conversational and in-depth explanations and to provide greater opportunities for asking questions, clarifying concepts, and interacting with their peers and teaching staff.

In the 2023 survey, students were similarly asked four final open-response questions to gauge their general opinions about the flexible learning approach. The questions asked were *'What do you like about the VetCloud platform? Please explain.'* (n = 46/46 responses), *'What do you dislike about the VetCloud platform? Do you have any suggestions for improvement? Please explain.'* (n = 20 responses, 43%), and *'Do you have any other comments about the VetCloud platform and/or how it has been used in VETS1003?'* (n = 9 responses, 20%). Students again praised the ease of use of the VetCloud platform and appreciated the provided resources, with suggestions for improvement largely based around technical aspects (e.g., requests for a greater variety of video playback controls) or requests for further resources (e.g., more quiz questions). Students liked having the option to attend face-to-face lectures, having access to video recordings of live lectures available for later viewing on VetCloud soon afterwards, and particularly having the other provided resources (short topic videos, learning outcomes, lecture slides, lecture slides with transcript notes, and self-assessment quizzes) available to them on VetCloud even before face-to-face lectures were held. Students felt that these factors allowed them greater flexibility in their learning, provided greater access to lecture content without the absolute requirement for commuting to campus, and positioned VetCloud as a one-stop 'hub' for learning resources that suit students' different learning preferences.

4. Discussion

There was a marked improvement in how well VetCloud supported students' work/study/life balance from 2022 to 2023, with the majority (56%) of students in 2023 rating the platform as excellent. Students in 2023 reported that they used their time much more efficiently when studying using VetCloud in the flexible learning approach, than the students in the flipped classroom approach in 2022. Similarly, students in 2023 also found that being able to use VetCloud in the flexible learning approach reduced their stress levels to a greater extent than the students in the flipped classroom approach in 2022.

It is an acknowledged limitation of this study that we are unable to compare student data from multiple learning cycles of VETS1003 that differed solely by one intervention (e.g., two iterations of a flipped classroom approach that included only changes to the online resources provided or our 2022 flipped classroom approach and a flexible learning approach that introduced face-to-face lectures without any other changes). However, this is active scholarship of teaching and learning (SoTL) research embedded in courses delivered in real time; fairness and justice in the impact of educational interventions on students is of paramount importance [22], and it is not ethical to repeat the recognized mistakes or limitations of a previous learning cycle and restrict student opportunities and/or benefits for the sake of having a repeatable study. The most ethical approach for us to take was to act on the clear, constructive student feedback from 2022 to improve the student learning experience into the next year rather than focusing on one single intervention, which resulted in the flexible learning approach we employed in 2023. Hence, our study is focused on the impacts of our employed flipped classroom and flexible learning approaches in two consecutive learning cycles on student experience from student perception data and feedback from 2022 and 2023. The incentive provided to students for survey participation—the opportunity to win one of a limited number of AUD 20 Coles-Myer retail gift cards if they identified themselves—potentially introduced enrolment bias into this study. Students were informed that all survey responses would remain anonymous to VETS1003 teaching staff, and that providing names and contact details with their otherwise-anonymous survey responses was strictly voluntary and only for gift card draw purposes. However, the perceived potential for survey responses to be identified could have resulted in some students declining to participate.

There is no single tool that meets all the curriculum requirements for teaching veterinary anatomy and physiology; every student has a unique learning style. This is consistent with an overall improvement in assessed parameters associated with the 2023 multi-modal presentation of content including online resources as well as face-to-face lectures—provision of resources in a format that offered students choice. Positive effects on both student performance and well-being of medical students using digital learning resources for self-directed study have been demonstrated in multiple disciplines, including anatomy [23], radiology [24], histology [25], ECG interpretation [26], and ultrasound training [27]. There is a significant positive relationship between psychological characteristics and academic fit in veterinary students [28]. Veterinary students can experience high levels of anxiety, depression, and decreased overall life satisfaction [29–32]; there is a positive relationship between psychological characteristics and engagement, and a negative relationship with exhaustion [28]. VetCloud is a practical intervention that supports the academic experience of veterinary students by addressing both their academic needs—by 2023 students felt that VetCloud provided them with sufficient learning materials to support their learning—and importantly also their psychological needs. Use of VetCloud in the flexible learning approach in 2023 improved students' work/study/life balance, reduced their stress levels, and enabled a more efficient use of their study time, compared to the flipped classroom approach used in 2022. VetCloud therefore offers educators a more holistic educational tool to support veterinary education.

While active teaching and learning approaches such as the flipped classroom are generally reported to be beneficial, such teaching approaches have not been implemented widely in veterinary science education because of the inherent challenges posed by the integrated nature of the curriculum [12] and by consistently poor student feedback. While a variety of offline and online teaching resources and activities have been developed worldwide for teaching veterinary science in recent years [13–18,33–40], the manner in which they are used can vary significantly based on specific institutional, ethical, disciplinary, or other requirements—including barriers to the implementation of flipped classroom-type approaches [12]. Multiple small changes to teaching methods employed in tandem, as we employed in 2023, can thus be very beneficial for student experience, student efficiency, and learning quality. The importance of seeking and considering student perspectives when evaluating the efficacy of teaching methods in veterinary science [15,39,40] and medicine [23,24,41] has been highlighted.

In 2022, when face-to-face anatomy and physiology lectures were not held and no recordings of full-length live lectures from previous years were available for reference, 49% of students stated that they would have preferred to have lectures delivered face-to-face, indicating a solid demand for a return to face-to-face learning. However, almost one-quarter of students (23%) did not engage with tutorials at all, largely because they either had not been able to complete watching the relevant lecture content videos on VetCloud on Friday morning prior to the scheduled tutorial time on Friday afternoon or they had watched the relevant videos but had not had sufficient time to 'digest' the content. Students who answered open-ended general feedback questions in the 2022 survey clearly explained that they did not appreciate the late release of online content/resources on Thursdays and that they found the same-day engagement/delivery of lecture content, tutorials, and practicals on Fridays too overwhelming, fast-paced, and stressful. Constructively, students requested the earlier release of online content/resources on VetCloud before scheduled classes, alongside slower, more in-depth explanations of complicated concepts in videos delivered in a less formal and more conversational manner and the addition of face-to-face lectures.

Responding to this feedback from 2022 students, face-to-face lectures were introduced for the anatomy and physiology modules of VETS1003 in 2023 and they were scheduled on Monday mornings, prior to face-to-face tutorials on Tuesday afternoons and practical classes on Friday afternoons. As part of the new flexible learning approach, the resources on VetCloud were this time provided to students from week 1 of the semester, facilitated by the development of the bulk of these resources in 2022, instead of progressive weekly release. Additionally, complete lecture recording videos of the live lectures were made available on VetCloud within one week of each lecture being held in 2023. This response to student feedback was associated with a stronger preference for VetCloud resources as a lecture delivery format, with 67% of students reporting a liking for full-length (50 min) lecture videos and 65% of students liking the short topic videos provided on VetCloud. Students who answered open-response questions in the 2023 survey appreciated having the option to attend face-to-face lectures and/or watch the video recordings of these live lectures on VetCloud soon afterwards, and particularly appreciated having the other provided resources (short topic videos, learning outcomes, lecture slides, lecture slides with transcript notes, and self-assessment quizzes) available to them on VetCloud even before face-to-face lectures were held. Students largely enjoyed the greater flexibility in their learning and greater access to lecture content provided by the changes made to the timing and provision of resources on VetCloud and the scheduling of learning activities in going from the flipped classroom approach in 2022 to the flexible learning approach in 2023.

While lectures are an effective method of conveying information [42], a benefit of the VetCloud platform is the provision of both short topic videos and full-length (50 min) lecture recordings, which provides students with diverse learning styles the advantage of choice regarding how they would prefer to engage with core knowledge content. It has been argued that there is an inverse relationship between the length of a lecture and the retention of material covered due to 'attention lapses' [43], supporting the justification of shorter modularized content; although issues with the analysis undertaken preclude broader extrapolation of the data presented [42]. However, in the context of modern veterinary education, there are additional benefits regarding modularized delivery of content beyond the potential for improved retention of knowledge. Veterinary students are a highly diverse cohort, with students ranging in age from 17 to 50+ years, and many students are currently under significant financial constraints. Attendance at a regional campus can raise conflicts with work, children, and caring responsibilities. VetCloud supports learning in a way that influences, motivates, and inspires students to learn, while embracing and highlighting inclusivity, catering to the diverse learning styles and life situations of our students. Examples of this include anecdotal feedback from students with learning disabilities who have explained that the modularization of content on VetCloud helped them clearly understand what needed to be taken away from each lecture, and breaking down concepts into small chunks meant they did not 'zone out'. In contrast, general feedback from veterinary science students across year levels at The University of Queensland over the past few years has indicated a strong collective dislike for being provided with only short, modularized videos. Indeed, our VETS1003 students did not find the modularized, short topic videos to be beneficial to their learning until they were offered in conjunction with complete full-length lecture recordings. This combination of modularized, short topic videos with the slower-paced explanations provided in full-length lectures were required by our first-year students for them to perceive that they had been provided with sufficient learning materials to meet their learning needs.

In the flipped classroom approach employed in VETS1003 in 2022, which involved the progressive provision of modularized content on the VetCloud platform, the majority of students felt they were not provided with sufficient learning materials, their work/study/life balance and stress levels were not supported, their use of study time was inefficient, and they did not find the employed approach to be more flexible or convenient than traditional, didactic teaching. Students thus asked for changes to the types and provision time of the offered online learning resources and the introduction of face-to-face lectures. Following the requested changes being integrated in the 2023 flexible learning approach, students largely felt that they were provided with sufficient learning materials and that the employed approach was more flexible and convenient for them, appreciating both having the online resources available to them earlier in the semester and the option to attend face-to-face lectures and/or watch the video recordings of these as it suited them best. The 2023 students reported that their work/study/life balance was supported, stress levels were reduced, and their study time was more efficiently used. This outcome highlights the positive impacts of applying iterative student feedback in teaching, and the importance of considering student perceptions and the student experience when implementing educational interventions.

5. Conclusions

Flexible teaching where online learning resources are offered in addition to in-class instruction can be successfully applied to teaching veterinary anatomy and physiology. Applying iterative student feedback regarding the provision of multi-modal learning resources and how they were utilized in teaching across flipped classroom and flexible teaching approaches had a positive impact on veterinary students' learning experience. In 2023, the use of VetCloud in the flexible learning approach improved students' work/study/life balance, reduced their stress levels, and enabled them to use their time much more efficiently when studying, compared to the flipped classroom approach used in 2022. This teaching method offers veterinary educators an innovative and efficient approach to veterinary student education in anatomy and physiology.

Supplementary Materials: The following supporting information can be downloaded at: https://www.mdpi.com/article/10.3390/ani14162335/s1, Supplementary File S1: 2022 Student survey; Supplementary File S2: 2023 Student survey.

Author Contributions: Conceptualization, F.M.S., M.G.H., P.S.W. and S.L.B.; Data curation, A.A.S.; Formal analysis, A.A.S. and A.B.; Funding acquisition, F.M.S., M.G.H., P.S.W. and S.L.B.; Methodology, A.A.S., F.M.S. and S.L.B.; Project administration, A.A.S., M.G.H., P.S.W. and S.L.B.; Resources, M.G.H. and P.S.W.; Software, P.S.W.; Supervision, M.G.H. and S.L.B.; Visualization, A.A.S.; Writing—original draft, A.A.S., A.B. and S.L.B.; Writing—review and editing, A.A.S., F.M.S., D.J.W. and S.L.B. All authors have read and agreed to the published version of the manuscript.

Funding: This research was funded by The University of Queensland Faculty of Science Teaching and Learning Grants scheme (2022 and 2023) and Faculty of Science funding to the Student-Led Observation for Course Improvement (SLOCI) Team (2022 and 2023).

Institutional Review Board Statement: This study was conducted in accordance with the Declaration of Helsinki and approved by the Human Ethics Committee of The University of Queensland (project number 2019/HE001666).

Informed Consent Statement: Implied consent was obtained from all students involved in this study by their voluntary choice to respond to surveys. Students were advised that survey responses would remain anonymous to teaching team members.

Data Availability Statement: The data presented in this study are available in the article.

Acknowledgments: We acknowledge the following people at The University of Queensland for their involvement in the development and implementation of the VetCloud platform and in the gathering of student feedback about VetCloud: the eLearning Innovations and Partnerships in Science and Engineering (eLIPSE) Team; Malcolm Jones; Paul Mills; and Julia Buczynski, Mikki Doonan, Mitchell Field, Mia Forsingdal, Aaron Netto, Samara Ranie, Alice Sewell, Susan Shanyn-Miller, Khristine Grace Valdellon, and Louise Manitzky (members of the Science SLOCI Team involved in partnerships with VetCloud-using courses in 2022 and 2023 alongside author A.A.S. [Arti Singh] in 2023). We also thank all student survey participants for their responses and input for this study.

Conflicts of Interest: The authors declare no conflicts of interest. The funders had no role in the design of the study; in the collection, analyses, or interpretation of data; in the writing of the manuscript; or in the decision to publish the results.

References

1. Mercer-Mapstone, L.; Dvorakova, S.L.; Matthews, K.E.; Abbot, S.; Cheng, B.; Felten, P.; Knorr, K.; Marquis, E.; Shammas, R.; Swaim, K. A systematic literature review of students as partners in higher education. *IJSaP* **2017**, *1*, 15–37. [CrossRef]
2. Hodges, C.; Moore, S.; Lockee, B.; Trust, T.; Bond, A. The Difference Between Emergency Remote Teaching and Online Learning. 2020. Available online: https://er.educause.edu/articles/2020/3/the-difference-between-emergency-remote-teaching-and-online-learning (accessed on 27 March 2024).
3. Slade, C.; Lawrie, G.; Taptamat, N.; Browne, E.; Sheppard, K.; Matthews, K.E. Insights into how academics reframed their assessment during a pandemic: Disciplinary variation and assessment as afterthought. *Assess. Eval. High. Educ.* **2022**, *47*, 588–605. [CrossRef]
4. Goyal, M.; Krishnamurthi, R.; Yadav, D. *E-Learning Methodologies—Fundamentals, Technologies and Applications*; Institution of Engineering and Technology: London, UK, 2021.
5. Reidsema, C.; Kavanagh, L.; Hadgraft, R.; Smith, N. *The Flipped Classroom: Practice and Practices in Higher Education*, 1st ed.; Springer: Singapore, 2017. [CrossRef]
6. Abeysekera, L.; Dawson, P. Motivation and cognitive load in the flipped classroom: Definition, rationale and a call for research. *High. Educ. Res. Dev.* **2015**, *34*, 1–14. [CrossRef]
7. O'Flaherty, J.; Phillips, C. The use of flipped classrooms in higher education: A scoping review. *Internet High. Educ.* **2015**, *25*, 85–95. [CrossRef]
8. Kazeminia, M.; Salehi, L.; Khosravipour, M.; Rajati, F. Investigation flipped classroom effectiveness in teaching anatomy: A systematic review. *J. Prof. Nurs.* **2022**, *42*, 15–25. [CrossRef] [PubMed]
9. Gopalan, C.; Klann, M.C. The effect of flipped teaching combined with modified team-based learning on student performance in physiology. *Adv. Physiol. Educ.* **2017**, *41*, 363–367. [CrossRef]
10. Megaw, P.L.; Zimanyi, M.A. Redesigning first year anatomy and physiology subjects for allied health students: Introducing active learning experiences for physiology in a first semester subject. *Int. J. Innov. Sci. Math. Educ.* **2019**, *27*, 26–35. [CrossRef]
11. Williams, D.E. The future of medical education: Flipping the classroom and education technology. *Ochsner J.* **2016**, *16*, 14–15.
12. Matthew, S.M.; Schoenfeld-Tacher, R.M.; Danielson, J.A.; Warman, S.M. Flipped classroom use in veterinary education: A multinational survey of faculty experiences. *J. Vet. Med. Educ.* **2019**, *46*, 97–107. [CrossRef]
13. Dooley, L.M.; Frankland, S.; Boller, E.; Tudor, E. Implementing the flipped classroom in a veterinary pre-clinical science course: Student engagement, performance, and satisfaction. *J. Vet. Med. Educ.* **2018**, *45*, 195–203. [CrossRef] [PubMed]
14. López-Úbeda, R.; García-Vázquez, F.A. Self-directed learning using computer simulations to study veterinary physiology: Comparing individual and collaborative learning approaches. *Vet. Record* **2022**, *191*, e1732. [CrossRef] [PubMed]
15. Gómez, O.; García-Manzanares, M.; Chicharro, D.; Juárez, M.; Llamazares-Martín, C.; Soriano, E.; Terrado, J. Application of blended learning to veterinary gross anatomy practical sessions: Students' perceptions of their learning experience and academic outcomes. *Animals* **2023**, *13*, 1666. [CrossRef] [PubMed]
16. Moffett, J.; Mill, A.C. Evaluation of the flipped classroom approach in a veterinary professional skills course. *Adv. Med. Educ. Pract.* **2014**, *5*, 415–425. [CrossRef] [PubMed]
17. Kelly, R.F.; Mihm-Carmichael, M.; Hammond, J.A. Students' engagement in and perceptions of blended learning in a clinical module in a veterinary degree program. *J. Vet. Med. Educ.* **2021**, *48*, 181–195. [CrossRef] [PubMed]
18. Duijvestijn, M.B.H.M.; Van der Wiel, B.M.W.K.; Vinke, C.M.; Diaz Espineira, M.M.; Bok, H.G.J.; Vernooij, J.C.M. Implementation of a blended learning module to teach handling, restraint, and physical examination of cats in undergraduate veterinary training. *J. Vet. Med. Educ.* **2022**, *49*, 537–546. [CrossRef] [PubMed]

19. George, P.P.; Papachristou, N.; Belisario, J.M.; Wang, W.; Wark, P.A.; Cotic, Z.; Rasmussen, K.; Sluiter, R.; Riboli-Sasco, E.; Tudor Car, L.; et al. Online eLearning for undergraduates in health professions: A systematic review of the impact on knowledge, skills, attitudes and satisfaction. *J. Glob. Health* **2014**, *4*, 010406. [CrossRef] [PubMed]
20. McAnally, S.; Buczynski, J.; Kavanagh, L. Student-led observations for course improvement (SLOCI): Closing the loop in course enhancement. *IJSaP* **2024**, accepted.
21. R Core Team. *R: A Language and Environment for Statistical Computing*; R Foundation for Statistical Computing: Vienna, Austria, 2024; Available online: https://www.R-project.org/ (accessed on 1 June 2024).
22. Yeo, M.; Miller-Young, J.; Manarin, K. Understanding SoTL. In *SoTL Research Methodologies*, 1st ed.; Routledge: New York, NY, USA, 2023; pp. 3–13.
23. El Sadik, A.; Al Abdulmonem, W. Improvement in student performance and perceptions through a flipped anatomy classroom: Shifting from passive traditional to active blended learning. *Anat. Sci. Educ.* **2021**, *14*, 482–490. [CrossRef] [PubMed]
24. Belfi, L.M.; Bartolotta, R.J.; Giambrone, A.E.; Davi, C.; Min, R.J. "Flipping" the introductory clerkship in radiology: Impact on medical student performance and perceptions. *Acad. Radiol.* **2015**, *22*, 794–801. [CrossRef]
25. Cheng, X.; Ka Ho Lee, K.; Chang, E.Y.; Yang, X. The "flipped classroom" approach: Stimulating positive learning attitudes and improving mastery of histology among medical students. *Anat. Sci. Educ.* **2017**, *10*, 317–327. [CrossRef]
26. Montassier, E.; Hardouin, J.-B.; Segard, J.; Batard, E.; Potel, G.; Planchon, B.; Trochu, J.-N.; Pottier, P. e-Learning versus lecture-based courses in ECG interpretation for undergraduate medical students. *Eur. J. Emerg. Med.* **2016**, *23*, 108–113. [CrossRef]
27. Beaulieu, Y.; Laprise, R.; Drolet, P.; Thivierge, R.L.; Serri, K.; Albert, M.; Lamontagne, A.; Bélliveau, M.; Denault, A.-Y.; Patenaude, J.-V. Bedside ultrasound training using web-based e-learning and simulation early in the curriculum of residents. *Crit. Ultrasound J.* **2015**, *7*, 1. [CrossRef]
28. Muca, E.; Molino, M.; Ghislieri, C.; Baratta, M.; Odore, R.; Bergero, D.; Valle, E. Relationships between psychological characteristics, academic fit and engagement with academic performance in veterinary medical students. *BMC Vet. Res.* **2023**, *19*, 132. [CrossRef] [PubMed]
29. Reisbig, A.M.J.; Danielson, J.A.; Wu, T.-F.; Hafen, M.; Krienert, A.; Girard, D.; Garlock, J. A study of depression and anxiety, general health, and academic performance in three cohorts of veterinary medical students across the first three semesters of veterinary school. *J. Vet. Med. Educ.* **2012**, *39*, 341–358. [CrossRef] [PubMed]
30. Killinger, S.L.; Flanagan, S.; Castine, E.; Howard, K.A.S. Stress and depression among veterinary medical students. *J. Vet. Med. Educ.* **2017**, *44*, 3–8. [CrossRef] [PubMed]
31. Ilić Živojinović, J.; Backović, D.; Belojević, G.; Valčić, O.; Soldatović, I.; Janković, J. Predictors of burnout among Belgrade veterinary students: A cross-sectional study. *PLoS ONE* **2020**, *15*, e0230685. [CrossRef]
32. Nahm, S.-S.; Chun, M.-S. Stressors predicting depression, anxiety, and stress in Korean veterinary students. *J. Vet. Med. Educ.* **2021**, *48*, 470–476. [CrossRef] [PubMed]
33. Kapoor, K.; Singh, A. Veterinary anatomy teaching from real to virtual reality: An unprecedented shift during COVID-19 in socially distant era. *Anat. Histol. Embryol.* **2022**, *51*, 163–169. [CrossRef] [PubMed]
34. Muca, E.; Cavallini, D.; Odore, R.; Baratta, M.; Bergero, D.; Valle, E. Are veterinary students using technologies and online learning resources for didactic training? A mini-meta analysis. *Educ. Sci.* **2022**, *12*, 573. [CrossRef]
35. Seddon, J.M.; Vo, A.T.T.; Kempster, S.R.; Lee, H.J.; Nguyen, T.T.; Munce, K.; Bianco, A.D.; Chakitdee, V.; Quang, T.; Shapter, F.M. Simulated clinical skills for veterinary students supplement limited animal and clinical resources in developing countries. *J. Vet. Med. Educ.* **2020**, *47*, 92–98. [CrossRef]
36. Wichtel, J.; zur Linden, A.; Khosa, D.; Singh, A.; Sears, W.; Phillips, J. Validation of a novel ultrasound simulation model for teaching foundation-level ultrasonography skills to veterinary students. *J. Vet. Med. Educ.* **2022**, *49*, 473–483. [CrossRef] [PubMed]
37. da Costa, B.N.; Sousa, M.G.; Tanji, F.N.; Ulanin, M.; Wolf, M.; Stedile, S.T.O. The use of 3-D models of echocardiographic imaging planes for teaching echocardiography techniques for use in dogs and cats. *Altern. Lab. Anim.* **2022**, *50*, 208–220. [CrossRef] [PubMed]
38. Linton, A.; Garrett, A.C.; Ivie, K.R., Jr.; Jones, J.D.; Martin, J.F.; Delcambre, J.J.; Magee, C. Enhancing anatomical instruction: Impact of a virtual canine anatomy program on student outcomes. *Anat. Sci. Educ.* **2022**, *15*, 330–340. [CrossRef] [PubMed]
39. Mahdy, M.A.A.; Sayed, R.K.A. Evaluation of the online learning of veterinary anatomy education during the COVID-19 pandemic lockdown in Egypt: Students' perceptions. *Anat. Sci. Educ.* **2022**, *15*, 67–82. [CrossRef] [PubMed]
40. Muca, E.; Cavallini, D.; Raspa, F.; Bordin, C.; Bergero, D.; Valle, E. Integrating new learning methods into equine nutrition classrooms: The importance of students' perceptions. *J. Equine Vet. Sci.* **2023**, *126*, 104537. [CrossRef] [PubMed]
41. Nasr El-Din, W.A.; Atwa, H.; Potu, B.K.; Deifalla, A.; Fadel, R.A. Checklist-based active learning in anatomy demonstration sessions during the COVID-19 pandemic: Perception of medical students. *Morphologie* **2023**, *107*, 219–227. [CrossRef] [PubMed]
42. Bradbury, N.A. Attention span during lectures: 8 seconds, 10 minutes, or more? *Adv. Physiol. Educ.* **2016**, *40*, 509–513. [CrossRef]
43. Johnstone, A.H.; Percival, F. Attention breaks in lectures. *Educ. Chem.* **1976**, *13*, 49–50.

animals

Article

Risk Communication on Zoonoses and Antimicrobial Resistance—How Do Exotic Pet Owners Perceive the Communication of Their Veterinarians?

Amelie Lisa Arnecke [1,*], Stefan Schwarz [2,3], Antina Lübke-Becker [2,3], Katharina Charlotte Jensen [4], Christina Herre [1] and Mahtab Bahramsoltani [1]

1 Institute of Veterinary Anatomy, School of Veterinary Medicine, Freie Universität Berlin, Koserstraße 20, 14195 Berlin, Germany; christina.herre@fu-berlin.de (C.H.); mahtab.bahramsoltani@fu-berlin.de (M.B.)
2 Institute of Microbiology and Epizootics, School of Veterinary Medicine, Freie Universität Berlin, Robert-von-Ostertag-Straße 7, 14163 Berlin, Germany; stefan.schwarz@fu-berlin.de (S.S.); antina.luebke-becker@fu-berlin.de (A.L.-B.)
3 Veterinary Centre for Resistance Research (TZR), School of Veterinary Medicine, Freie Universität Berlin, Robert-von-Ostertag-Straße 8, 14163 Berlin, Germany
4 Institute for Veterinary Epidemiology and Biostatistics, School of Veterinary Medicine, Freie Universität Berlin, Königsweg 67, 14163 Berlin, Germany; charlotte.jensen@fu-berlin.de
* Correspondence: al.arnecke@fu-berlin.de

Simple Summary: Exotic animals can carry pathogens that may spread to humans and other animals. When traded and kept as pets, the risk of disease transmission increases as there is a higher potential of close contact and stress involved that can weaken the animals' immune system, making them more likely to shed pathogens. This becomes especially important for households with children younger than five years, elderly and pregnant people or immunocompromised individuals. Thus, this survey investigated how exotic pets are kept, the advice given by veterinarians and how well veterinarians communicate the risks of zoonoses and antimicrobial resistance. The results showed that owning exotic pets comes with several health risks. However, pet owners generally felt satisfied with their veterinarians' communication, especially when they had consulted a veterinarian for a longer time. Despite this, pet owners expressed a desire for more frequent information on these topics. Therefore, it is important to provide more educational resources. Enhancing education and training for veterinarians, particularly in universities, could improve their communication with pet owners about the risks associated with exotic pets. This study highlights the important role of veterinarians in the prevention of pathogen transmission from animals to humans through targeted risk communication.

Abstract: Exotic animals traded and kept as pets can transmit a variety of diseases to humans and other animals, and vice versa. Therefore, it is essential for pet owners, particularly vulnerable groups, to be informed about associated risks. Veterinarians play a crucial role in informing pet owners about health risks associated with zoonotic pathogens and antimicrobial resistance (AMR) and should, therefore, have good communication skills to effectively transfer information to pet owners. Thus, exotic pet owners in Germany were surveyed on animal husbandry, veterinary consultation and risk communication. To evaluate the perception of communication, a self-developed questionnaire was used to derive a communication score. The perception of veterinarian communication received a high average score showing a high level of satisfaction. The duration of the veterinarian–client relationship was associated with better communication perception, and the frequency of communication on zoonoses and AMR was associated with the presence of a permanent veterinarian. However, the results indicated that the frequency of disseminated information on zoonoses and/or AMR from veterinarians was lower than desired by the pet owners. Therefore, more educational material on zoonoses and AMR should be made available, and the awareness concerning risk communication should be increased by further education and training at universities.

Keywords: risk communication; risk perception; risk awareness; zoonoses; antimicrobial resistance (AMR); pathogen transmission; one health; exotic pets

1. Introduction

Over the last decades, there has been an emergence of more than 100 different human diseases originating from wild animals, posing significant concerns for human health [1]. In this context, the live animal trade, including the exotic pet trade, was identified as one of five major contributors to the spread of pathogens within the wildlife trade [2]. Zoonotic pathogens are relevant for both humans and animals as they can be transmitted between and among them, leading to illness and fatalities, posing a threat to public health, veterinary health and wildlife populations [3–5].

Private pet ownership, including exotic pet animals, is widespread in Germany and is particularly common among families with children [6,7]. Contact with pets is linked to people's mental and physical wellbeing [8,9]. However, contact with exotic pets especially is associated with specific risks, as they can transmit a variety of diseases to humans [4,10–14]. In addition, bacterial pathogens exhibiting antimicrobial resistance (AMR) pose a significant health threat by reducing the effectiveness of antimicrobial agents in treating infections [15]. Previous studies support the theory on potential cross-transmission of antimicrobial-resistant bacteria between animals and humans [16–22]. As antimicrobial-resistant pathogens are found in small and exotic animals, pets can be considered as potential reservoirs [23–25]. Consequently, there is a high likelihood of resistant bacteria transferring between pets and humans [26].

This undermines efforts to control infectious diseases in both humans and animals, emphasizing the interconnectedness of health across different species and ecosystems [27]. Due to the close interaction between humans and animals, it is vital to acknowledge the different routes of infection transmission but also to be aware of the individual risks connected to vulnerable groups, such as children younger than five years, adults older than 65 years, people with weakened immune systems and pregnant people [28]. Besides this, the population of immunocompromised individuals has experienced a steep exponential rise over the past few decades [29].

Thus, the role of medical professionals is crucial to translate risk communication messages into clinical practice [30]. However, previous findings have revealed that physicians tend to consider veterinarians as having a superior knowledge and understanding of zoonoses [31,32]. Studies suggest that veterinarians have indeed a superior comprehension of zoonotic pathogens and demonstrate higher proficiency in diagnosing zoonoses when compared to physicians [33]. As veterinarians hold specialized knowledge and expertise in animal health but also have a unique position at the human–animal interface, they bear a distinct responsibility to the public health sector [34]. In contrast to physicians, veterinarians are required to have a broad understanding of many species, which could lead to gaps in specialized knowledge. Furthermore, their expertise with wildlife species and exotic pets is often limited due to the focus on common domestic animals in primary training and practice. Specialisations require additional postgraduate training beyond the scope of the standard veterinary education [35–37]. Nevertheless, veterinarian communication plays a significant role strengthening the bond between veterinarians and pet owners by amplifying the clients' willingness to follow recommendations given by the veterinarian [38]. However, low compliance with deworming protocols and gaps in pets' immunization indicate a noticeable decrease in the utilization of preventive medicine among pet owners, thereby prompting the need for improved communication and information strategies [39–41]. Furthermore, emerging zoonoses are unpredictable events that require special communication strategies. This issue should be addressed and practiced in training programs, so that the veterinary community is prepared for an outbreak situation [42]. Previous studies have shown that veterinary practitioners can further benefit from training on specific communication skills [43]. Research supports the idea that strong communication skills, particularly in veterinary science and related health sectors are vital [44]. Despite this, veterinarians face a distinct challenge in interacting and communicating effectively with pet owners [45,46], and the perception of risk depends not only on the objective reality but also on the people's needs, goals, past experiences, expectations and reference points [47]. Thus, it is important to assess pet owners on their perception of veterinarian communication in order to adapt the risk communication strategies [48].

The aim of this study was to gain insights into exotic pet owners' perception of veterinarian communication on zoonoses and AMR. In particular, the frequency of risk communication and the perception of communication in relation to risk factors and risk behaviours should be assessed. Furthermore, the association between risk communication and the veterinarian–client relationship as well as the reason for the consultation should be determined. Thus, the findings can provide important insights for practicing veterinarians, since they have an important role in risk communication to strengthen global health at the human–animal interface.

2. Participants, Materials and Methods

2.1. Participants

For this study, exotic pet owners in Germany were surveyed. The survey, conducted via Lime-Survey Cloud Version 5.6.56® from December 2022 to April 2023, was promoted on social media (Facebook and Instagram). Participants could access the survey by using a link or scanning a QR code. The participation was voluntary, and participants were given the freedom to withdraw from the study at any point without facing consequences. Before starting the survey, participants had to read the legal notice and agree to our privacy policy. In addition, they had to confirm that they are at least 18 years old. The study concept was approved by the Ethics Committee (ZEA-Nr. 2022-018) of the Freie Universität Berlin.

2.2. Questionnaire

The questionnaire consisted of six sections. Every participant was queried on risk factors, their pet(s) and associated risk behaviour, the veterinarian–client relationship and if/why veterinarian consultation took place within the past 12 months. A distinction was made between routine (routine visit or preventive check-up, e.g., immunisation, blood, or dental control) and specific (specific symptoms and pathogen detection). If they stated having visited the veterinarian, they were asked if communication on zoonoses and/or AMR took place. If so, they were asked for their perception of the communication with veterinarians on zoonoses and/or AMR. If not, they proceeded directly to the section containing the final questions on veterinary advice and needs. To avoid misunderstandings or misinterpretations, all technical terms were explained beforehand and repeated in the description section of the specific question. The definitions of zoonoses and AMR were based on the definition of the World Health Organisation [15,49]. Furthermore, the classification of exotic pets (bird, fish, mammal and terrarium animal including reptile, amphibian, insect and arachnid) was based on the data from the Zentralverband Zoologischer Fachbetriebe Deutschlands e.V. (ZZF) [6].

2.2.1. Risk Factors

The questions on risk factors gathered information on vulnerable groups in the participants household, including immunocompromised individuals, children under six years, elderly people over 65 years and pregnant individuals (Table 1). The variable 'children under six' was created, combining the variables 'infant' and 'toddler'. The variable 'immunocompromised individuals' was created by adding the variables 'cancer, chronically ill, diabetes and immunosuppressed'.

Table 1. Questions on risk factors (vulnerable groups) in the household. (multiple answers possible: 1. and 2.).

1. Which age groups of people live in your household? (infant [1], toddler [2], school-aged children, teenagers, adults, elderly [3]) 2. Do any individuals of these groups live in your household? (pregnant, cancer, chronical ill, diabetes, immunosuppressed [4])

[1] under two years, [2] two to five years, [3] over 65 years, [4] congenital or acquired (e.g., medical treatments like chemotherapy and radiation therapy).

2.2.2. Pet(s) and Associated Risk Behaviours

The second section of the questionnaire focused on information related to the respondent's pet(s) (animal classes/species) and risk behaviours connected to the origin (wild-caught and/or import from abroad), access to shared living spaces and risky feeding practices (raw meat/fish, offal, uncooked bones, frozen and/or live prey) (Table 2).

Table 2. Questions on the pet(s) and associated risk behaviours. (multiple answers possible: 1. and 2.).

1. Which type of pet(s) do you currently have, or have kept in the last year? (reptile, amphibian, bird, fish, arachnid, insect, exotic mammal, others) 2. Which is the origin of your pet? (breeder, private purchase, pet fair, internet portal, animal shelter or organisation, garden centre or pet store, wild-caught, others) 3. Is your pet imported from abroad? (yes, no) 4. Does your pet have access to shared living spaces? (yes, no) 5. Do you feed raw meat/fish, fresh offal, uncooked bones, frozen and/or live prey? (yes, no)

2.2.3. Veterinarian–Client Relationship

The section on the veterinarian–client relationship assessed the permanency, duration of the respondents' relationship with their veterinarians and the satisfaction of care. If participants indicated that they did not have a permanent veterinarian, they were inquired about the reasons behind this decision. Information was assessed using the following questions (Table 3).

Table 3. Questions on veterinarian–client relationship. (multiple answers possible: 4.).

1. Do you have a permanent veterinarian? (yes, no) if yes: 2. How long have you been a regular client of your veterinarian? (<1 year, 1–3 years, 3–6 years, >6 years) 3. Are you satisfied with the care you receive from your veterinarian? (disagree, rather disagree, rather agree, agree) if no: 4. Which is the reason why you do not have a permanent veterinarian? (no need, multiple, dissatisfaction with quality, distance, others)

2.2.4. Veterinary Consultation

In the veterinary consultation section, participants were asked if and why they visited the veterinarian during the past 12 months (Table 4). Regarding the reasons for the consultation, a distinction was made between routine visits including preventive check-ups (e.g., immunisation, blood or dental control) and consultations due to specific symptoms with pathogen detection. The variable 'specific' was combined from the different variables of the question assessing specific symptoms (gastrointestinal, urinary, skin, respiratory and others). Furthermore, the detection of pathogens was assessed using a list of the most relevant pathogens (Supplement S1), which was compiled through the literature research and in dialogue with practicing veterinarians. The skin and gastrointestinal tract have been identified as the most significant areas for zoonotic concerns [4,29,42,43]. Conversely, concerns about AMR are often linked to surgery but also to chronic conditions associated with various organ tracts, such as the gastrointestinal, urinary, skin and respiratory system [50–52].

Table 4. Questions on veterinary consultation. (multiple answers possible: 2., 3., 5.).

1. Have you visited a veterinarian within the past 12 months?
(yes, no)
if yes: 2. For which reason have you consulted the veterinarian?
(routine check-up, acute or chronic illness, emergency, surgery, others)
3. Does or did your pet have symptoms?
(gastrointestinal, skin, respiratory, urinary, others)
4. Was a pathogen detected?
(yes, no)
if yes: 5. The following pathogen(s) was/were detected during the examination.
(Supplement S1)

2.2.5. Veterinarian Communication

2.2.5.1. Frequency of Veterinarian Communication

If participants selected that they visited the veterinarian for routine or specific reasons, they were asked whether communication on zoonoses and/or AMR took place (Table 5).

Table 5. Questions on communication frequencies. (multiple answers possible: 3.).

1. The veterinarian spoke with me in this context about zoonoses.
(yes, no)
2. The veterinarian spoke with me in this context about AMR.
(yes, no)
3. The veterinarian spoke with me about following pathogen(s).
(Supplement S1)

2.2.5.2. Perception of Veterinarian Communication

A questionnaire was developed and validated to measure the perception of veterinarian communication by pet owners.

Development of the Questionnaire

The generated items relate to Friedemann Schulz von Thun's four-sides model. This communication model is based on the assumption that every message always has four facets, which are referred to as the sides of the message, i.e., factual level, appeal level, relationship level and self-disclosure. The factual level indicates the information provided. The facet of the message that gives an indication of what the sender of the message wants the recipient to do is called the appeal level. The relationship level is the facet of the message that shows what the sender of the message thinks of the recipient and the relationship between them. The fourth facet of the message, self-disclosure, contains the aspects that the sender discloses about him- or herself in the message [53]. Four items were formulated for each side of the communication, which were assessed by the participants on a 4-point Likert scale ranging from 1 (disagree), 2 (rather disagree), 3 (rather agree) to 4 (agree).In addition, they had the option to choose 'no answer'. The items regarding the factual level were aimed at whether the relevant information was given and whether it was formulated in a way that the pet owner could understand. To assess the communication at appeal level, the items related to whether appeals were made and explained in a comprehensive manner and if consequences for complying or not complying with the appeals were pointed out. Regarding the relationship level, the items were intended to determine the pet owners' perception of the veterinarian's appreciation, trust and empathy. For the assessment of self-disclosure, items were formulated to find out whether the veterinarian's self-presentation led pet owners to perceive the veterinarian as professionally competent (Table 6).

Table 6. Items on pet owners' perception of veterinarian communication.

Side of the Message [53]	Items (Specific)	Items (Routine)
factual level	The veterinarian explained the cause and transmission of my pet's infection (e.g., pathogen characteristics).	The veterinarian explained the cause and transmission of zoonoses/AMR (e.g., pathogen characteristics).
factual level	I was able to follow the veterinarian's explanations on the cause and transmission of my pet's infection (e.g., language, choice of words, pace of speech).	I was able to follow the veterinarian's explanations on the cause and transmission of zoonoses/AMR (e.g., language, choice of words, pace of speech).
factual level	The veterinarian's explanations of the cause and transmission of my pet's infection were formulated in a language I could understand.	The veterinarian's explanations of the cause and transmission of zoonoses/AMR were formulated in a language I could understand.
factual level	The veterinarian emphasised the most important points about the cause and transmission of my pet's infection (e.g., transmission mechanism, pathogen characteristics).	The veterinarian emphasised the most important points on the cause and transmission of zoonoses/AMR (e.g., transmission mechanism, pathogen characteristics).
appeal level	The veterinarian provided me with instructions to prevent the transmission of my pet's infection (e.g., cleaning and disinfecting hands, food bowls, toys, pet beds, baskets, blankets and pet toilets).	The veterinarian provided me with instructions to prevent the transmission of zoonoses/AMR (e.g., cleaning and disinfecting hands, food bowls, toys, pet beds, baskets, blankets and pet toilets).
appeal level	The veterinarian explained the reasons for the recommended behavioural instructions connected to my pet's infection (e.g., preventing the transmission of the pathogen to me, maintaining the infection and reinfection of the pet).	The veterinarian explained the reasons for the recommended behavioural instructions connected to zoonoses/AMR (e.g., preventing the transmission of the pathogen to me, maintaining the infection and reinfection of the pet).
appeal level	The veterinarian explained to me the advantages of the behavioural instructions connected to my pet's infection (e.g., prevention of new outbreaks of disease, health care and health protection, cost savings).	The veterinarian explained to me the advantages of the behavioural instructions connected to zoonoses/AMR (e.g., prevention of new outbreaks of disease, health care and health protection, cost savings).
appeal level	The veterinarian provided me with informational material on my pet's infection (e.g., information sheets, magazines, websites).	The veterinarian provided me with informational material on zoonoses/AMR (e.g., information sheets, magazines, websites).
relationship level	The veterinarian demonstrated understanding towards me during the conversation on my pet's infection.	The veterinarian demonstrated understanding towards me during the conversation on zoonoses/AMR.
relationship level	I had the feeling that the veterinarian took my questions serious during the conversation on my pet's infection.	I had the feeling that the veterinarian took my questions serious during the conversation on zoonoses/AMR.
relationship level	The veterinarian was able to understand what the behavioural instructions, connected to my pet's infection, mean to me.	The veterinarian was able to understand what the behavioural instructions, connected to zoonoses/AMR, mean to me.
relationship level	I trust the veterinarian's advice connected to my pet's infection.	I trust the veterinarian's advice connected to zoonoses/AMR.
self-disclosure	I felt that the veterinarian gave me competent advice connected to my pet's infection.	I felt that the veterinarian gave me competent advice connected to zoonoses/AMR.
self-disclosure	I had the feeling that the conversation with the veterinarian on my pet's infection, took place at eye level.	I had the feeling that the conversation with the veterinarian on zoonoses/AMR took place at eye level.
self-disclosure	I had the feeling that I could ask the veterinarian questions about my pet's infection at any time.	I had the feeling that I could ask the veterinarian questions about zoonoses/AMR at any time.
self-disclosure	I had the feeling that it was important to the veterinarian that I understand the causes and consequences of my pet's infection.	I had the feeling that it was important to the veterinarian that I understand the causes and consequences of zoonoses/AMR.

Validation of the Questionnaire

To assess the validity of the self-developed questionnaire structure, a factor analysis based on the four-sides model was conducted, incorporating four items corresponding to each side. This analysis aimed at determining if the four sides would be an adequate instrument to assess communication in our questionnaire. Sensitivity controls revealed that the sides were not distinct: Cronbach's Alpha was 0.891 for the 16 items indicating a high internal consistency. In addition, an exploratory factor analysis did not allow a distinction of the four sides into four factors. The Kaiser–Meyer–Olkin Measure of Sampling Adequacy of 0.567 and Bartlett's test of sphericity ($p < 0.001$) already indicated a high correlation of communication variables. The resulting structure also pointed towards a one-factor solution with all items except the item 'The veterinarian provided me with info material' depicting high loadings upon the first factor extracted. As the Eigenvalue and Scree Plot also indicated a one-factor solution, the expected structure of the four sides could not be confirmed and was rejected. Therefore, it was decided to calculate a one-dimensional score from the mean value to represent the perceived communication.

2.2.6. Veterinary Advice and Needs

The final chapter focused on the respondent's final thoughts regarding veterinary advice. It assessed the respondent's interest and needs for specific advice or guidance in the following areas: zoonoses, AMR, nutrition, behaviour, husbandry, immunisation, hygiene measurements and the treatment of endo- and ectoparasites (Table 7).

Table 7. Questions on veterinary advice and needs. (multiple answers possible: 3.).

1. Would you like to receive veterinary advice on zoonoses? (yes, no)
2. Would you like to receive veterinary advice on AMR? (yes, no)
3. Would you like to receive veterinary advice on any of the following topics: (nutrition, behaviour, husbandry, immunisation, treatment of endoparasites and application of deworming medication, treatment of ectoparasites and application of tick and flea control products, hygiene measurements)

2.3. *Statistical Analysis*

Data were exported in Microsoft Excel 2024®, and the statistical analyses were carried out with IBM SPSS Statistics Version 29®. Only participants who finished the questionnaire were included in the analyses. Descriptive analyses were carried out.

2.3.1. Analysis of Communication Frequencies

To gain an understanding of risk communication regarding zoonoses and AMR, we examined whether communication occurs and whether risk factors (the existence of vulnerable groups in the household and pathogen detection) and risk behaviours (feeding of raw meat/fish, offal, uncooked bones, frozen and/or live prey, free access to shared living spaces, imported and wild-caught animals) have an impact on the frequency. When correlating two categorical variables, a Chi^2-Test was applied. If the assumption of having an expected count of at least 5 within each cell was violated, Fisher's exact test was used.

2.3.2. Analysis of Communication Perception

The mean score of the specific communication (specific symptom with pathogen detection) was compared with that of the routine communication (routine consultation and preventive health check-up) using the Mann–Whitney-U-Test. For the analysis, a distinction was not made between pathogens with zoonotic potential and those with multidrug-resistant potential; instead, the cases of confirmed pathogens were aggregated and compared with the communication during routine visits. The differences in communication (mean scores) to the duration of veterinary care were tested by calculating the

Kruskal–Wallis-Test. For the pairwise comparison of groups (<1 year, 1–3 years, 3–6 years, >6 years), *p*-values were adjusted for multiple testing (Bonferroni correction). Besides that, the differences (mean scores) regarding risk factors and behaviours were tested. For all inferential analyses, a significance level of 5% was chosen.

3. Results

A total of 547 exotic pet owners participated. Out of those, 344 completed the survey.

3.1. Presence of Risk Factors in the Household

Among the participants, almost one-third (32%, n = 111 of 344) stated having individuals from at least one vulnerable group in their household, including immunocompromised individuals, children younger than six years, elderly and pregnant people (Figure 1).

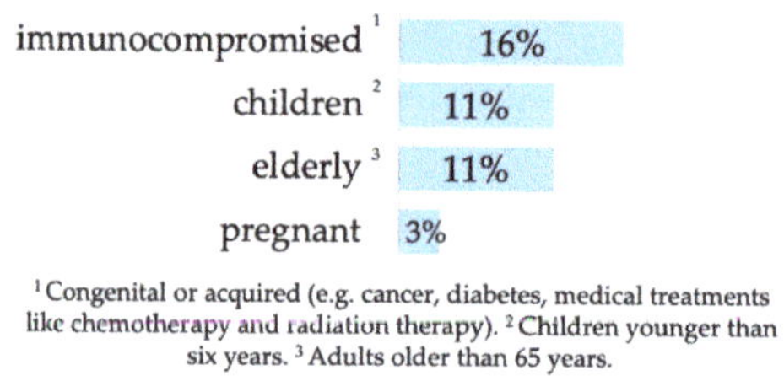

Figure 1. Presence of risk factors (vulnerable groups) in the household (immunocompromised n = 56, children n = 37, elderly n = 36, pregnant n = 10 of 344) multiple answers were possible.

3.2. Pet(s) and Associated Risk Behaviours

Participants reported owning a variety of different exotic animals (reptiles 58%, exotic mammals 33%, birds 20%, insects 15%, arachnids 13%, fishes 13%, amphibians 8%, others 4%).

Furthermore, 80% (n = 276 of 344) of the participants reported engaging in activities that could pose an increased risk of pathogen transmission (Figure 2). Nearly half of all participants fed raw meat/fish, offal, uncooked bones and frozen and/or live prey and allowed free access to shared living spaces. Besides this, about one quarter of the participants stated that at least one of their animals was imported from abroad, while a concerning 4% (n = 12 of 344) acknowledged owning a wild-caught animal.

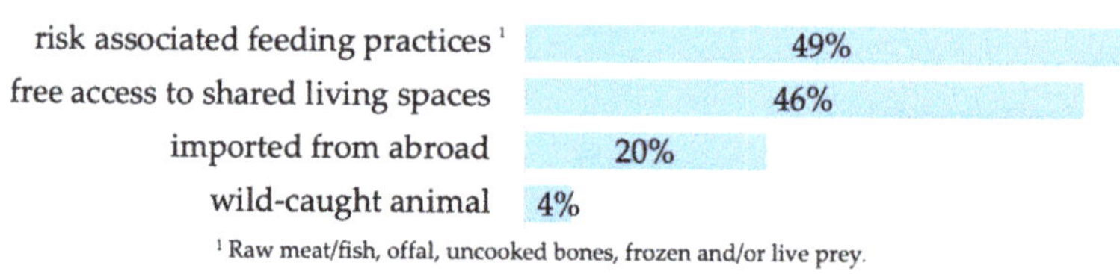

Figure 2. Presence of risk behaviour (risk-associated feeding practice n = 161 of 327, free access to shared living spaces n = 154 of 333, imported from abroad n = 64 of 326, wild-caught animal n = 12 of 344; multiple answers were possible).

3.3. Veterinarian–Client Relationship

The results show that 85% (n = 283 of 335) of the participants had a permanent veterinarian (11% <1 year, 27% 1–3 years, 20% 3–6 years, 42% >6 years). A notable level of customer satisfaction is indicated by the fact that 74% (n = 208 of 281) chose 'agree' for the item 'Are you satisfied with the care you receive from your veterinarian?'. The reasons for not having a permanent veterinarian (16%, n = 52 of 335) were no perceived need, dissatisfaction with the quality of care, distance from available veterinarians, lack of specialised veterinary services, consulting multiple veterinarians and other reasons (Figure 3).

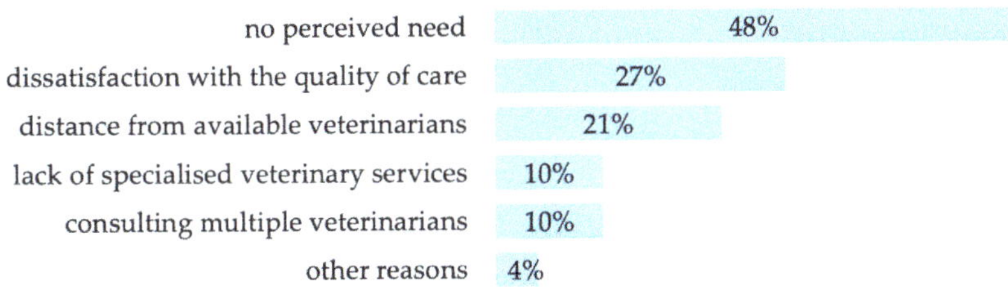

Figure 3. Reasons for not having a permanent veterinarian (no perceived need n = 25, dissatisfaction with the quality of care n = 14, distance from available veterinarians n = 11, lack of specialised veterinary services n = 5, consulting multiple veterinarians n = 5, other reasons n = 2 of 52; multiple answers were possible).

3.4. *Reasons for Veterinary Consultation*

Within the past 12 months, 66% (n = 227 of 343) of the participants consulted a veterinarian. Among those participants who stated having visited a veterinarian, 64% (n = 146 of 227) did so due to a routine visit or preventive check-up, while 48% (n = 109 of 227) consulted the veterinarian due to specific symptoms. Out of these consultations, 38% (n = 87) were only due to specific symptoms, 22% (n = 50) were only for routine consultations, and 26% (n = 59) involved both specific symptoms and routine consultations.

The primary concerns prompting veterinary consultation revolved around the respiratory tract, followed by the skin, gastrointestinal and urinary tract. Additionally, they cited other symptoms of concern such as neurological, dental and ocular.

Among the participants who visited a veterinarian within the past 12 months, 11% (n = 25 of 227) of the participants reported the detection of pathogens with zoonotic (9%, n = 20 of 227) or/and AMR (4%, n = 9 of 227) potential. A total of 43 cases—including bacteria, fungi, protozoa, ectoparasites and endoparasites—were reported.

3.5. *Veterinarian Communication on Zoonoses and AMR*

3.5.1. Frequencies of Veterinarian Communication

The frequency of communication on zoonoses and AMR was associated with the presence of a permanent veterinarian ($p = 0.002$). Among participants who consulted the veterinarian within the past 12 months, 20% (n = 46 of 227) reported receiving information on zoonoses and 17% (n = 39 of 227) on AMR. An association of the existence of vulnerable groups in the household ($p = 0.454$) or with other risk behaviours was not proven ($p = 0.292$).

Information on zoonoses was statistically significantly more frequently given ($p < 0.001$) during consultations due to specific reasons (50%, n = 25 of 50) compared to those who visited a veterinarian for routine reasons (22%, n = 31 of 144). Furthermore, during consultations prompted by specific reasons, pet owners received statistically more frequently ($p < 0.001$) information on zoonoses (50%, n = 25 of 50) than on AMR (18%, n = 24 of 132). During routine consultations, pet owners received information on zoonoses (22%, n = 31 of 144) with a similar frequency to AMR (17%, n = 24 of 144).

3.5.2. Participant's Perception of Veterinarian Communication

In general, the perception of veterinarian communication received a high average score of 3.7 out of a maximum 4.0 (mean; n = 72), most choosing 'rather agree' and 'agree' for the given items (Table 8). The second item of the relationship level, 'I had the feeling that the veterinarian took my questions serious', and the third item of the self-disclosure received 'agree' most frequently. The only exception was the fourth item of the appeal level: 'The veterinarian provided me with informational material', which received a high frequency of 'disagree', showing that informational material was distributed in less than half of the cases.

Table 8. Communication perception. Connected to the four levels of communication (factual level, appeal level, relationship level, self-disclosure) based on Schulz von Thun's four-sides model. Four items were formulated for each level of the communication, which were assessed by the participants on a 4-point Likert scale ranging from 1 (disagree), 2 (rather disagree), 3 (rather agree) to 4 (agree).

Item	Perception (Specific)	Perception (Routine)
factual level:	missing/disagree/rather disagree/rather agree/agree $n = 20$	missing/disagree/rather disagree/rather agree/agree $n = 52$
The veterinarian explained the cause and transmission.	1/1/2/6/10	0/0/4/8/40
I was able to follow the veterinarian's explanations.	3/0/0/3/14	1/0/0/7/44
The veterinarian's explanations were formulated in a language I could understand.	3/0/1/3/13	0/0/2/6/43
The veterinarian emphasises the most important points about the cause and transmission	5/1/1/5/8	1/0/3/5/43
appeal level:		
The veterinarian provided me with instructions to prevent the transmission.	4/2/1/1/12	1/1/2/7/41
The veterinarian explained the reasons for the recommended behavioural instructions	3/1/1/1/14	1/1/2/6/42
The veterinarian explained me the advantages of the behavioural instructions.	4/1/1/2/12	2/1/4/6/39
The veterinarian provided me with information material.	4/11/2/0/3	0/24/4/5/19
relationship level:		
The veterinarian demonstrates understanding towards me.	2/0/0/5/13	4/0/0/6/42
I had the feeling that the veterinarian took my questions serious.	1/0/0/2/17	0/0/0/2/50
The veterinarian was able to understand what the behavioural instructions mean to me.	4/0/0/4/12	6/0/0/8/38
I trust the veterinarian's advice.	2/0/0/3/15	0/0/0/4/48
self-disclosure:		
I felt that the veterinarian gave me competent advice.	2/0/1/2/15	0/1/2/3/46
I had the feeling that the conversation took place at eye level.	0/0/0/4/16	0/0/1/3/48
I had the feeling that I could ask the veterinarian questions at any time.	0/0/0/2/18	0/0/1/1/50
I had the feeling that it was important to the veterinarian that I could understand the causes and consequences.	4/0/0/2/14	2/0/2/4/44

Perception of Communication Connected to Risk Factors and Risk Behaviours

The presence of vulnerable groups in the household resulted in a higher average communication score of 3.8 (n = 19) in comparison to households with no vulnerable groups of 3.6 (n = 53). This result was not statistically significant, but a trend could be detected (p = 0.052).

The presence of risk behaviour resulted in a slightly higher average score of 3.7 (n = 59) in comparison to households with no risk behaviours of 3.6 (n = 12), with no statistically significant difference (p = 0.635).

Perception of Communication Connected to Duration of Veterinary Care

Among all participants who answered the communication model and stated having a permanent veterinarian, the following observation was made: the longer the pet owners were clients, the better they rated the communication (under one year: mean = 3.5, n = 5; one to two years: mean = 3.4, n = 7; three to six years: mean = 3.7, n = 16; over six years: mean = 3.7, n = 44) (Figure 4). This result was not statistically significant, but a trend could be detected ($p = 0.057$). Post hoc tests revealed that there was an improvement in perceived communication for pet owners being clients for three to six years compared to those who were clients for less than one year (z= −1.869, $p = 0.062$) and for those being clients for more than six years compared to the ones who were clients for one to three years (z= −2.213, $p = 0.027$).

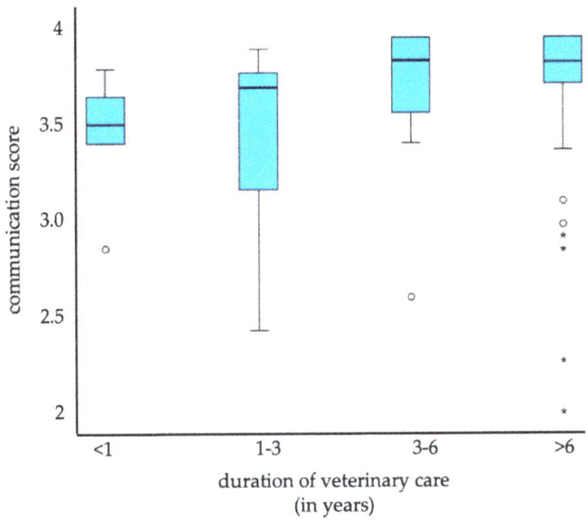

Figure 4. Average communication perception in relation to the duration of veterinary care (under one year: mean = 3.5, n = 5; one to two years: mean = 3.4, n = 7; three to six years: mean = 3.7, n = 16; over six years: mean = 3.7, n = 44; o = outlier, * = extreme value).

Perception of Communication Connected to Reason of Consultation

The perceived communication during a routine visit revealed a slightly higher average score (mean = 3.7, n = 52) than the specific communication (mean = 3.6, n = 20), with no statistically significant difference ($p = 0.113$). The average score was slightly lower when a pathogen was detected (mean = 3.6, n = 31) compared to no detected pathogen (mean = 3.7, n = 41) but was not statistically significant ($p = 0.103$). Furthermore, the communication of zoonoses (mean = 3.7, n = 42) perceived a slightly higher average score than AMR (mean = 3.6, n = 30) but was not statistically significant ($p = 0.707$).

3.6. Veterinary Advice and Needs

More than half (66%, n = 195 of 296) of the participants indicated that they would like veterinary advice on zoonoses and on AMR (64%, n = 193 of 301). Besides this, pet owners also wanted the veterinarian to provide information on nutrition, behaviour, animal husbandry, immunisation, treatment of endoparasites and ectoparasites, hygiene measures and other topics (Figure 5).

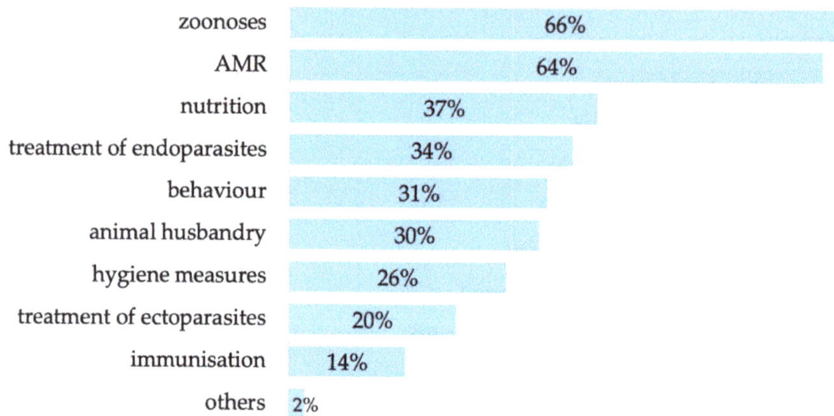

Figure 5. Topics for veterinary advice (zoonoses n = 195 of 296, AMR n = 193 of 301, nutrition n = 126, treatment of endoparasites n = 116, behaviour n = 105, animal husbandry n = 103, hygiene measures n = 90, treatment of ectoparasites n = 69, immunisation n = 48, others n = 7 of 344; multiple answers possible).

4. Discussion

Since the husbandry of exotic pets can lead to infections with zoonotic and antimicrobial-resistant pathogens [16–25], it is an essential task of veterinarians to provide pet owners with information about these risks [34]. The veterinarians' communication skills as well as their knowledge and awareness play a significant role in the extent to which this information is distributed to and understood by pet owners and whether the veterinarians' instructions are followed [38]. Therefore, the aims of this study were to assess (i) the role of veterinary practitioners in communicating risks of zoonoses and AMR as well as (ii) exotic pet owners' perception of their veterinarian communication.

Previous studies have shown the presence of zoonotic and antimicrobial-resistant pathogens in exotic pets [4,10–14]. In the present study, 11% of the pet owners, who had consulted a veterinarian within the past 12 months, reported the detection of pathogens with zoonotic (9%) or/and AMR (4%) potential in their pet(s).

Cohort and case–control studies have indicated that certain groups—young children (under six years), older adults (65 years and older), immunocompromised individuals and pregnant individuals—are at a higher risk for zoonotic diseases. As their immune system is either impaired or not fully developed yet, these groups have an increased risk of falling ill and may experience more severe symptoms or disease progression compared to other patients [28,32,54–56]. Among the participants, 32% reported having individuals from such vulnerable groups in their household. In addition, 80% of the participants reported activities that could pose an increased risk of pathogen transmission. Nearly half of all participants reported feeding raw meat, fish, offal, bones and frozen and/or live prey. Investigations of various raw meat feeding approaches have validated the presence of pathogens, including antimicrobial-resistant pathogens, capable of causing severe human illnesses, and pets consuming raw meat may harbour these pathogens without exhibiting symptoms, serving as carriers and potential sources of transmission [57,58]. Especially vulnerable groups, who are more likely than others to fall seriously ill, face an elevated risk handling such products [59,60]. Besides this, about one quarter of the participants stated that at least one of their animals was imported from abroad, while, concerningly, 4% acknowledged owning a wild-caught animal. Those animals may pose a health risk to humans and other animals due to their potential to carry specific pathogens [61–64]. The stress of capture and transport, combined with a lack of strict health regulations, increases the risk of introducing new diseases and antibiotic-resistant bacteria into local ecosystems [65,66].

Therefore, a tailored risk communication is required for raising awareness and potentially preventing pathogen transmission [67–70]. The results show that the frequency of communication on zoonoses and AMR during veterinary consultation was higher when a pathogen was detected as during routine visits and was associated with the presence of a permanent veterinarian. Even though the overall perception of veterinarian communication received a high average score showing a high level of satisfaction, also the duration of the veterinarian–client relationship was positively associated with a better communication perception. These findings align well with previous studies, as they also underscore the significant role of the veterinarian–client relationship for successful communication [31], resulting in higher compliance and thus improved patient outcomes [49].

The results indicate a gap between the wish to be informed on zoonoses (66%) or AMR (64%) and the frequency of disseminated information from veterinarians to pet owners, as 20% of the participants who consulted the veterinarian within the past 12 months received information on zoonoses and 17% on AMR. The gap between the wish to be informed and the actual frequency of information distributed to the pet owners might be connected to the fact that COVID-19 has raised awareness about zoonoses, connected health risks and the importance of preventive measures [71–73]. In addition, the veterinary community has several concerns, including the clients' intent to adhere, the perception that adherence is redundant, misunderstanding or denial of risks, costs, rural culture, fear for reputation and the emotional state of the client [42]. These could be reasons why there is a gap between the good perception of veterinarian communication and the limited frequency of risk communication. However, it is important to pet owners that they receive the desired information in the necessary scope, in understandable language and ideally in several formats [74]. However, the pet owners surveyed in this study assessed the veterinarians' communication regarding explanations of the cause and transmission of infections slightly, although not significantly, worse after pathogen detection compared to no pathogen detection. In addition, pet owners rarely reported having received information material on the pet's infection. Additional information media, such as flyers that can be taken and read at home at leisure, could be a helpful alternative for people of distinct ages and academic backgrounds [74]. Therefore, increased efforts should be made to produce information material on zoonoses and AMR, tailored to pet owners and their pets in order to support veterinarians in the important task of maintaining the health of animals and humans. In addition, increasing the communication skills of veterinarians contributes to the effective education of pet owners about zoonoses and AMR. Thus, future veterinarians could significantly benefit from learning communication skills at a university level, not just for conveying complex medical information to pet owners, fostering trust and ensuring the compliance of pet owners with treatment plans but also to collaborate more efficiently with colleagues and other professionals in the public health sector [43,75–77].

Future studies and research could focus on assessing the effectiveness of information materials on zoonoses and AMR, understanding the factors influencing veterinarian selection and evaluating pet owners' feeding practices. These areas could help to build a more detailed understanding of the veterinarian–client dynamic, ultimately improving pet care and health outcomes. Additionally investigating the impact of communication techniques of veterinarians and physicians and conducting longitudinal studies on pets' and their owners' health could provide valuable insights for improving not only veterinary care but also moving in the direction towards One Health.

There are some limitations connected to participant engagement in this study. The distribution method via the internet posed a barrier for some individuals, potentially leading to selection bias. Moreover, those persons who accessed the internet and were part of the groups where the survey was promoted and read the invitation might differ from the target population, as participation needs time, a general willingness to participate in surveys and the impression that the topic of the survey is appealing. Even though we limited the timeframe to 12 months, memory bias remains a potential limitation, as respondents might inaccurately recall their consultations or base their responses on more recent experiences or emotional states, thereby reducing the reliability and validity of the collected data. Another limitation factor is that veterinary consultations are stressful, which is why the message sent is not always the message received. Furthermore, the use of a 4-point Likert scale in the communication perception questionnaire may have provided too few gradations to yield distinct results, suggesting that the questionnaire should be retested with a Likert scale that has more gradations.

5. Conclusions

This survey of pet owners has shown that risk factors and risk behaviour in relation to zoonoses and AMR are of particular relevance to the husbandry of exotic pets. Veterinarians play a crucial role in communicating risks ofzoonoses and AMR associated with exotic pets to their owners. The results of this study have revealed that the duration of the veterinarian–client relationship contributes both to a higher frequency of communication on zoonoses and AMR and to pet owners' perceptions of better veterinarian communication. However, since pet owners would prefer to receive significantly more information on zoonoses and AMR, more target-group-specific information materials should be made available to veterinarians for distribution to their clients. Here, the awareness of veterinarians should be increased by further education and the implementation of communication teaching during veterinary education at universities.

Supplementary Materials: The following supporting information can be downloaded at: https://www.mdpi.com/article/10.3390/ani14142035/s1, Supplement S1: List of Pathogens; Supplement S2: Raw Data.

Author Contributions: Conceptualization, A.L.A., M.B., S.S. and A.L.-B.; methodology, A.L.A., M.B. and K.C.J.; formal analysis, A.L.A. and K.C.J.; investigation, A.L.A.; visualization, A.L.A.; supervision and project administration, M.B. and S.S.; writing—original draft, A.L.A., M.B., K.C.J. and C.H.; writing—review and editing, A.L.A., M.B., K.C.J. and S.S. All authors have read and agreed to the published version of the manuscript.

Funding: This research received no external funding.

Institutional Review Board Statement: The study was conducted according to the guidelines of the Declaration of Helsinki and approved by the Ethics Committee of Freie Universität Berlin (ZEA-Nr. 2022-018, 1 December 2022).

Informed Consent Statement: Informed consent was obtained from all subjects involved in the study.

Data Availability Statement: Data are contained within the article or Supplementary Materials.

Acknowledgments: Special thanks go to Alina Pohl for support with the development of the questionnaire on communication perception and to all participants for their contribution in the survey. The publication of this article was funded by Freie Universität Berlin.

Conflicts of Interest: The authors declare no conflicts of interest.

References

1. WOAH—World Organisation for Animal Health. Wildlife Health—WOAH—World Organisation for Animal Health. Available online: https://www.woah.org/en/what-we-do/animal-health-and-welfare/wildlife-health/ (accessed on 30 May 2024).
2. Travis, D.A.; Watson, R.P.; Tauer, A. The spread of pathogens through trade in wildlife. *Rev. Sci. Tech.* **2011**, *30*, 219–239. [CrossRef] [PubMed]
3. Elsohaby, I.; Villa, L. Zoonotic diseases: Understanding the risks and mitigating the threats. *BMC Vet. Res.* **2023**, *19*, 186. [CrossRef] [PubMed]
4. Rahman, M.T.; Sobur, M.A.; Islam, M.S.; Ievy, S.; Hossain, M.J.; El Zowalaty, M.E.; Rahman, A.T.; Ashour, H.M. Zoonotic Diseases: Etiology, Impact, and Control. *Microorganisms* **2020**, *8*, 1405. [CrossRef] [PubMed]
5. Namusisi, S.; Mahero, M.; Travis, D.; Pelican, K.; Robertson, C.; Mugisha, L. A descriptive study of zoonotic disease risk at the human-wildlife interface in a biodiversity hot spot in South Western Uganda. *PLoS Negl. Trop. Dis.* **2021**, *15*, e0008633. [CrossRef]

6. ZZF. Anzahl der Haustiere in Privaten Haushalten in Deustchland in den Jahren 2007 bis 2022. Available online: https://de.statista.com/statistik/daten/studie/859229/umfrage/anteil-der-haushalte-in-deutschland-mit-haustieren/ (accessed on 28 March 2024).
7. Zentralverband Zoologischer Fachbetriebe Deutschlands e.V. der Deutsche Heimtiermarkt 2022. Available online: https://www.zzf.de/fileadmin/ZZF/Dokumente/Heimtiermarkt/ZZF_IVH_Der_Deutsche_Heimtiermarkt_Anzahl_Heimtiere_2022.pdf (accessed on 28 March 2024).
8. Purewal, R.; Christley, R.; Kordas, K.; Joinson, C.; Meints, K.; Gee, N.; Westgarth, C. Companion Animals and Child/Adolescent Development: A Systematic Review of the Evidence. *Int. J. Environ. Res. Public Health* **2017**, *14*, 234. [CrossRef]
9. Vagnoli, L.; Caprilli, S.; Vernucci, C.; Zagni, S.; Mugnai, F.; Messeri, A. Can presence of a dog reduce pain and distress in children during venipuncture? *Pain Manag. Nurs.* **2015**, *16*, 89–95. [CrossRef]
10. Nosanchuk, J.D.; Shoham, S.; Fries, B.C.; Shapiro, D.S.; Levitz, S.M.; Casadevall, A. Evidence of zoonotic transmission of *Cryptococcus neoformans* from a pet cockatoo to an immunocompromised patient. *Ann. Intern. Med.* **2000**, *132*, 205–208. [CrossRef]
11. Boseret, G.; Losson, B.; Mainil, J.G.; Thiry, E.; Saegerman, C. Zoonoses in pet birds: Review and perspectives. *Vet. Res.* **2013**, *44*, 36. [CrossRef] [PubMed]
12. Souza, M.J. One health: Zoonoses in the exotic animal practice. *Vet. Clin. N. Am. Exot. Anim. Pract.* **2011**, *14*, 421–426. [CrossRef]
13. Varela, K.; Brown, J.A.; Lipton, B.; Dunn, J.; Stanek, D.; Behravesh, C.B.; Chapman, H.; Conger, T.H.; Vanover, T.; Edling, T.; et al. A Review of Zoonotic Disease Threats to Pet Owners: A Compendium of Measures to Prevent Zoonotic Diseases Associated with Non-Traditional Pets: Rodents and Other Small Mammals, Reptiles, Amphibians, Backyard Poultry, and Other Selected Animals. *Vector Borne Zoonotic Dis.* **2022**, *22*, 303–360. [CrossRef]
14. Ziarati, M.; Zorriehzahra, M.J.; Hassantabar, F.; Mehrabi, Z.; Dhawan, M.; Sharun, K.; Emran, T.B.; Dhama, K.; Chaicumpa, W.; Shamsi, S. Zoonotic diseases of fish and their prevention and control. *Vet. Q.* **2022**, *42*, 95–118. [CrossRef] [PubMed]
15. WHO—World Health Organization. Antimicrobial Resistance. Available online: https://www.who.int/news-room/fact-sheets/detail/antimicrobial-resistance (accessed on 30 May 2024).
16. Strommenger, B.; Kehrenberg, C.; Kettlitz, C.; Cuny, C.; Verspohl, J.; Witte, W.; Schwarz, S. Molecular characterization of methicillin-resistant *Staphylococcus aureus* strains from pet animals and their relationship to human isolates. *J. Antimicrob. Chemother.* **2006**, *57*, 461–465. [CrossRef] [PubMed]
17. van Duijkeren, E.; Wolfhagen, M.J.H.M.; Box, A.T.A.; Heck, M.E.O.C.; Wannet, W.J.B.; Fluit, A.C. Human-to-dog transmission of methicillin-resistant *Staphylococcus aureus*. *Emerg. Infect. Dis.* **2004**, *10*, 2235–2237. [CrossRef]
18. Jin, M.; Osman, M.; Green, B.A.; Yang, Y.; Ahuja, A.; Lu, Z.; Cazer, C.L. Evidence for the transmission of antimicrobial resistant bacteria between humans and companion animals: A scoping review. *One Health* **2023**, *17*, 100593. [CrossRef]
19. Nienhoff, U.; Kadlec, K.; Chaberny, I.F.; Verspohl, J.; Gerlach, G.-F.; Schwarz, S.; Simon, D.; Nolte, I. Transmission of methicillin-resistant *Staphylococcus aureus* strains between humans and dogs: Two case reports. *J. Antimicrob. Chemother.* **2009**, *64*, 660–662. [CrossRef] [PubMed]
20. Gao, Y.; Wang, Z.; Fu, J.; Cai, J.; Ma, T.; Xie, N.; Fan, R.; Zhai, W.; Feßler, A.T.; Sun, C.; et al. Spreading of *cfr*-Carrying Plasmids among Staphylococci from Humans and Animals. *Microbiol. Spectr.* **2022**, *10*, e0246122. [CrossRef]
21. Cuny, C.; Arnold, P.; Hermes, J.; Eckmanns, T.; Mehraj, J.; Schoenfelder, S.; Ziebuhr, W.; Zhao, Q.; Wang, Y.; Feßler, A.T.; et al. Occurrence of *cfr*-mediated multiresistance in staphylococci from veal calves and pigs, from humans at the corresponding farms, and from veterinarians and their family members. *Vet. Microbiol.* **2017**, *200*, 88–94. [CrossRef] [PubMed]
22. Alonso, C.A.; Michael, G.B.; Li, J.; Somalo, S.; Simón, C.; Wang, Y.; Kaspar, H.; Kadlec, K.; Torres, C.; Schwarz, S. Analysis of bla_{SHV-12}-carrying *Escherichia coli* clones and plasmids from human, animal and food sources. *J. Antimicrob. Chemother.* **2017**, *72*, 1589–1596. [CrossRef] [PubMed]
23. Walther, B.; Wieler, L.H.; Friedrich, A.W.; Hanssen, A.-M.; Kohn, B.; Brunnberg, L.; Lübke-Becker, A. Methicillin-resistant *Staphylococcus aureus* (MRSA) isolated from small and exotic animals at a university hospital during routine microbiological examinations. *Vet. Microbiol.* **2008**, *127*, 171–178. [CrossRef]
24. Muñoz-Ibarra, E.; Molina-López, R.A.; Durán, I.; Garcias, B.; Martín, M.; Darwich, L. Antimicrobial Resistance in Bacteria Isolated from Exotic Pets: The Situation in the Iberian Peninsula. *Animals* **2022**, *12*, 1912. [CrossRef]
25. Wieler, L.H.; Ewers, C.; Guenther, S.; Walther, B.; Lübke-Becker, A. Methicillin-resistant staphylococci (MRS) and extended-spectrum beta-lactamases (ESBL)-producing Enterobacteriaceae in companion animals: Nosocomial infections as one reason for the rising prevalence of these potential zoonotic pathogens in clinical samples. *Int. J. Med. Microbiol.* **2011**, *301*, 635–641. [CrossRef] [PubMed]
26. Guardabassi, L.; Schwarz, S.; Lloyd, D.H. Pet animals as reservoirs of antimicrobial-resistant bacteria. *J. Antimicrob. Chemother.* **2004**, *54*, 321–332. [CrossRef] [PubMed]
27. Mackenzie, J.S.; Jeggo, M. The One Health Approach—Why Is It So Important? *Trop. Med. Infect. Dis.* **2019**, *4*, 88. [CrossRef] [PubMed]
28. CDC—Centers for Disease Control and Prevention. About Zoonotic Diseases. Available online: https://www.cdc.gov/one-health/about/about-zoonotic-diseases.html?CDC_AAref_Val=https://www.cdc.gov/onehealth/basics/zoonotic-diseases.html (accessed on 30 May 2024).
29. Wallace, B.I.; Kenney, B.; Malani, P.N.; Clauw, D.J.; Nallamothu, B.K.; Waljee, A.K. Prevalence of Immunosuppressive Drug Use Among Commercially Insured US Adults, 2018–2019. *JAMA Netw. Open* **2021**, *4*, e214920. [CrossRef] [PubMed]

30. Alharbi, A.B.; Berrou, I.; Umaru, N.; Al Hamid, A.; Shebl, N.A. Factors influencing the implementation of medicine risk communications by healthcare professionals in clinical practice: A systematic review. *Res. Soc. Adm. Pharm.* **2023**, *19*, 28–56. [CrossRef] [PubMed]
31. Grant, S.; Olsen, C.W. Preventing zoonotic diseases in immunocompromised persons: The role of physicians and veterinarians. *Emerg. Infect. Dis.* **1999**, *5*, 159–163. [CrossRef] [PubMed]
32. Hill, W.A.; Petty, G.C.; Erwin, P.C.; Souza, M.J. A survey of Tennessee veterinarian and physician attitudes, knowledge, and practices regarding zoonoses prevention among animal owners with HIV infection or AIDS. *J. Am. Vet. Med. Assoc.* **2012**, *240*, 1432–1440. [CrossRef] [PubMed]
33. Garcia-Sanchez, P.; Romero-Trancón, D.; Sainz, T.; Calvo, C.; Iglesias, I.; Perez-Hernando, B.; Hurtado-Gallego, J.; Sánchez, R.; Alcolea, S.; Moya, L.; et al. The role of veterinarians in zoonosis prevention: Advising families of immunocompromised children with pets. *One Health* **2024**, *18*, 100662. [CrossRef] [PubMed]
34. de Melo, R.T.; Rossi, D.A.; Monteiro, G.P.; Fernandez, H. Veterinarians and One Health in the Fight Against Zoonoses Such as COVID-19. *Front. Vet. Sci.* **2020**, *7*, 576262. [CrossRef]
35. Aguirre, A.A. Essential veterinary education in zoological and wildlife medicine: A global perspective. *Rev. Sci. Tech.* **2009**, *28*, 605–610. [CrossRef]
36. Espinosa García-San Román, J.; Quesada-Canales, Ó.; Arbelo Hernández, M.; Déniz Suárez, S.; Castro-Alonso, A. Veterinary Education and Training on Non-Traditional Companion Animals, Exotic, Zoo, and Wild Animals: Concepts Review and Challenging Perspective on Zoological Medicine. *Vet. Sci.* **2023**, *10*, 357. [CrossRef] [PubMed]
37. Frölich, K.; Grabitzky, S.E.; Walzer, C.; Delahay, R.J.; Dorrestein, G.M.; Hatt, J.-M. Zoo and wildlife medical education: A European perspective. *J. Vet. Med. Educ.* **2006**, *33*, 401–407. [CrossRef]
38. Lue, T.W.; Pantenburg, D.P.; Crawford, P.M. Impact of the owner-pet and client-veterinarian bond on the care that pets receive. *J. Am. Vet. Med. Assoc.* **2008**, *232*, 531–540. [CrossRef]
39. Belshaw, Z.; Robinson, N.J.; Dean, R.S.; Brennan, M.L. Motivators and barriers for dog and cat owners and veterinary surgeons in the United Kingdom to using preventative medicines. *Prev. Vet. Med.* **2018**, *154*, 95–101. [CrossRef]
40. Evason, M.; McGrath, M.; Stull, J. Companion animal preventive care at a veterinary teaching hospital—Knowledge, attitudes, and practices of clients. *Can. Vet. J.* **2021**, *62*, 484–490. [PubMed]
41. Garcia-Sanchez, P.; Aguilar-Valero, E.; Sainz, T.; Calvo, C.; Iglesias, I.; Bueno, D.; Frauca, E.; Ramos-Boluda, E.; Alcolea-Sanchez, A.; García-Guereta, L.; et al. Immunocompromised Children and Young Patients Living with Pets: Gaps in Knowledge to Avoid Zoonosis. *Transbound. Emerg. Dis.* **2023**, *2023*, 2151761. [CrossRef]
42. Mendez, D.H.; Büttner, P.; Kelly, J.; Nowak, M.; Speare Posthumously, R. Difficulties experienced by veterinarians when communicating about emerging zoonotic risks with animal owners: The case of Hendra virus. *BMC Vet. Res.* **2017**, *13*, 56. [CrossRef]
43. Pun, J.K.H. An integrated review of the role of communication in veterinary clinical practice. *BMC Vet. Res.* **2020**, *16*, 394. [CrossRef] [PubMed]
44. Cake, M.A.; Bell, M.A.; Williams, J.C.; Brown, F.J.L.; Dozier, M.; Rhind, S.M.; Baillie, S. Which professional (non-technical) competencies are most important to the success of graduate veterinarians? A Best Evidence Medical Education (BEME) systematic review: BEME Guide No. 38. *Med. Teach.* **2016**, *38*, 550–563. [CrossRef]
45. Emmett, L.; Aden, J.; Bunina, A.; Klaps, A.; Stetina, B.U. Feminization and Stress in the Veterinary Profession: A Systematic Diagnostic Approach and Associated Management. *Behav. Sci.* **2019**, *9*, 114. [CrossRef]
46. Stetina, B.U.; Krouzecky, C. Reviewing a Decade of Change for Veterinarians: Past, Present and Gaps in Researching Stress, Coping and Mental Health Risks. *Animals* **2022**, *12*, 3199. [CrossRef] [PubMed]
47. Weber, E.U.; Johnson, E.J. Mindful judgment and decision making. *Annu. Rev. Psychol.* **2009**, *60*, 53–85. [CrossRef] [PubMed]
48. Coe, J.B.; Adams, C.L.; Bonnett, B.N. A focus group study of veterinarians' and pet owners' perceptions of veterinarian-client communication in companion animal practice. *J. Am. Vet. Med. Assoc.* **2008**, *233*, 1072–1080. [CrossRef] [PubMed]
49. WHO—World Health Organization. Zoonoses. Available online: https://www.who.int/news-room/fact-sheets/detail/zoonoses (accessed on 27 June 2024).
50. Costelloe, C.; Metcalfe, C.; Lovering, A.; Mant, D.; Hay, A.D. Effect of antibiotic prescribing in primary care on antimicrobial resistance in individual patients: Systematic review and meta-analysis. *BMJ* **2010**, *340*, c2096. [CrossRef] [PubMed]
51. Chatterjee, A.; Modarai, M.; Naylor, N.R.; Boyd, S.E.; Atun, R.; Barlow, J.; Holmes, A.H.; Johnson, A.; Robotham, J.V. Quantifying drivers of antibiotic resistance in humans: A systematic review. *Lancet Infect. Dis.* **2018**, *18*, e368–e378. [CrossRef] [PubMed]
52. European Centre for Disease Prevention and Control. Antimicrobial Resistance Surveillance in Europe 2014. Available online: https://www.ecdc.europa.eu/en/publications-data/antimicrobial-resistance-surveillance-europe-2014 (accessed on 20 May 2024).
53. von Thun, F.S. *Miteinander Reden 1: Störungen und Klärungen. Allgemeine Psychologie der Kommunikation*; 1. Aufl.; Rowohlt E-Book: Reinbek, Germany, 2013; ISBN 9783644446410.
54. Hung, C.-C.; Hung, M.-N.; Hsueh, P.-R.; Chang, S.-Y.; Chen, M.-Y.; Hsieh, S.-M.; Sheng, W.-H.; Sun, H.-Y.; Huang, Y.-T.; Lo, Y.-C.; et al. Risk of recurrent nontyphoid *Salmonella* bacteremia in HIV-infected patients in the era of highly active antiretroviral therapy and an increasing trend of fluoroquinolone resistance. *Clin. Infect. Dis.* **2007**, *45*, e60–e67. [CrossRef] [PubMed]

55. Mani, I.; Maguire, J.H. Small animal zoonoses and immuncompromised pet owners. *Top. Companion Anim. Med.* **2009**, *24*, 164–174. [CrossRef] [PubMed]
56. Kourtis, A.P.; Read, J.S.; Jamieson, D.J. Pregnancy and infection. *N. Engl. J. Med.* **2014**, *370*, 2211–2218. [CrossRef] [PubMed]
57. van Bree, F.P.J.; Bokken, G.C.A.M.; Mineur, R.; Franssen, F.; Opsteegh, M.; van der Giessen, J.W.B.; Lipman, L.J.A.; Overgaauw, P.A.M. Zoonotic bacteria and parasites found in raw meat-based diets for cats and dogs. *Vet. Rec.* **2018**, *182*, 50. [CrossRef]
58. Wu, Y.; Fan, R.; Wang, Y.; Lei, L.; Feßler, A.T.; Wang, Z.; Wu, C.; Schwarz, S.; Wang, Y. Analysis of combined resistance to oxazolidinones and phenicols among bacteria from dogs fed with raw meat/vegetables and the respective food items. *Sci. Rep.* **2019**, *9*, 15500. [CrossRef]
59. CDC—Centers for Disease Control and Prevention. Health Communication Gateway. Available online: https://www.cdc.gov/healthcommunication/index.html?CDC_AA_refVal=https://www.cdc.gov/healthcommunication/healthbasics/WhatIsHC.html (accessed on 24 May 2024).
60. German Federal Institute for Risk Assessment. *Safe Food—Especially Vulnerable Groups in Communal Facilities*; [Leaflet] BfR Press Office: Berlin, Germany, 2024.
61. Fooks, A.R.; Johnson, N. Jet set pets: Examining the zoonosis risk in animal import and travel across the European Union. *Vet. Med.* **2015**, *6*, 17–25. [CrossRef]
62. Avashia, S.B.; Petersen, J.M.; Lindley, C.M.; Schriefer, M.E.; Gage, K.L.; Cetron, M.; DeMarcus, T.A.; Kim, D.K.; Buck, J.; Montenieri, J.A.; et al. First reported prairie dog-to-human tularemia transmission, Texas, 2002. *Emerg. Infect. Dis.* **2004**, *10*, 483–486. [CrossRef] [PubMed]
63. Riley, P.Y.; Chomel, B.B. Hedgehog zoonoses. *Emerg. Infect. Dis.* **2005**, *11*, 1–5. [CrossRef] [PubMed]
64. Petrovan, S.O.; Aldridge, D.C.; Bartlett, H.; Bladon, A.J.; Booth, H.; Broad, S.; Broom, D.M.; Burgess, N.D.; Cleaveland, S.; Cunningham, A.A.; et al. Post COVID-19: A solution scan of options for preventing future zoonotic epidemics. *Biol. Rev. Camb. Philos. Soc.* **2021**, *96*, 2694–2715. [CrossRef]
65. Davy, C.M.; Donaldson, M.E.; Subudhi, S.; Rapin, N.; Warnecke, L.; Turner, J.M.; Bollinger, T.K.; Kyle, C.J.; Dorville, N.A.S.-Y.; Kunkel, E.L.; et al. White-nose syndrome is associated with increased replication of a naturally persisting coronaviruses in bats. *Sci. Rep.* **2018**, *8*, 15508. [CrossRef] [PubMed]
66. Fèvre, E.M.; Bronsvoort, B.M.d.C.; Hamilton, K.A.; Cleaveland, S. Animal movements and the spread of infectious diseases. *Trends Microbiol.* **2006**, *14*, 125–131. [CrossRef] [PubMed]
67. Mulderij-Jansen, V.; Elsinga, J.; Gerstenbluth, I.; Duits, A.; Tami, A.; Bailey, A. Understanding risk communication for prevention and control of vector-borne diseases: A mixed-method study in Curaçao. *PLoS Negl. Trop. Dis.* **2020**, *14*, e0008136. [CrossRef] [PubMed]
68. Refaei, S.A.; El-Gilany, A.-H. Risk communication during infectious diseases pandemics. *Int. J. Health Sci.* **2022**, *6*, 4450–4470. [CrossRef]
69. Amer, F.; Khalil, H.E.S.; Elahmady, M.; El Badawy, N.E.; Zahran, W.A.; Abdelnasser, M.; Rodríguez-Morales, A.J.; Wegdan, A.A.; Tash, R.M.E. Mpox: Risks and approaches to prevention. *J. Infect. Public Health* **2023**, *16*, 901–910. [CrossRef] [PubMed]
70. Hara, M.R.; Kovacs, J.J.; Whalen, E.J.; Rajagopal, S.; Strachan, R.T.; Grant, W.; Towers, A.J.; Williams, B.; Lam, C.M.; Xiao, K.; et al. A stress response pathway regulates DNA damage through β2-adrenoreceptors and β-arrestin-1. *Nature* **2011**, *477*, 349–353. [CrossRef]
71. Halabowski, D.; Rzymski, P. Taking a lesson from the COVID-19 pandemic: Preventing the future outbreaks of viral zoonoses through a multi-faceted approach. *Sci. Total Environ.* **2021**, *757*, 143723. [CrossRef] [PubMed]
72. Wu, C., Astbury, C.C.; Lee, K.M.; Cong, Z.; Chen, S.; Li, A.; Tsasis, P.; Penney, T. Public awareness of One Health in China. *One Health* **2023**, *17*, 100603. [CrossRef] [PubMed]
73. Powell, L.; Lavender, T.M.; Reinhard, C.L.; Watson, B. Pet Owners' Perceptions of COVID-19, Zoonotic Disease, and Veterinary Medicine: The Impact of Demographic Characteristics. *Vet. Sci.* **2022**, *9*, 195. [CrossRef] [PubMed]
74. Stoewen, D.L.; Coe, J.B.; MacMartin, C.; Stone, E.A.; Dewey, C.E. Qualitative study of the communication expectations of clients accessing oncology care at a tertiary referral center for dogs with life-limiting cancer. *J. Am. Vet. Med. Assoc.* **2014**, *245*, 785–795. [CrossRef] [PubMed]
75. Tvarijonaviciute, A.; Roca, D.; Escribano, D.; Franco-Martínez, L.; Bernal, L.J.; Ceron, J.J.; Martínez-Subiela, S.; Rojo-Villada, P.A. Interdisciplinary Collaboration Between Veterinary and Communication Students to Promote Communication Skills: A Qualitative Pilot Study. *Front. Vet. Sci.* **2020**, *7*, 586086. [CrossRef]
76. Adams, C.L.; Kurtz, S. Coaching and feedback: Enhancing communication teaching and learning in veterinary practice settings. *J. Vet. Med. Educ.* **2012**, *39*, 217–228. [CrossRef]
77. Gibbs, S.E.J.; Gibbs, E.P.J. The historical, present, and future role of veterinarians in One Health. *Curr. Top. Microbiol. Immunol.* **2013**, *365*, 31–47. [CrossRef]

animals

MDPI

Article

Assessment of a Teaching Module for Cardiac Auscultation of Horses by Veterinary Students

Alyse Wood †, Frances Marie Shapter † and Allison J. Stewart *,†

School of Veterinary Science, University of Queensland Gatton, 5391 Warrego Highway, Gatton, QLD 4343, Australia; alyse.wood@uqconnect.edu.au (A.W.); f.shapter@uq.edu.au (F.M.S.)
* Correspondence: allison.stewart@uq.edu.au
† These authors contributed equally to this work.

Simple Summary: Veterinary students are required to determine an animal's heart rate and diagnose heart murmurs and arrhythmias by the time of graduation. Accurate assessment of the heart sounds of horses is considered as a day one clinical competency. Limited opportunities exist in the veterinary curriculum to develop these competencies, especially during COVID-19 times. This research aimed to determine if a multimodal learning resource consisting of diagrams, heart sound recordings and visual representation of the sounds would assist in the development of veterinary students' confidence and ability to recognize normal and abnormal heart sounds of horses. Students were invited to utilize the teaching resource and voluntarily complete surveys about their confidence in recognizing normal heart sounds as well as various murmurs and important arrhythmias of horses. The survey results were analyzed by qualitative and quantitative means. Over a two-year period, 231 fourth-year and 222 fifth-year veterinary students had access to the resource; 89 completed the initial survey and 57 completed a second survey after using the resource. Results confirmed that after access to the resource students' understanding and perception of their auscultation abilities improved.

Abstract: Auscultation of heart sounds is an important veterinary skill requiring an understanding of anatomy, physiology, pathophysiology and pattern recognition. This cross-sectional study was developed to evaluate a targeted, audio-visual training resource for veterinary students to improve their understanding and auscultation of common heart conditions in horses. Fourth- and fifth-year 2021 and 2022 Bachelor of Veterinary Science students at the University of Queensland (UQ) were provided the learning resource and surveyed via online pre- and post-intervention surveys. Results were quantitatively analyzed using descriptive statistics and Mann–Whitney U tests. Open-ended survey questions were qualitatively analyzed by thematic analysis and Leximancer™ Version 4 program software analysis. Over the two-year period, 231 fourth-year and 222 fifth-year veterinary students had access to the resource; 89 completed the pre-intervention survey and 57 completed the post-intervention survey. Quantitative results showed the resource helped students prepare for practicals and their perception of competency and confidence when auscultating equine cardiac sounds improved ($p < 0.05$). Compared to fifth-year students, fourth-year students felt less competent at identifying murmurs and arrythmias prior to accessing the learning resource ($p < 0.05$). Fourth-year and fifth-year students' familiarity with detection of murmurs improved after completing the learning resource ($p < 0.001$). Qualitative analysis demonstrated a limited number of opportunities to practice equine cardiac auscultation throughout the veterinary degree, especially during the COVID-19 pandemic, and that integrated audio-visual resources are an effective means of teaching auscultation.

Keywords: self-directed learning; equine; education; COVID-19; on-line learning; cardiology; murmur; arrhythmia; electronic stethoscope; thematic analysis

1. Introduction

The development of strong practical skills is an important component of veterinary medicine [1–4]. Skills training is optimized by a multidimensional approach, which creates a safe environment for active learning, provides students with a scaffold to guide their self-directed learning (SDL), encourages students to self-assess their development, is relevant and facilitates students taking responsibility for their learning and tailoring it to their individual strengths and weaknesses [2,5–8]. A recent study conducted by Muca et al. (2023) also determined that flipped classroom (FC) and peer-assisted learning methods helped veterinary students engage more in nutritional classes [9]. The flipped classroom technique incorporates self-directed learning components that enhance a student's engagement and willingness to learn, and use time more effectively in class [9,10].

Due to costs, safety and animal welfare considerations, during a five-year Bachelor of Veterinary Science degree, opportunities to practice equine auscultatory skills are finite, with the bulk of equine auscultations occurring during final year rotations. Students obtain cardiac auscultation experiences across many species, which supports comparative learning between, and cumulative learning across, all species taught. However, while most auscultation skills are transferable between species, some aspects of diagnostic equine auscultation are specific to horses. The conventional approach to learning equine cardiac auscultation is through the delivery of lecture content, practical sessions and participating in rotations involving client-owned animals. UQ students' first exposure to cardiac anatomy and physiology content is in the first semester of their second year. This is followed by physical examination practicals in their third year, where students practice multi-species heart auscultation, including horses. In the first semester of their fourth year, equine cardiology theory is reviewed, followed by a forty-minute practical in the second semester focusing on equine cardiac auscultation. Finally, in their fifth year, students spend a minimum of one month on an equine rotation and have the option to competitively apply to enroll in an additional four-week rotation in the specialist equine hospital. However, in 2020 and 2021 the third- and fourth-year practical classes, as well as fifth-year rotations, were severely impacted by the COVID-19 pandemic, requiring the addition of new supporting resources to bridge the gaps in face-to-face teaching. The 2020 to 2022 graduating cohorts may have only been exposed to live auscultation of the equine heart during their final year rotations. Across many disciplines, graduates whose practical education was affected by the COVID-19 pandemic teaching constraints are cognizant of perceived and actual deficiencies in their learning.

Veterinary licensure allows a veterinarian to treat any patient within their capabilities. However, it is difficult for students and new graduates to determine what they do not know, and if physical examination competencies are underdeveloped, then the health of the patient may suffer [11,12]. Veterinary and medical educators agree that students benefit from a multidimensional approach to teaching auscultation techniques [4,13,14]. Therefore, it is paramount that during their training, students receive as many varied learning and self-assessment opportunities as possible to improve their competency and self-efficacy prior to graduation. UQ students who have an interest in equine or mixed practice can become involved in a student led Equine Special Interest Group, assist with an annual equine practitioner's conference and can complete two to four weeks of additional elective rotations involving horses. Additionally, many students appreciate self-directed learning (SDL) opportunities to increase their skills, especially when the availability of practical sessions or clinical rotations is curtailed, as occurred during the COVID-19 pandemic.

When creating SDL resources for auscultation skills, electronic stethoscopes allow recordings of heart, lung and gastrointestinal (GIT) sounds and their graphical representation (phonograph) to be saved as media files that can be incorporated into digital training resources [15]. Electronic stethoscopes allow for the recording of heart, lung and gastrointestinal (GIT) sounds and their graphical representation (phonograph). The sounds and phonographs can be saved as media files that can be incorporated into training resources. Some studies have shown that pairing sounds from electronic stethoscopes, digitally or in real-time, with phonographs assists with the identification of heart sounds to a greater degree than using conventional stethoscopes [13,16]. Integration of multidimensional teaching tools also improves animal health and well-being, as the students are better prepared during live animal interactions [1,17,18]. Hence an audio-visual equine cardiac auscultation resource was developed for veterinary students at UQ to integrate theoretical and practical content (Figure 1).

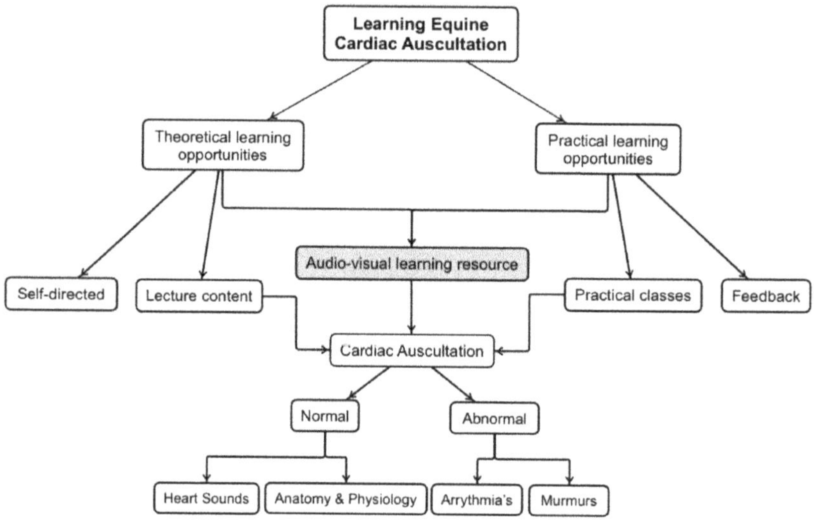

Figure 1. Equine cardiac auscultation learning pathway for veterinary science students at the University of Queensland.

This study was designed to determine whether there would be an uptake of an additional learning SDL tool by already time-poor students, and whether the resource aided in the development of students' perceived equine cardiac auscultatory confidence and improved practical training of fourth- and final-year veterinary students at UQ. Feedback was collected from pre- and post-intervention surveys, which is essential to understand the value of further development of multimodal learning resources and models for veterinary students nationally and internationally.

2. Methodology

2.1. Live Animal Recordings

This study was conducted in compliance with the animal ethics guidelines (certificate number SVS/214/20). Thirty-five adult horses (University of Queensland Australian Stock Horse Stud and client owned), ten foals/juvenile (University of Queensland Australian Stock Horse Stud) and six client-owned horses with cardiac pathologies (with written consent) had their heart sounds recorded utilizing the Eko CORE™ (Oakland, CA, USA) digital stethoscope. Heart sounds were recorded on the left side over the pulmonary (3rd intercostal space), aortic (4th intercostal space) and mitral valves (5th intercostal space), as well as on the right side over the tricuspid valve (4th intercostal space). Recordings were made under field conditions.

2.2. Resource Development and Distribution

Sound recordings and phonographs of normal and abnormal auscultatory findings were downloaded from the Eko CORE™ Digital Stethoscope application (App, https://app.ekodevices.com (accessed on the 2 December 2019)) and uploaded to a cloud-based data manager. Normal and abnormal heart auscultatory findings were selected to create a PowerPoint™ (Microsoft, Redmond, WA, USA) learning resource. The resource included recordings of normal heart sounds, sounds with background interference from other internal sounds (gastrointestinal sounds) and interference from external sources (tractors, wild birds). Examples of classic equine cardiac abnormalities that were utilized as recordings included second-degree atrioventricular blocks, atrial fibrillation and murmurs (mitral, aortic and tricuspid, ventricular septal defect and pentalogy of Fallot). An example of the visual presentation of slides can be seen in Figure 2 and the full presentation can be viewed in Supplementary File S1.

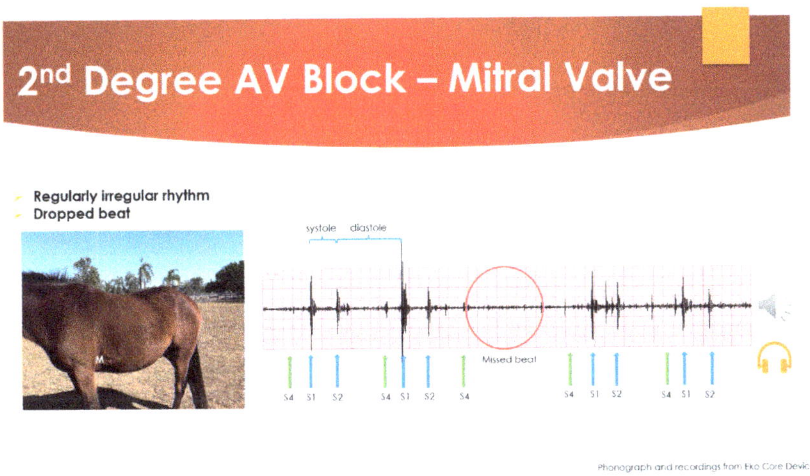

Figure 2. Example slide from the audio-visual resource (PowerPoint™ slide 53).

2.3. Survey Data Capture

The usefulness of the resource was assessed using qualitative means and quantitative statistics based on pre- and post-intervention surveys, which included an assessment of pre- and post-perceived knowledge (Supplementary File S2). Utilizing the PowerPoint™ presentation learning resource was not a curriculum requirement; however, all fourth- and fifth-year veterinary students were encouraged to access it via the online learning management system (Blackboard™; Reston, VI, USA). With ethical approval (project number 2020/HE002986), students who engaged with the learning resource were given the additional option of undertaking online, anonymous, pre- and post-intervention surveys. Human ethics required that students could utilize the resource without completing the surveys as it would likely enhance the grades of all students who did use the resource. All student responses had to be kept anonymous and lecturers that graded the students were not allowed to directly determine which students had utilized the resource. Therefore, it was impossible to test if student utilization of the resource directly improved the students' grades or abilities.

Overarching survey questions focused on establishing background information, the individual's diagnostic capabilities and the importance of targeted, audio-visual training resources in the development of students' practical skills in the auscultation of heart sounds. Surveys captured mainly dichotomized or ordinal responses (e.g., Likert scale or yes/no questions). Students were encouraged to complete the surveys for future study and resource purposes; however, students didn't need to complete either survey due to human ethics constraints.

2.4. Method of Data Analysis

Responses from the anonymous, pre- and post-intervention surveys were collated in Microsoft Excel™ (Microsoft, Redmond, WA, USA) spreadsheets and GraphPad Prism™

(GraphPad Software Version 10, San Diego, CA, USA). The Likert-style questions (Supplementary File S2) of both surveys were coded (strongly agree = 5, agree = 4, neutral = 3, disagree = 2, strongly disagree = 1). Simple descriptive statistics such as the number of respondents, the mean, standard deviation, median, inter-quartile ranges and confidence intervals (as appropriate for parametric and non-parametric data) were calculated for the coded responses of the pooled, fourth-year and fifth-year responses, on both software platforms for both surveys. The normality of distribution was assessed using the Shapiro–Wilk test on GraphPad Prism™. As all the data was non-parametric, GraphPad Prism™ was utilized to perform a Mann–Whitney U test on questions 8 to 14 of the pooled data comparing both surveys and comparing the fourth- and fifth-year responses for each question. The p value was set at <0.05 [19].

Qualitative analysis of the open-ended pre- and post-intervention survey questions was conducted by manual thematic analysis, the findings of which were compared with those generated by the Leximancer™ Version 4 software data analysis program (Brisbane, Queensland, Australia). The first step of the manual analysis was to examine the raw data and inductively develop a set of codes to represent patterns in the data (themes) [20,21]. This 'coding template' was utilized to code each response individually [20]. Once coded, key themes were identified based on salience to the research project and how prevalent they were across the dataset [20]. Leximancer™, a qualitative analysis software platform that statistically analyses a document's text for keywords and concepts through the use of algorithms then displays these in a visual concept map without subjectivity and bias when qualitatively analyzing the data set [22–25]. The comparison of manually-coded and Leximancer analyses constitutes a form of triangulation and strengthens the reliability of this study's qualitative findings [22,26,27].

3. Results

3.1. Quantitative Data

Utilizing the learning resource was not mandatory, and additional surveys were optional even if students used the resource. Students were time-poor; therefore, completion rates of pre- and post-intervention surveys demonstrated positive student engagement with this training resource (Table 1). When completing the survey, there were specific questions asked that were compulsory to answer, for example, "What is the name of your first pet?" This enabled results from the individual students who responded in consecutive years to remain anonymous, yet be identified and excluded from further analysis, ensuring the data represented equaled the number of individuals surveyed. Two students completed the surveys in both their fourth and fifth years and their responses from their fifth year were excluded. Pooled responses for the pre-intervention surveys showed that the majority of respondents strongly agreed to being interested in more audio-visual learning resources for cardiac auscultation, and they thought these resources would benefit their practical studies and they would feel more competent in practicals if they had access to such a learning resource beforehand (Q1, Q2 and Q4, Figure 3a). For questions 1 to 4, the median score was five, which further indicated strong agreement with these statements (Figure 4a). For question 5, 47% of participants disagreed that they were already competent at auscultating sounds over each of the heart valves (Figure 3a). This was supported by a median score of two (Figure 4a). The majority of respondents agreed that they were familiar with identifying normal heart sounds (Q6, Figure 3a). Finally, respondents had a median score of two (Figure 4b) and disagreed that they were able to identify murmurs and arrythmias (Q8–14, Figure 3a).

Table 1. Audio-visual Auscultation Resource Survey Response Rates.

Year & Total Responses		Pre-Intervention Cohort		Post-Intervention Cohort	
Year & Cohort	Total	Responses	Percentage	Responses	Percentage
2021 4th year	112	35	31%	26	23%
2021 5th year	110	16	15%	9	8%
2022 4th year	119	14	12%	8	7%
2022 5th year	112	24	21%	14	13%

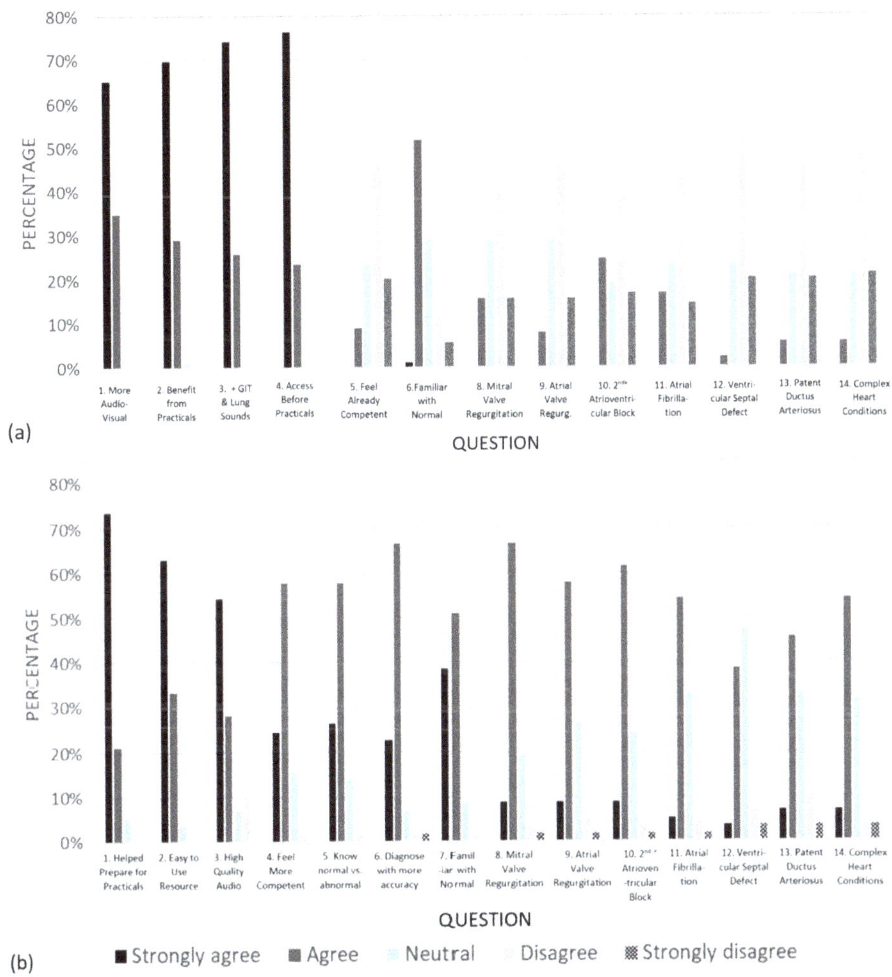

Figure 3. Response rates for the audio-visual auscultation resource surveys comparing pooled data for pre- and post-survey questions; (**a**) Pre-intervention survey Likert response rates, (**b**) post-intervention survey Likert response rates.

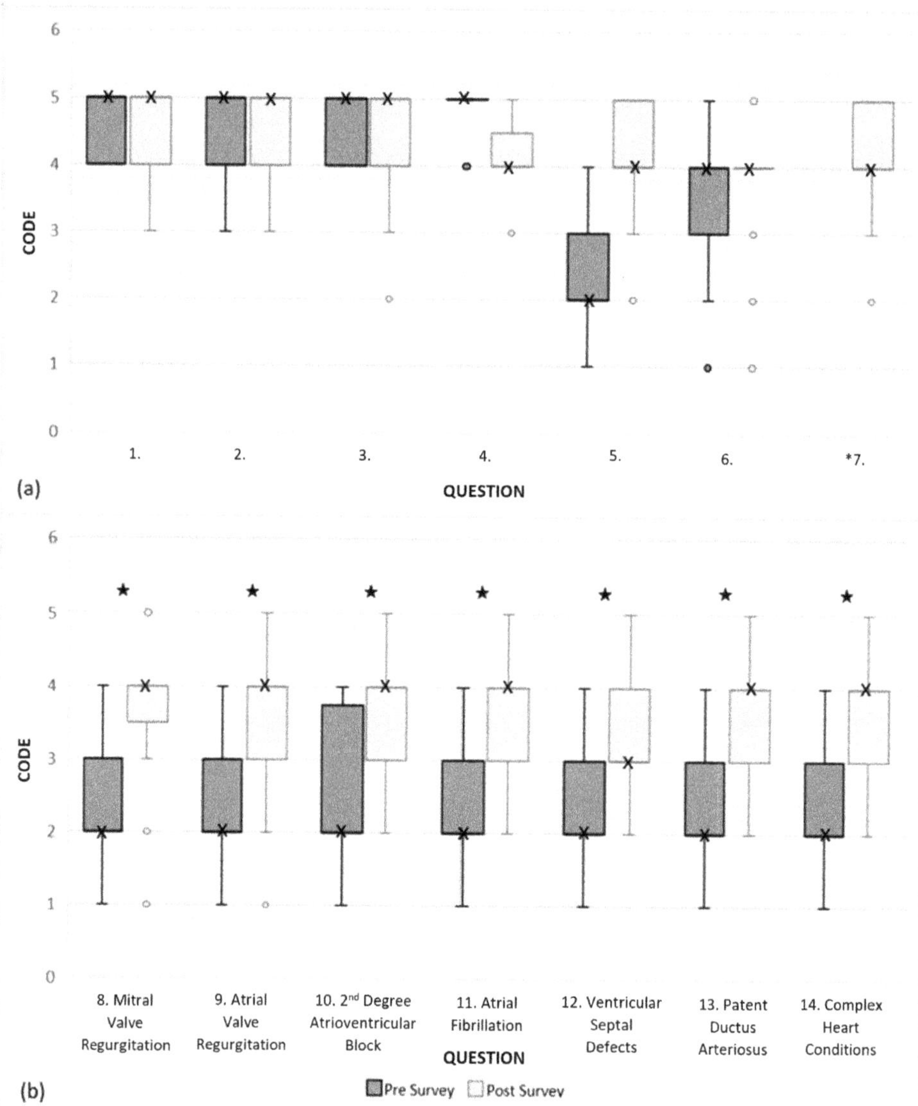

Figure 4. Comparison of the Likert values of Box and whisker plots comparing pre-intervention and post-intervention survey results for questions 8 to 14 (median and IQR). Sub-figure (**a**) shows comparison of responses to questions 1–7 and sub-figure (**b**) shows comparison of responses 8–14 of both surveys. The Y-axis score shows the student's perceived ability to recognize the auscultatory findings associated with specific cardiac pathology using a 1–5 scale. For abbreviations, refer to Figure 3. ★ $p < 0.0001$; o Outliers; X Median. * There was no equivalent question for Q7 of the post-intervention survey in the pre-intervention survey.

Pooled responses for the pre-intervention surveys identified that the majority of respondents strongly agreed that they were interested in more audio-visual learning resources for cardiac auscultation, and that they thought these resources would benefit their practical studies and would feel more competent in practicals if they had access to such learning resources beforehand (Q1, Q2 and Q4.). Almost half of the participants did not feel competent at auscultating sounds over each of the heart valves (Q5). The majority of respondents agreed that they felt familiar with identifying normal heart sounds (Q6), but felt unable to identify murmurs and arrhythmias (Q8–14). Likert scale percentages and median values for each question are presented in Figures 3a and 4a, respectively.

Pooled responses for the post-intervention survey showed that most participants strongly agreed that the resource helped them prepare for practicals, that the resource was easy to work with and that they prefer high-quality audio without background noise and artifacts for learning auscultation techniques (Q1–3, Figure 3b). The median score for each of these questions was five, supporting strong agreeance (Figure 4a). Additionally, students agreed that they felt more competent with their practical and diagnostic skills, that they could differentiate between normal and abnormal equine heart sounds, that they believed they could diagnose heart sounds with more accuracy and that they were familiar with identifying normal heart sounds after utilizing the resource (Q4–7, Figure 3b). Respondents also agreed that they believed that they could now identify murmurs and arrhythmias (Q8–14, Figure 3b). This was supported by a median of four for questions 8 to 11, 13 and 14 (Figure 4).

Data from all questions (Table 2) from the pooled data sets and year level responses were not normally distributed. Graphs showing responses for questions 8 to 14 (median and interquartile ranges (IQR)) for the fourth- and fifth-year cohorts are shown (Figure 5). Comparative analysis ($p < 0.05$) of the pre-intervention survey data identified that fourth-year students believed they were less competent at auscultating sounds over each of the heart valves and less able to identify arrhythmias and murmurs when compared to fifth-year students (Table 2 and Figure 5). No differences were detected in the post-survey questions between the two year levels ($p > 0.05$). Comparing the pooled data for pre- and post-survey questions 8 to 14, an improvement in students' abilities to identify equine cardiac murmurs and arrhythmias after access to the learning resource was detected ($p < 0.0001$).

3.2. Qualitative Data

A summary of the coded responses to the open-ended survey questions is shown in Table 3 and Supplementary File S3. The codes represent patterns in the data. For example, a participant's response to the pre-intervention survey question: 'What do you find most difficult about developing auscultation skills?' was "I struggle to find the proper landmarks or perhaps do not have the proper technique for my auscultation to be of diagnostic quality". This was coded under 'understanding anatomy, physiology and placement of stethoscope' (A&P) and 'lack of opportunity to develop practical skills' (PRAC). As a further example, the response "unless I can hear something, and be told/figure out—what I'm hearing is 'this', then it's tricky to develop an ear for it" was coded under 'having supervision when auscultating, teachers or learning resources' (TEACH).

In relation to what students find most difficult about developing auscultation skills, most participants responded that having few opportunities to practice equine cardiac auscultation in the program was problematic. This perception was exemplified in responses such as "practical training in this area is extremely lacking in this program" and "lack of hands-on experience, we learn so much theory, but I had probably only heard 8 murmurs before 5th year". Finding it hard to distinguish between normal and abnormal heart sounds, especially low-grade heart murmurs, was also a concern for many respondents. For example, a coded response for this was "hearing low grade heart murmurs" and "developing confidence to confidently identify mildly abnormal changes".

Leximancer analysis of this question grouped responses similarly (Figure 6). The three dominant themes from the Leximancer analysis were "practice", "sounds" and "murmurs". The analysis found that students perceive it as difficult to distinguish between normal and abnormal, especially with subtle differences. Additionally, students reported it is difficult to diagnose low-grade murmurs and there is therefore a need for exposure to many different murmurs before they could feel competent with equine cardiac auscultation.

Table 2. Differences between fourth- and fifth-year responses for pre- and post-intervention surveys.

Pre-Intervention Survey Difference for 4th versus 5th Year Responses		**Post-Intervention Survey Difference for 4th and 5th Year Responses**		**Pre and Post-Survey Comparison of Pooled Responses**	
Question	***p* Value**	**Question**	***p* Value**	**Question**	***p* Value**
1. I am interested in more audio-visual learning resources for cardiac auscultation	0.66	1. This resource helped me prepare for practicals/training	0.50	Questions 1–7 are not comparable between the pooled pre-and post-intervention responses	
2. I think these resources would benefit practical studies immensely	0.99	2. The resource was easy to work with	0.11		
3. I would like to see more resources with recordings of GIT and lung sounds also	0.14	3. I prefer clear high-quality audio without background noise and artefacts for learning new auscultation techniques,	0.87		
4. I/students would feel more competent in practicals if we/they had access to such learning resources beforehand	0.46	4. I feel more competent with my practical and diagnostic skills	0.28		
5. I am already competent at auscultating sounds over each of the heart valves	0.005 *	5. I can differentiate between normal and abnormal equine heart sounds	0.30		
6. I am familiar with identifying normal heart sounds	0.72	6. I believe I can diagnose heart sounds with more accuracy after using the resource	0.14		
7. #		7. I am familiar with identifying normal heart sounds	0.32		
8. I am able to identify mitral valve regurgitation (systolic murmur)	0.0001 *	8. I am able to identify mitral valve regurgitation (systolic murmur)	0.11	8.	<0.0001 √
9. I am able to identify aortic valve regurgitation (diastolic murmur)	0.007 *	9. I am able to identify aortic valve regurgitation (diastolic murmur)	0.36	9.	<0.0001 √
10. I am able to identify second degree atrioventricular blocks (AVB)	0.0001 *	10. I am able to identify second degree atrioventricular blocks (AVB)	0.24	10.	<0.0001 √
11. I am able to identify atrial fibrillation	0.0008 *	11. I am able to identify atrial fibrillation	0.55	11.	<0.0001 √
12. I am able to identify ventricular septal defects (VSD)	0.005 *	12. I am able to identify ventricular septal defects (VSD)	0.17	12.	<0.0001 √
13. I am able to identify a patent ductus arteriosus (PDA)	0.008 *	13. I am able to identify a patent ductus arteriosus (PDA)	0.05	13.	<0.0001 √
14. I understand how to diagnose complex heart conditions	0.01*	14. I understand how to diagnose complex heart conditions	0.29	14.	<0.0001 √

* $p < 0.05$ = difference between the fourth and fifth-year student responses; √ $p < 0.0001$ = difference between pre- and post-intervention pooled survey responses; # Notes: One less question was asked on the pre-intervention survey, and question numbers were re-calibrated for simplicity in results. The full original data set is provided in Supplementary Data.

In relation to the second open-ended question 'What was the most helpful about the learning resource?', thematic analysis showed that the audio-visual nature of the learning resource was most helpful to respondents. Some examples of responses included "the audios were very helpful, and the animations were very good to follow along with" and it was helpful to have "realistic sounds with gut sounds in background—useful for in practice to know what these sound like". Many students also appreciated the access to a complete resource that was easy to use and had clear explanations and clear recordings embedded. Examples of correlated responses included "excellently presented and easy to use—very straightforward" and it was also helpful "having audio files and all the information in one place, it was very clearly structured and written".

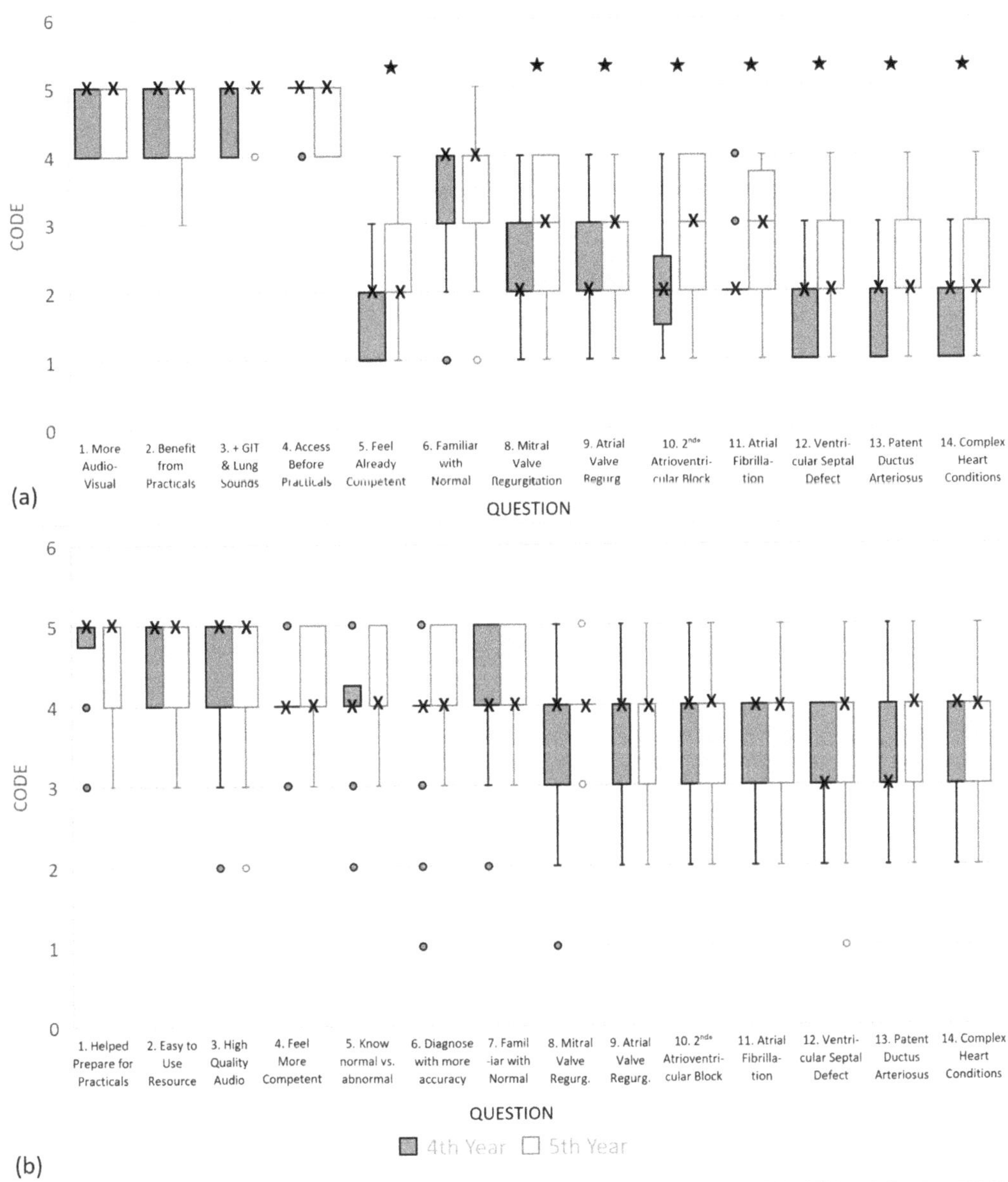

Figure 5. (**a**) Box and whisker plots comparing fourth- and fifth-year student's pre-intervention Likert survey responses (median and IQR) (**b**) Box and whisker plots comparing fourth- and fifth-year students' post-intervention Likert survey responses (median and IQR). The *y*-axis score shows student's survey responses using a 1–5 scale for questions 1–14. For abbreviations, refer to Figure 3. ★ $p < 0.05$; o Outliers; X Median.

Table 3. Definitions of coding nodes for efficacy of audio-visual resource survey questions.

Pre-Intervention Survey Question: 'What Do You Find Most Difficult about Developing Auscultation Skills?'			
Title	**Code**	**Attributes**	**Responses**
Practical skills	PRAC	Few opportunities to gain practical skills in auscultation	41
Abnormal versus normal	A&N	Difficulty in distinguishing between normal and abnormal cardiac sounds/pathologies to make a diagnosis	23
Anatomy and physiology	A&P	Understanding anatomy, physiology and placement of stethoscope for auscultation	16
Heart murmur	MUR	Heart murmurs specifically subtle/low-grade heart murmurs	13
Teaching and learning	TEA	Having supervision when auscultating, teachers or learning resources	11
GIT auscultation	GIT	GIT auscultation	3
Other	OTH	Anything that doesn't fit any of the above	4
Post-intervention survey question: 'What was most helpful about the learning resource?'			
Title	**Code**	**Attributes**	**Responses**
Complete resource	RES	The helpfulness of having the material condensed into a single resource	5
Audio visual	AV	The audio or visuals being helpful or the inclusion of audio recordings and/or ECG's in the resource	46
Abnormal	ABN	Including information regarding abnormalities or pathologies	6
Nothing	NOT	The resource not being helpful	1
Revision	REV	Anatomy and/or revision	5
Heart murmur	MUR	Heart murmurs specifically	5
Clear explanation	CLE	Clear explanations and descriptions	13
Ease of use	EASE	Ease of use	2
Understanding	UN	Understanding information presented in the resource	5
Other	OTH	Anything that doesn't fit any of the above	1
Post-intervention survey question: 'What would improve the learning resource?'			
Title	**Code**	**Attributes**	**Responses**
Clearer explanations	CLA	The explanations and clarity of information in the resource	3
Audio	AUD	The clearness of audio recordings or inclusion of more recordings	17
Concise	CON	Improving the conciseness of the slides	5
Nothing	NOT	The resource not needing any improvements	1
Cases	CAS	More cases and/or inclusion of more quiz questions	5
More interaction	INT	Technology and improved graphics to make it even more interactive	17
Accessibility	ACC	More accessibility to the resource and/or incorporation in more areas of the curriculum	2
Additional information	INFO	Additional information to include	6
Other	OTH	Anything that doesn't fit any of the above	2

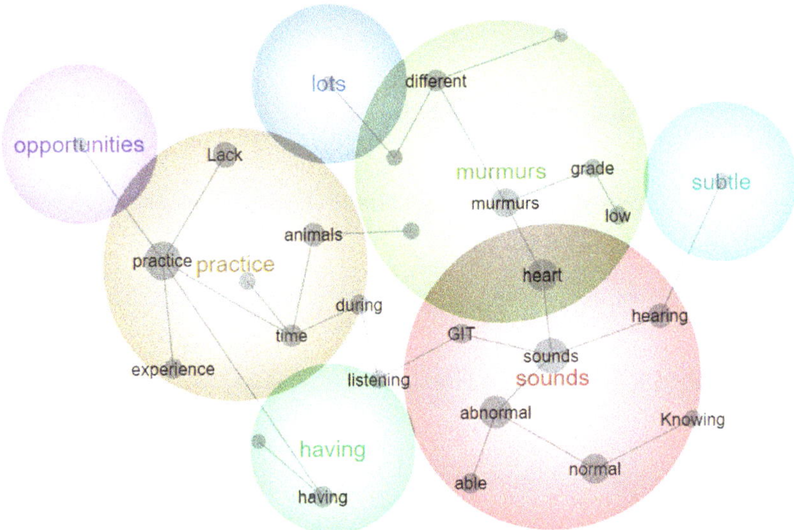

Figure 6. Leximancer concept map for 'What do you find most difficult about developing auscultation skills?' The large, colored circles are the overarching themes, whilst the words within are the concepts linking the themes.

The Leximancer Version 4 software analysis of this question was again very similar to the manual thematic analysis (Figure 7). Students found the explanations of abnormalities, ECG's and heart sounds to be clear, helpful and easy to understand. From the visual representation of the program analysis (Figure 7), it was also clear that the audio-visual resource was easy to use and could also be utilized for revision purposes.

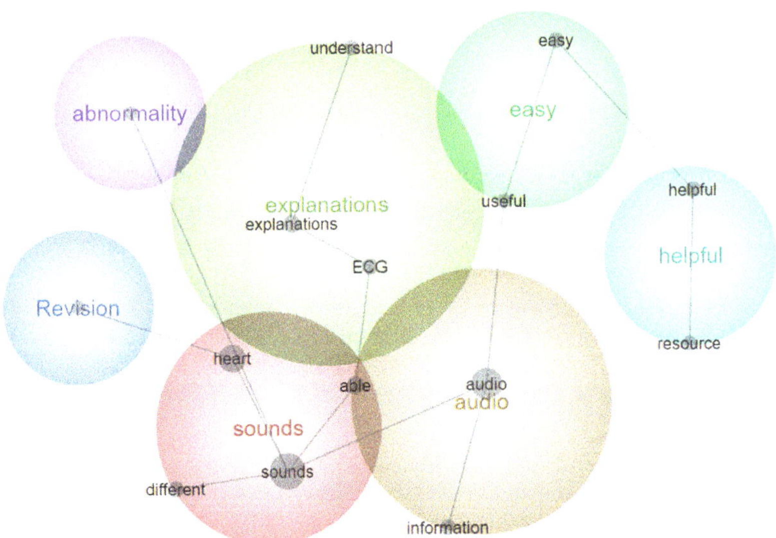

Figure 7. Leximancer concept map for 'What was the most helpful about the learning resource?' The large, colored circles are the overarching themes, whilst the words within are the concepts linking the themes.

The thematic analysis of responses to the final question 'What would improve this learning resource?' centered around further content development: inclusion of more recordings; clearer audio and the inclusion of more technology and graphics on the slides of the resource. Examples of correlating responses include "slightly clearer sound examples", "different recordings of the same problem as every case is different and hearing the same problem on different horses would sound different", and digitally mapping the "corresponding position on ECG as the audio is playing".

Leximancer software analysis identified similar themes for this question (Figure 8). The key themes the program found were recordings, audio and ECG. The inclusion of additional and higher quality audio recordings was the main suggestion for improvement of the learning resource. Additionally, different horse recordings, the inclusion of background ECG traces and embedding the YouTube recordings were suggested improvements.

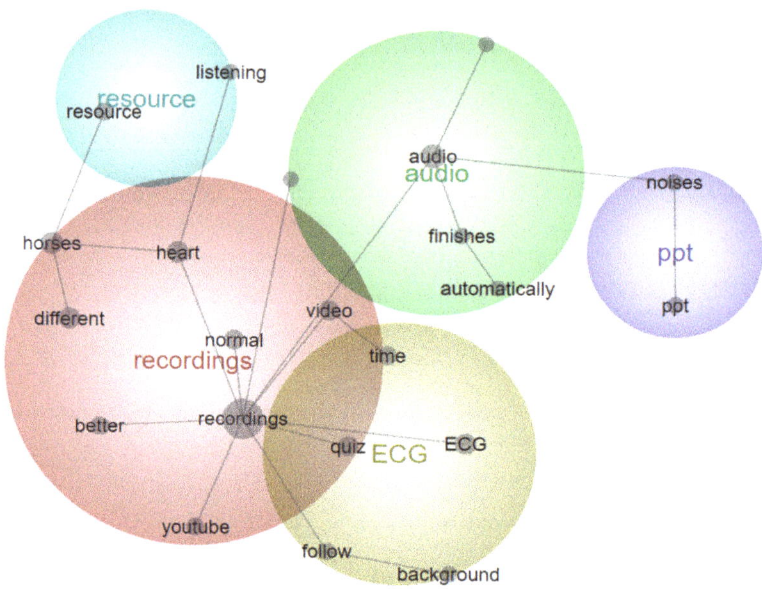

Figure 8. Leximancer concept map for 'What would improve this learning resource?' The large, colored circles are the overarching themes, whilst the words within are the concepts linking the themes; ppt = PowerPoint.

4. Discussion

Analysis of pre- and post-intervention survey data showed that before accessing the resource, most respondents had a low perception of their ability to identify cardiac murmurs (mitral valve regurgitation, aortic valve regurgitation, tricuspid valve regurgitation, VSDs, PDAs and murmurs from complex congenital abnormalities) or common arrhythmias (second degree AVBs and atrial fibrillation). Their perceptions of competency for distinguishing between normal and abnormal cardiology findings, equine cardiology diagnostics and auscultation of murmurs and arrythmias improved after utilizing the learning resource. Respondents also appreciated the usability of the resource, the compilation of all information in one location, and believed that the use of the audio-visual resource assisted with their understanding of the auscultation of cardiac abnormalities. Additionally, thematic analysis and Leximancer software analysis revealed that students would like more practical opportunities to practice their auscultation and to be able to better differentiate between normal and abnormal heart sounds. Adequate cardiac auscultation is also a day-one clinical competency that medical students must meet [28]. "Simulation-based medical education" can improve students' cardiac auscultation knowledge and practical skills [29]. Similar results were found when third-year medical students were examined after access to an online cardiac auscultation tutorial and simulation [28]. Access to online multimodal learning databases has been demonstrated to improve medical students' abilities to distinguish murmurs [30–32].

Although the learning resource was highly recommended to all fourth- and fifth-year students, as we believed it would improve their knowledge, prepare them for the fourth-year equine auscultation practical class and clinical cases and likely improve their grades, it was not compulsory or directly assessed. Use of the learning resource and completion of the surveys was voluntary, and our human ethics required that the resource be made available to all students irrespective of whether they volunteered their time to complete the surveys. As the use of the resource and completion of the surveys had to be anonymous, we could not test if its utilization improved the student's grades. It was our impression that most of the students did ultimately utilize the resource (often after the practical class, once they heard from their colleagues how useful it was). Unfortunately, as with most surveys, the number of students who gave up their time to complete the surveys was much lower than the number that utilized the resource.

A higher percentage of students filled out the pre-intervention survey compared to the post-intervention survey, and fourth-year students had the highest response rate for both surveys. The COVID-19 pandemic impacted many teaching modalities, especially practical classes, across different professions [33–37], including the graduating class of 2022's cardiac auscultation practicals (2021 fourth-year cohort). There has been a general shift to incorporating more online learning opportunities for veterinary students in recent years [37]. Veterinary students have also had more access to portable devices in COVID times, and due to social distancing restrictions, there has been an inability to conduct face-to-face lectures or even access hard-copy textbooks [37]. Potentially, fourth-year student response rates were higher due to willingness to view and complete surveys for the audio-visual resource during SDL, whereas fifth-year students were on clinical rotations and had less SDL time available. This cohort had their third-year physical examination practical canceled due to COVID-19 restrictions for face-to-face learning and were only exposed to one (40 min) fourth-year equine cardiac auscultation practical before beginning their fifth-year rotations in 2022. The two highest response rates were from the cohorts that undertook their fourth-year training, where the bulk of the auscultation was taught, under stricter COVID protocols and reduced practical training opportunities. It was theorized that because the students felt like their learning had been compromised, they were more willing to engage in additional SDL opportunities in preparation for their fifth-year clinical placements.

Quantitative analysis showed that before undertaking the learning resource, fourth-year students felt less competent at auscultating over each of the heart valves and were less able to identify murmurs and arrhythmias (questions 5, and 8 through to 14) compared to fifth-year students. This is to be expected, as fifth-year students should be further advanced in their veterinary degree. However, after completion of the learning resource, no difference was detected between the fourth- and fifth-year responses for questions 5 and 8 to 14 on the post-intervention survey. The use of the learning resource appeared to equalize their perceived knowledge. There was a significant improvement in perceived competencies for both fourth- and fifth-year students when comparing the pre- and post-intervention survey responses (p value < 0.0001 for Questions 6–8), suggesting that the audio-visual resource helped with students' understanding of equine cardiology and perceived competency of auscultation. Finally, there was also a strong interest in more resources for auscultation, as 100% of respondents either strongly agreed (65%) or agreed (35%) that audio-visual resources would benefit practical studies and students would be more competent if they had accessed the learning resource before practical classes.

Thematic analysis can be criticized as being highly subjective and lacking in scientific rigor when measured against quantitative evaluative criteria [20,21,26,38]. However, qualitative research strategies, such as thematic analysis, allow researchers to generate a granularity of findings that cannot be obtained through quantitative means [20,21,26]. Participants can give voice to their individual perspectives and are not constrained by the researcher's hypotheses [20,21,26]. Qualitative researchers can then take the full breadth of these individual perceptions and analyze them to describe and report patterns within data sets [20,21,26]. If the thematic analysis codes are well defined and representative, then a high intercoder agreement will be achieved [39]. In this study, the qualitative findings provided valuable insights into what students perceived to be particularly challenging about developing equine auscultation skills and how they perceived the learning resource could be improved.

Through both comparative analyses of the open-ended survey questions utilizing a thematic analysis technique and the Leximancer software program, it was evident that students desired more practical opportunities to improve their auscultation skills throughout their studies. Respondents also relayed that the learning resource helped distinguish normal from abnormal sounds, and also identified common internal and external background noises. Some students believed that this made the identification of abnormalities more difficult, but most appreciated that these noises were reflective of real-world clinical practice. The utilization of both methods of qualitative analysis offered quality control of results and reduced the likelihood of individual bias [24,38].

Qualitative analysis determined that students found it difficult to diagnose low-grade murmurs and needed exposure to lots of different murmurs before they could feel competent with equine cardiac auscultation. New graduates are not expected to be competent at differentiating all murmurs by auscultation [40]. Expected day one competencies include identifying between normal and abnormal, the location of the point of maximum intensity of the murmur, the timing of the murmur (systolic/diastolic), grade of the murmur and the formulation of a differential list [40]. To understand the sound, students need to understand the anatomy and physiology/pathophysiology. Characteristic sounds allow the detection of an abnormality for further investigation by electrocardiogram or echocardiology to determine the appropriate prognosis and necessity of treatment or safety recommendations. Day one competencies can be improved after many years of practice, continuing education, ongoing case-based reading, internships, residencies, post-graduate competency courses, exams and board certification [31,41].

One of the limitations of this study was the moderate completion rate of both surveys. The overall community survey completion rates of the cohorts were approximately 20% for the pre-intervention survey and 13% for the post-intervention survey. The voluntary completion rate of student evaluations of fourth- and fifth-year veterinary students at UQ is between 10% and 25%; therefore, the completion rates for this study were comparable. To enhance program learning outcomes, particularly in the light of COVID restrictions on practical teaching, all students were provided equal access to the learning resource irrespective of whether they elected to complete one or both surveys. Therefore, it was not possible to have a control group that did not have access to the learning resource and test the difference in knowledge between students who did or did not utilize the resource. The surveys were completed voluntarily with no incentive or benefit from survey completion. The low response rate to the post-intervention survey is acknowledged; however, completion was dependent on the student's generosity to donate their time to assist with this study. Although we did not detect a difference in perceived competencies between fourth- and fifth-year students after utilizing the resource, this may have been a true lack of difference (with the resource equalizing their knowledge), or failure to detect a difference due to inadequate power. It should also be noted that whilst the resource indicates where to auscultate heart sounds on a horse, it does not replace practically finding the heart sounds on a live horse, it just better prepares students before practicals.

During practical classes and clinical rotations, it was noted by lecturers and tutors that individual students frequently commented on how useful the learning resource was and encouraged their colleagues to utilize the resource. The resource was likely utilized more frequently than the completion of the actual surveys. As students' learning is cumulative across the curriculum with ongoing overlapping multispecies courses, it was not possible to determine the exact improvement in students' perceived abilities attributable solely to this learning resource. Clinical equine rotation occurs throughout their final year, and students likely had greater knowledge at the end of their clinical year when compared to the start of the clinical year. Anecdotally, most students completed the post-survey questions immediately after utilizing the resource, but some students did complete it within the two-week equine medicine rotation and their knowledge may have improved during the rotation. Highly motivated students were more likely to make time to participate in voluntary additional learning opportunities, and the results of the surveys may not be representative of the entire cohort. Students with an interest in equine medicine or previous horse experience may have had improved perceptions of their abilities before utilizing the resource. A question in the pre-survey regarding the level of previous experience with horses to determine if there was any difference in the pre- and post-survey results for students with prior equine experience would be a valuable addition to future work.

This study determined that the students' perception of knowledge improved after the utilization of the targeted, audio-visual training resource. However, actual diagnostic capabilities before or after utilizing the learning resource, or between students who did or did not utilize the resource, were not determined because no form of physical assessment was able to be implemented during COVID restrictions and managing their ongoing impacts. It is well illustrated by Cook et al. (2012) that one must be careful about the claims made about whether an educational intervention worked or not [42]. However, as the perception of the resource was very positive, then it appears worthwhile to embed the resource within the curriculum, possibly incorporating more quiz questions within the resource and continuing to encourage students to use the resource before practical classes and as a means to prepare for examinations in earlier years. High-quality, audio-based quiz questions before and after using the resource, or in end-of-semester equine cardiology exams, could be used to assess the effectiveness of the resource; however, as a clinical skill, this should ideally be measured via a structured skills exam.

Traditionally, veterinary students learn about cardiology based on a foundation in physiology and pathophysiology. Auscultation skills are practiced on a variety of species, comparatively providing cumulative knowledge. Although this learning resource was centered around equine cardiology, the basic skills learned would benefit all students irrespective of their interest in equine practice. As horses have large hearts and slow heart rates, in addition to lack of panting (dogs) or purring (cats), horses with a placid temperament provide an ideal species for students to learn to auscultate normal heart sounds over different valves, in addition to common murmurs and arrhythmias. This resource was tested in students affected by COVID lockdowns and its benefits were proven within a framework of limited other opportunities that disrupted the usual cumulative teaching program. Student feedback indicated that this multimodal teaching resource should be deployed repeatedly to third-, fourth- and fifth-year students. Our resource is provided for download in an open-access platform to benefit veterinary students worldwide.

Electronic stethoscopes have the potential for artificial intelligence and algorithm-generated diagnoses [16]. As more recordings are taken of abnormal and normal sounds, the algorithms can be improved with greater accuracy [43]. The audio data collected during this project will be utilized to assist with engineering stethoscope algorithms tailored for use in horses to benefit clinical examinations. The development of such algorithms will assist the veterinary profession on a global scale and aid in creating algorithms for other species. This will ultimately result in increased telemedicine capabilities to assist rural, remote and even third-world veterinarians [13,44]. Adding recordings to a patient's electronic medical record also helps to document future disease progression [13].

5. Conclusions

This research sought to improve the quality of the learning resources available to the veterinary science program at UQ, and through presentations and publications to assist the National and International veterinary education community. There is a plethora of teaching resources available, but few have quantitative data to support their efficacy as a teaching device. Results established that the targeted, audio-visual training resource helped veterinary students improve their understanding and perception of competency and confidence when auscultating equine cardiac sounds. This improved perception of auscultatory competency may assist in communicating clinical findings with clients in the future. Similar to all studies that rely on voluntary completion of surveys, there are limitations due to volunteer bias and a moderate participation rate. However, forcing survey participation is unethical, only providing the resource to a subset of students is not equitable and the workload required to implement pre- and post-intervention skills exams during clinical training for large cohorts is unmanageable. The post-intervention survey responses indicated that the audio-visual learning resource helped students prepare for practical classes and rotations and was easy to utilize. Respondents agreed that they could differentiate between normal and abnormal equine heart sounds and could recognize various murmurs and arrhythmias after accessing the resource. Irrespective of future testing, it was clear that students found this resource helpful to their learning, and sharing this resource would likely benefit the wider veterinary population. The use of this audio-visual resource shows the effectiveness of the implementation of such multimodal presentations for use in furthering veterinary education. The ultimate impact is increased confidence in the diagnostic capabilities of future veterinarians when auscultating cardiac abnormalities.

Supplementary Materials: The following supporting information can be downloaded at: https://www.mdpi.com/article/10.3390/ani14091341/s1. File S1. Learning Resource; File S2. Pre-intervention Survey; File S3. Post-intervention Survey; File S4. Thematic analysis coding and questions.

Author Contributions: Conceptualization, A.J.S., A.W. and F.M.S.; methodology, A.J.S., A.W. and F.M.S.; software, A.J.S., A.W. and F.M.S.; validation, A.J.S., A.W. and F.M.S.; formal analysis, A.J.S., A.W. and F.M.S.; investigation, A.J.S., A.W. and F.M.S.; resources, A.J.S., A.W. and F.M.S.; data curation, A.J.S., A.W. and F.M.S.; writing—original draft, A.W.; writing—review and editing, A.J.S., A.W. and F.M.S.; visualization, A.J.S., A.W. and F.M.S.; supervision, A.J.S. and F.M.S.; project administration, A.J.S., A.W. and F.M.S.; funding acquisition, A.J.S. All authors have read and agreed to the published version of the manuscript.

Funding: Student summer scholarship funding was provided by The University of Queensland Faculty of Science and M3DICINE Pty Ltd. Recipient; M3DICINE Pty Ltd. ABN 46 602 099 329 of 88 Brandl St, Eight Mile Plains QLD 4113. Commencement Date; 1 November 2020. Research Services; Using a Stethee Vet Stethoscope, record heart, lung and gastrointestinal sounds from 50 horses to create a library of sounds. Initial Material; 4 Stethee Vet Stethoscope(s) and 4 access(es) to Stethee Vet Portal.

Institutional Review Board Statement: The study was conducted according to the guidelines of the Declaration of Helsinki, and approved by the Human and Animal Ethics Committee of The University of Queensland (human ethics project number 2020/HE002986 approved on the 11th of February 2021, animal ethics certificate number SVS/214/20 approved on the 16th of July 2020).

Informed Consent Statement: Informed consent was obtained from all subjects involved in the study.

Data Availability Statement: The data presented in this study are available on request from the corresponding author. The data are not publicly available due to ethical restrictions.

Acknowledgments: Eva King for guidance on processes of qualitative analysis. Abbey Cox and research students for assisting with recording the heart sounds and creating the learning resource. The author also thanks all survey participants for their responses and input for this study.

Conflicts of Interest: The authors declare no conflict of interest. The funders had no role in the design of the study; in the collection, analyses, or interpretation of data; in the writing of the manuscript; or in the decision to publish the results.

References

1. Eichel, J.-C.; Korb, W.; Schlenker, A.; Bausch, G.; Brehm, W.; Delling, U. Evaluation of a training model to teach veterinary students a technique for injecting the jugular vein in horses. *J. Vet. Med. Educ.* **2013**, *40*, 288–295. [CrossRef] [PubMed]
2. Duijvestijn, M.B.H.M.; Van der Wiel, B.M.W.K.; Vinke, C.M.; Diaz Espineira, M.M.; Bok, H.G.J.; Vernooij, J.C.M. Implementation of a Blended Learning Module to Teach Handling, Restraint, and Physical Examination of Cats in Undergraduate Veterinary Training. *J. Vet. Med. Educ.* **2021**, *49*, 537–546. [CrossRef]
3. Voin, V.; Oskouian, R.J.; Loukas, M.; Tubbs, R.S. Auscultation of the heart. *Clin. Anat.* **2017**, *30*, 58–60. [CrossRef] [PubMed]
4. Travis, L.D. Auscultation Resources. *J. Electron. Resour. Med. Libr.* **2015**, *12*, 190–197. [CrossRef]
5. Dilly, M.; Read, E.K.; Baillie, S. A Survey of Established Veterinary Clinical Skills Laboratories from Europe and North America: Present Practices and Recent Developments. *J. Vet. Med. Educ.* **2017**, *44*, 580–589. [CrossRef]
6. George, J.H.; Doto, F.X. A simple five-step method for teaching clinical skills. *Fam. Med.* **2001**, *33*, 577–578.
7. Silva-Fletcher, A. The modern outcome-based curriculum and the role of the clinical skills laboratory. In *Veterinary Clinical Skills Manual*; Coombes, N., Silva-Fletcher, A., Eds.; CAB International: Wallingford, UK, 2018; pp. 9–15.
8. Lake, F.R.; Hamdorf, J.M. Teaching a skill. In *Teaching on the Run*; Australasian Medical Publishing Company: Pyrmont, Australia, 2007; pp. 15–18.
9. Muca, E.; Cavallini, D.; Raspa, F.; Bordin, C.; Bergero, D.; Valle, E. Integrating New Learning Methods into Equine Nutrition Classrooms: The Importance of Students' Perceptions. *J. Equine Vet. Sci.* **2023**, *126*, 104537. [CrossRef] [PubMed]
10. Baillie, S.; Decloedt, A.; Londgren, M.F. Designing Flipped Classrooms to Enhance Learning in the Clinical Skills Laboratory. *J. Vet. Med. Educ.* **2021**, *49*, 699–704. [CrossRef] [PubMed]
11. Bok, H.G.J.; Jaarsma, D.A.D.C.; Teunissen, P.W.; van der Vleuten, C.P.M.; van Beukelen, P. Development and Validation of a Competency Framework for Veterinarians. *J. Vet. Med. Educ.* **2011**, *38*, 262–269. [CrossRef] [PubMed]
12. Danielson, J.A. Key Assumptions Underlying a Competency-Based Approach to Medical Sciences Education, and Their Applicability to Veterinary Medical Education. *Front. Vet. Sci.* **2021**, *8*, 688457. [CrossRef]
13. Jani, V.; Danford, D.A.; Thompson, W.R.; Schuster, A.; Manlhiot, C.; Kutty, S. The discerning ear: Cardiac auscultation in the era of artificial intelligence and telemedicine. *Eur. Heart J. Digit. Health* **2021**, *2*, 456–466. [CrossRef] [PubMed]
14. Barrett, M.J.; Mackie, A.S.; Finley, J.P. Cardiac Auscultation in the Modern Era: Premature Requiem or Phoenix Rising? *Cardiol. Rev.* **2017**, *25*, 205–210. [CrossRef] [PubMed]
15. Machado, A.; Oliveira, A.; Jácome, C.; Pereira, M.; Moreira, J.; Rodrigues, J.; Aparício, J.; Jesus, L.M.T.; Marques, A. Usability of Computerized Lung Auscultation–Sound Software (CLASS) for learning pulmonary auscultation. *Med. Biol. Eng. Comput.* **2018**, *56*, 623–633. [CrossRef] [PubMed]
16. Kelmenson, D.A.; Heath, J.K.; Ball, S.A.; Kaafarani, H.M.A.; Baker, E.M.; Yeh, D.D.; Bittner, E.A.; Eikermann, M.; Lee, J. Prototype electronic stethoscope vs conventional stethoscope for auscultation of heart sounds. *J. Med. Eng. Technol.* **2014**, *38*, 307–310. [CrossRef] [PubMed]
17. Jones, J.L.; Rinehart, J.; Spiegel, J.J.; Englar, R.E.; Sidaway, B.K.; Rowles, J. Development of Veterinary Anesthesia Simulations for Pre-Clinical Training: Design, Implementation, and Evaluation Based on Student Perspectives. *J. Vet. Med. Educ.* **2018**, *45*, 232–240. [CrossRef] [PubMed]
18. Read, E.K.; Vallevand, A.; Farrell, R.M. Evaluation of veterinary student surgical skills preparation for ovariohysterectomy using simulators: A pilot study. *J. Vet. Med. Educ.* **2016**, *43*, 190–213. [CrossRef] [PubMed]
19. Panagiotakos, D.B. Value of *p*-value in biomedical research. *Open Cardiovasc. Med. J.* **2008**, *2*, 97–99. [CrossRef] [PubMed]
20. Braun, V.; Clarke, V. Using thematic analysis in psychology. *Qual. Res. Psychol.* **2006**, *3*, 77–101. [CrossRef]
21. King, E.; Norman, E.J.; Mossop, L.H.; Cobb, K.A.; Matthew, S.M.; Scholz, E.C.; Schull, D.N. Qualitative Research in Veterinary Medical Education: Part 1—Principles of Qualitative Design. *J. Vet. Med. Educ.* **2021**, *48*, 511–518. [CrossRef]
22. Myers, S.A.; Blackmore, M.J.; Smith, T.F.; Carter, R.W.B. Climate change and stewardship: Strategies to build community resilience in the Capricorn Coast. *Australas. J. Environ. Manag.* **2012**, *19*, 164–181. [CrossRef]
23. Leximancer User Guide. Available online: https://static1.squarespace.com/static/5e26633cfcf7d67bbd350a7f/t/61a84738789d220c1a865559/1638418279565/Leximancer-User-Guide-5.pdf (accessed on 1 November 2022).
24. Sotiriadou, P.; Brouwers, J.; Le, T.-A. Choosing a qualitative data analysis tool: A comparison of NVivo and Leximancer. *Ann. Leis. Res.* **2014**, *17*, 218–234. [CrossRef]
25. Crofts, K.; Bisman, J. Interrogating accountability: An illustration of the use of Leximancer software for qualitative data analysis. *Qual. Res. Account. Manag.* **2010**, *7*, 180–207. [CrossRef]
26. King, E.; Scholz, E.C.; Matthew, S.M.; Mossop, L.H.; Cobb, K.A.; Norman, E.J.; Schull, D.N. Qualitative Research in Veterinary Medical Education: Part 2—Carrying Out Research Projects. *J. Vet. Med. Educ.* **2021**, *48*, 519–527. [CrossRef] [PubMed]
27. Patton, M.Q. Enhancing the quality and credibility of qualitative analysis. *Health Serv. Res.* **1999**, *34*, 1189–1208. [PubMed]
28. Butter, J.; McGaghie, W.C.; Cohen, E.R.; Kaye, M.; Wayne, D.B. Simulation-based Mastery Learning Improves Cardiac Auscultation Skills in Medical Students. *J. Gen. Intern. Med.* **2010**, *25*, 780–785. [CrossRef]
29. McKinney, J.; Cook, D.A.; Wood, D.; Hatala, R. Simulation-Based Training for Cardiac Auscultation Skills: Systematic Review and Meta-Analysis. *J. Gen. Intern. Med.* **2013**, *28*, 283–291. [CrossRef] [PubMed]
30. Power, J.E.; Toft, L.E.B.; Barrett, M. The Murmur Online Learning Experience (MOLE) Curriculum Improves Medical Students' Ability to Correctly Identify Cardiac Murmurs. *MedEdPORTAL* **2020**, *16*, 10904. [CrossRef] [PubMed]

31. Ward, J.J.; Wattier, B.A. Technology for enhancing chest auscultation in clinical simulation. *Respir. Care* **2011**, *56*, 834–845. [CrossRef] [PubMed]
32. Finley, J.P.; Sharratt, G.P.; Nanton, M.A.; Chen, R.P.; Roy, D.L.; Paterson, G. Auscultation of the heart: A trial of classroom teaching versus computer-based independent learning. *Med. Educ.* **1998**, *32*, 357–361. [CrossRef]
33. Radu, M.-C.; Schnakovszky, C.; Herghelegiu, E.; Ciubotariu, V.-A.; Cristea, I. The Impact of the COVID-19 Pandemic on the Quality of Educational Process: A Student Survey. *Int. J. Env. Res. Public. Health* **2020**, *17*, 7770. [CrossRef]
34. Mahdy, M.A.A. The Impact of COVID-19 Pandemic on the Academic Performance of Veterinary Medical Students. *Front. Vet. Sci.* **2020**, *7*, 594261. [CrossRef] [PubMed]
35. Mahdy, M.A.A.; Sayed, R.K.A. Evaluation of the online learning of veterinary anatomy education during the COVID-19 pandemic lockdown in Egypt: Students' perceptions. *Anat. Sci. Educ.* **2022**, *15*, 67–82. [CrossRef] [PubMed]
36. Stoian, C.E.; Fărcașiu, M.A.; Dragomir, G.-M.; Gherheș, V. Transition from Online to Face-to-Face Education after COVID-19: The Benefits of Online Education from Students' Perspective. *Sustainability* **2022**, *14*, 12812. [CrossRef]
37. Muca, E.; Cavallini, D.; Odore, R.; Baratta, M.; Bergero, D.; Valle, E. Are Veterinary Students Using Technologies and Online Learning Resources for Didactic Training? A Mini-Meta Analysis. *Educ. Sci.* **2022**, *12*, 573. [CrossRef]
38. Christley, R.M.; Perkins, E. Researching hard to reach areas of knowledge: Qualitative research in veterinary science: Researching hard to reach areas of knowledge. *Equine Vet. J.* **2010**, *42*, 285–286. [CrossRef]
39. Henderson, D.; Baffour, T. Applying a Socio-Ecological Framework to Thematic Analysis Using a Statewide Assessment of Disproportionate Minority Contact in the United States. *Qual. Rep.* **2015**, *20*, 1960. [CrossRef]
40. Royal College of Veterinary Surgeons. Code of Professional Conduct for Veterinary Surgeons. Available online: https://www.rcvs.org.uk/setting-standards/advice-and-guidance/code-of-professional-conduct-for-veterinary-surgeons/ (accessed on 2 November 2022).
41. Mullowney, D.; Fuentes, V.L.; Barfield, D. Cardiac auscultation skills in final year veterinary students and recent veterinary graduates, referral hospital veterinary surgeons and veterinary cardiologists or cardiology residents. *Vet. Rec.* **2021**, *189*, e305. [CrossRef]
42. Cook, D.A. If you teach them, they will learn: Why medical education needs comparative effectiveness research. *Adv. Health Sci. Educ. Theory Pract.* **2012**, *17*, 305–310. [CrossRef] [PubMed]
43. Selek, M.; Duyar, M.; Isler, Y. Electronic Stethoscope Design. *J. Intell. Syst. Appl.* **2020**, *3*, 10–16. [CrossRef]
44. Fan, M.; Wang, Q.; Liu, J.; Su, L.; Wang, B.; Xu, H.; Li, Q.; Zhang, Z. Real-world evaluation of the Stemoscope electronic tele-auscultation system. *Biomed. Eng. Online* **2022**, *21*, 63. [CrossRef]

animals

MDPI

Article

Measuring Veterinarian Professions' Readiness for Interprofessional Learning in a Pre- and Post-Intervention Study

Sylva Agnete Charlotte Heise [1,*], Andrea Tipold [2], Karl Rohn [3] and Christin Kleinsorgen [1,*]

1 E-Learning-Consulting, Center for E-Learning, Didactics and Educational Research, University of Veterinary Medicine Hannover, 30559 Hannover, Germany
2 Clinic for Small Animals, University of Veterinary Medicine Hannover, 30559 Hannover, Germany; andrea.tipold@tiho-hannover.de
3 Institute of Biometrics, Epidemiology and Information Processing, University of Veterinary Medicine Hannover, 30559 Hannover, Germany
* Correspondence: sylva.heise@tiho-hannover.de (S.A.C.H.); christin.kleinsorgen@tiho-hannover.de (C.K.); Tel.: +49-511-953-8075 (S.A.C.H.)

Simple Summary: Interprofessional learning is increasingly important across all health care sectors, including veterinary medicine. Communication with animal owners and within the team is considered a core competency. As communication courses have been offered mostly on a voluntary basis, we conducted an interprofessional learning course for veterinary practice professions in this study with the aim of integrating such a course in the curriculum in the long term. We measured the readiness using the Readiness for Interprofessional Learning Scale before and after the course. While few significant changes emerged in the pre- and post-test comparison, more notable differences were observed in the evaluation of the 19 statements among different professions.

Abstract: The integration of interprofessional collaboration is becoming increasingly crucial in veterinary care settings, emphasising the need for interprofessional education (IPE) in veterinary programmes. This study explores the readiness for interprofessional learning among German veterinary students, apprentices and related occupations before and after an interprofessional communication course. It assesses the impact of this course on the participants' attitudes using the Readiness for Interprofessional Learning Scale (RIPLS). The course, offered in two iterations, combined asynchronous online modules, live seminars and practical training elements. The RIPLS was administered before and after the course to gauge attitude shifts towards interprofessional learning. Statistical analyses, including McNemar, Cohen's Kappa and exact Fisher tests, were employed to compare pre- and post-test responses. Despite challenges in participant linking, significant findings emerged between the student and apprentice groups in specific areas of the RIPLS, notably in the "Professional Identity" subscale post-course. However, correlations between face-to-face contact and RIPLS ratings were not observed, suggesting a need for more integrated interprofessional learning experiences. While some limitations in sample size and profession distribution hinder generalisability, this study indicates a high receptiveness to interprofessional learning in veterinary education, emphasising the potential for attitude changes with more interactive participation and programme adjustments.

Keywords: interprofessional; blended learning; teamwork; RIPLS; communication

1. Introduction

Patient care in veterinary practices is increasingly handled by persons from different professional groups who must work together to effectively care for patients [1] (Kinnison et al., 2014). In the German veterinary medicine degree study programme, the first intensive interprofessional contact typically occurs during the final year of study, the practical year. To facilitate the transition to professional life, interprofessional events during undergraduate education or apprenticeships could be beneficial.

Interprofessional teamwork is gaining importance in all health care sectors. Studies indicate that treatment success relies not only on expertise but also on effective collaboration [2] (Antoni, 2010). While communication and, in some cases, explicit interprofessional communication have already been integrated into learning objectives in many health care fields, communication training in the field of veterinary medicine is not embedded [3,4], but often conducted on a voluntary basis at the five veterinary institutions in Germany, typically in the form of elective courses with a focus on patient communication [5]. Previous needs assessments have indicated that adjustments are required in veterinary medicine, including the need for communication training [6]. Furthermore, there have been suggestions at a high level for curriculum adjustments in order to integrate interprofessional approaches [7]. In the training catalogue for veterinary assistants' communication with owners is also emphasised, but no interprofessional communication is mentioned [8].

Although the veterinary team may comprise various professions such as practice managers, physiotherapists, nutritionists, etc., this study specifically focuses on veterinary students, doctoral students, veterinary assistants and trainees, animal keepers and trainees and biology laboratory technicians. The occupations of veterinary assistants, animal keepers and biology laboratory technicians are nationally recognised and require certification in Germany, involving a three-year training period. Veterinary assistants aid veterinarians in animal examinations, treatments and care and provide guidance to the animal owners. They also handle organisational and administrative tasks. Animal keepers can also find employment in veterinary practices where they are responsible for animal care and provide support for procedures and treatments. Both professions frequently interact with clients as part of their daily professional responsibilities [1]. Biology laboratory technicians typically have less contact with the clients, although they sometimes communicate with owners about testing results. Nonetheless, they also play a crucial role in the diagnostic and analytical aspects of animal health. They need to work hand-in-hand with the other professions to collect samples, prepare them for diagnostic testing, interpret the results and prepare the reports. Veterinary medicine study courses in Germany take eleven terms (resulting in 5 ½ years), with most practical internships in veterinary practice occurring during the ninth and 10th term [9].

Hattie et al. [10] define learning interventions as extracurricular activities intentionally designed to improve academic performance. These activities go beyond mere content learning and also aim to instill learning-related skills such as self-efficacy and study techniques. Similarly, an interprofessional learning intervention includes learning outcomes beyond cognitive competences and addresses affective learning outcomes, involving attitudes, motivation and values [11].

The Readiness for Interprofessional Learning Scale (RIPLS) is a validated measurement instrument originally developed for human medicine to assess the readiness for interprofessional learning. It consists of 19 statements divided into three sections: (1) teamwork and collaboration, (2) professional identity and (3) roles and responsibilities [12]. It was initially developed for use with students in health care disciplines but has also been validated for graduates [13]. The originally English questionnaire has been translated into German by various institutions, including Heidelberg University and Martin Luther University Halle-Wittenberg [14]. Both versions were methodologically reviewed and compared, although not all sections yielded acceptable reliability values. The use of a German translation in the context of a bachelor's programme in "Interprofessional Health Care" showed limitations, particularly in the third section "Roles & Responsibilities" [15]. Nevertheless, the RIPLS and its translations provide a valuable starting point for interprofessional needs assessment. In human medicine, it has already been observed that professional identification has various effects on attitudes towards interprofessional learning [16]. Nursing students showed a more positive impact than medical students, and interprofessional contact with different professional groups did not significantly influence the results. The observations are also supported by social identity theory, which illustrates that social position in a social structure significantly contributes to a sense of belonging [17]. Members of groups with lower status tend to place more importance on their group identity compared to those with higher status if it can increase the value of their own group.

The RIPLS questionnaire has already been applied comparatively to medical doctors and veterinarians, with results indicating that the need for teamwork is higher in veterinary medicine [18]. In 2021, a high relevance of communication skills and a strong interest in teaching these skills as part of an interprofessional education were identified in veterinary medicine [19]. Based on these findings, an interprofessional learning intervention was developed and implemented at the University of Veterinary Medicine Hannover (TiHo Hannover), Germany. This study assesses the impact of an interprofessional learning course using the RIPLS to quantitatively measure readiness for interprofessional learning. The research question to be examined is how evaluation of the relevance of interprofessional learning, using the RIPLS, changes through the interprofessional communication intervention?

2. Materials and Methods

At the TiHo Hannover, an interprofessional learning intervention was conducted as an elective course in the winter term of 2022/2023. The course was made available for veterinary students and veterinary assistant trainees from the Veterinary University Hannover. It was designed as a blended learning course consisting of an asynchronous online course comprising nine modules on the learning management system Moodle. This course design should facilitate participation from individuals across different professional groups and accommodate their differing daily schedules accordingly. While most theoretical content was delivered within self-learning phases, interaction between participants and course directors was facilitated during online and in-person seminars. Within the modules, different theoretical content was delivered, supplemented with video materials and interactive tasks. The modules' topics were developed in alignment with the core competencies outlined by the WHO [7] and the recommendations provided by the Interprofessional Education Collaborative [20]. The IPEC core competencies were used as a basis, as they have been developed, revised and already incorporated into curricula and accreditation standards for several years. The processing time for each module was designed to be around two hours, whereas the processing period for participation ranged from one to three weeks depending on its scope. Upon completion of each module, participants were required to complete tasks to validate successful engagement. These tasks encompassed quizzes, interactive videos, audio recordings or text composition. As part of the course preparation, thematically relevant topics were collected and discussed by course facilitators. Videos were then produced as either best practice or worst case examples, with professional actors highlighting typical situations and conflicts encountered in the veterinary practice. Additionally, one synchronous online seminar on the topic of roles and responsibilities, prejudices and conflict potentials, one in-person seminar led by a communication coach on resilience and stress management and a simulation training with professional actors to apply the theoretically learned content were included (see Figure 1, Course 1). To assess the demand for interprofessional learning, the RIPLS was administered before and after the course using the survey tool LimeSurvey® (LimeSurvey GmbH, Version 3.23.1, Hamburg, Germany) in accordance with the translation by the Martin Luther University Halle-Wittenberg [14]. Instead of the four-point scale version used by the Martin Luther University Halle-Wittenberg, a five-point Likert scale, as in the version implemented by Heidelberg University, was used [14,21]. Furthermore, a comment was added that under the term "health care students", participants should include veterinarians, vet nurses, vet technicians and others. Moreover, under the term "doctor", they may also consider veterinarians. The items of the RIPLS are numbered from 1 to 19 in the following and belong to three subscales (Table 1). The RIPLS questionnaire was part of the pre- and post-test, which also included general questions about personal information and previous experiences, a knowledge test and self-assessment of their own communication skills. Additionally, expectations for the course were surveyed in advance, followed by a comprehensive evaluation in the post-test.

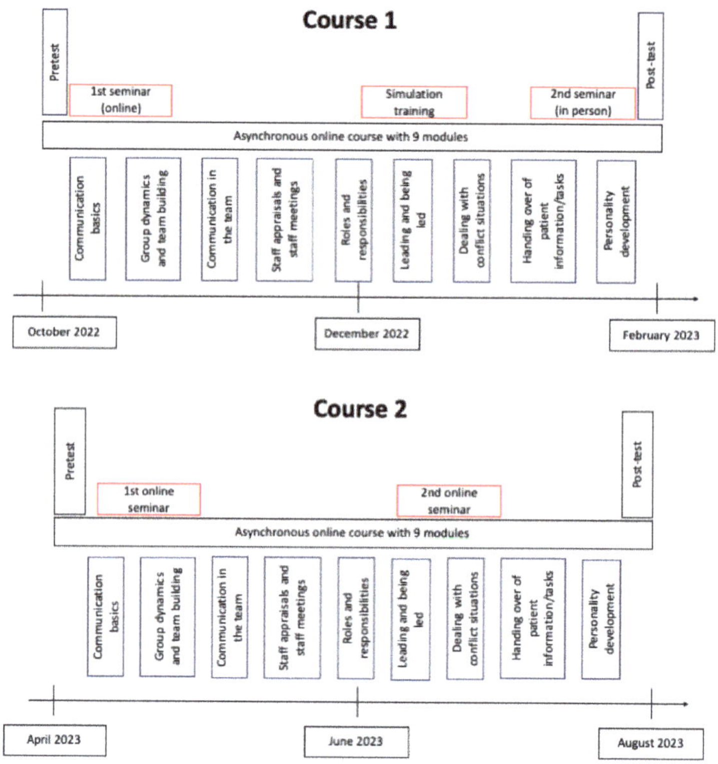

Figure 1. The blended learning course design for the winter term 2022/2023 (Course 1) and for the summer term 2023 (Course 2); differences in the design are highlighted in red.

Table 1. Median of the RIPLS item answers of the paired samples of both courses (n = 60).

Subscale	RIPL Item	Pretest	Post-Test
	1. Learning with students will help me become a more effective member of a health care team.	3.28	3.93
	2. Patients would ultimately benefit if health care students worked together to solve patient problems.	4.70	4.55
	3. Shared learning with other health care students will increase my ability to understand clinical problems.	4.05	3.83
	4. Learning with health care students before qualification would improve relationships after qualification.	3.83	4.17
Teamwork and collaboration	5. Communication skills should be learned with other health care students.	3.87	4.03
	6. Shared learning will help me to think positively about other professionals.	3.75	4.05
	7. For small group learning to work, students need to trust and respect each other.	4.55	4.52
	8. Teamwork skills are essential for all health care students to learn.	4.43	4.40
	9. Shared learning will help me to understand my own limitations.	3.62	3.80

Table 1. *Cont.*

Subscale	RIPL Item	Pretest	Post-Test
Professional identity	10. I do not want to waste my time learning with other health care students.	1.72	1.68
	11. It is not necessary for undergraduate health care students to learn together.	2.10	2.28
	12. Clinical problem-solving skills can only be learned with students from my own department.	2.33	2.25
	13. Shared learning with other health care students will help me to communicate better with patients and other professionals.	4.13	4.02
	14. I would welcome the opportunity to work on small-group projects with other health care students.	3.83	3.87
	15. Shared learning will help to clarify the nature of patient problems.	3.92	3.82
	16. Shared learning before qualification will help me become a better team worker.	3.83	4.07
Roles and responsibilities	17. The function of nurses and therapists is mainly to provide support for doctors.	3.07	3.13
	18. I am not sure what my professional role will be.	2.38	2.20
	19. I have to acquire much more knowledge and skills than other health care students.	3.22	3.02

In the summer of 2023, the course was offered again as an elective course, but without face-to-face events due to resource limitations (see Figure 1, Course 2). This meant that the simulation training was omitted and the second seminar was held online instead of in person. However, it was made available to all trainees and fully trained professionals in various veterinary practice occupations at the TiHo Hannover as well as to students and doctoral candidates. These changes in the course design may influence this study's results. Hereafter, we will group all of the vocational training professions that participated under "apprentices" (veterinary assistants and trainees, animal keepers and trainees, laboratory technicians and trainees) and all of the veterinary students and doctoral candidates under "students".

The surveys carried out were subject to general data protection regulations. Written consent to participate in the study was obtained from all participants before answering the questionnaires. Furthermore, an individualised code was self-generated by each participant following an instruction so that an anonymised, paired sample could be collected. Participation was voluntary and anonymous. Apart from the unprocessed IP address, no data were collected that would have allowed conclusions to be drawn about the identity of the respondents. Each question could be skipped or answered with "no answer".

Pre- and post-test data were exported from LimeSurvey® (Version 3.23.1+200825) as Microsoft Excel (Version 16.80 (23121017)) spreadsheets, and SAS 9.7M7 with Enterprise Guide 7.1 (SAS Institute Inc., Cary, NC, USA) was used for the analysis of the collected data.

To calculate intrarater reliability, the McNemar and Bowker tests and Cohen's kappa with PaBaK (prevalence and adjustment) were used for statistical analysis. Fisher's exact test was used to calculate the group differences. The statistical test McNemar was used for paired data in 2×2 tables (Bowker test for $n \times n$ tables, where n is greater than 2) and it was applied to examine situations where the same subjects or elements are measured under two different conditions, e.g., at two different time points. In our case, it was applied to examine the symmetry of responses given in the pre- and post-test and to identify any deviations. The probability of error for the McNemar test alpha was set to 5%, i.e., the assumption of the symmetrical bias is rejected with a p-value < 0.05.

To assess the agreement of the responses between the pretest and the post-test, the concordance index kappa was calculated. In our case, the prevalence- and bias-adjusted kappa coefficient (PaBaK) was calculated because it is more suitable for the asymmetric distributions between the cell frequencies than the simple kappa coefficient. For the interpretation of the concordance index kappa, we used the table by Landis and Koch [22] as a reference point.

- <0 no agreement.
- 0–0.20 slight agreement.
- 0.21–0.40 fair agreement.
- 0.41–0.60 moderate agreement.
- 0.61–0.80 substantial agreement.
- 0.81–1.0 perfect agreement.

Significant differences in the responses to the RIPLS were determined using Fisher's exact test. This test was used because the probability of the observed cell contents of the contingency table are often less than five and therefore the chi-square test may become inaccurate. The probability of error alpha for Fisher's exact test was set to 5%, i.e., the assumption of equality of both professions is rejected at a p-value < 0.05.

Due to focus of the research question of this study, the results of the knowledge test, self-assessment and course evaluation were not included; thus, in the following, only results regarding the assessments of the Readiness for Interprofessional Learning Scale are illustrated.

3. Results

3.1. Descriptive Analysis

In the first course, in the winter term 2022/2023, a total of 18 veterinary students and 13 prospective veterinary assistants were enrolled. In total, 22 questionnaires could be paired by individual codes. In the second course, in the summer term 2023, a total of 81 participants registered for the course, including 63 students, 2 doctoral candidates and 16 who had completed their apprenticeship training (1 of them had yet to complete their training) in veterinary practice occupations. For the evaluation, 59 questionnaires from the pretest and 54 from the post-test were analysable. In this course, a total of 38 paired samples were identified by individual codes. In the following, we will focus on the paired samples of both courses. The demographic data of the course participants with paired samples identified in pre- and post-tests from both courses are shown in Table 2. The majority of the participants had never been part of a communication training before (n = 44, 73.33%), but the majority had already worked in a team (n = 55, 91.67%) and a similar amount had already participated in team activities (e.g., sports, music) (n = 54, 90.00%).

Table 2. Demographic data of the paired samples from both courses (n = 60).

	Course 1		**Course 2**		**Total**
	Vet Students and Veterinarians	**Vet Nurses, Laboratory Assistants, etc.**	**Vet Students and Veterinarians**	**Vet Nurses, Laboratory Assistants, etc.**	
Female	15	6	30	7	58
Male	1	0	1	0	2
Previous communication training	7	1	7	1	16
Teamwork experience at work	16	5	29	6	59
Teamwork experience in free time	14	6	28	6	54

Descriptive statistics of the overall ratings of the RIPLS items in pre- and post-test during both courses are illustrated in Table 1. The statement that received the highest median approval in the pretest was the same as in the post-test, namely, item 2: "Patients ultimately benefit when health professionals work together to solve patients' health professions." Item 10—"I do not want to waste my time learning together with members of other care professions"—earned the least approval in both tests.

In Figure 2, the first nine items of the RIPLS are presented, covering the subscale "Teamwork and collaboration". For each question, the pretests and post-tests of both courses were combined and compared for all paired samples. This subscale consists of positive statements regarding interprofessional learning, and statements were predominantly rated in agreement by the participants.

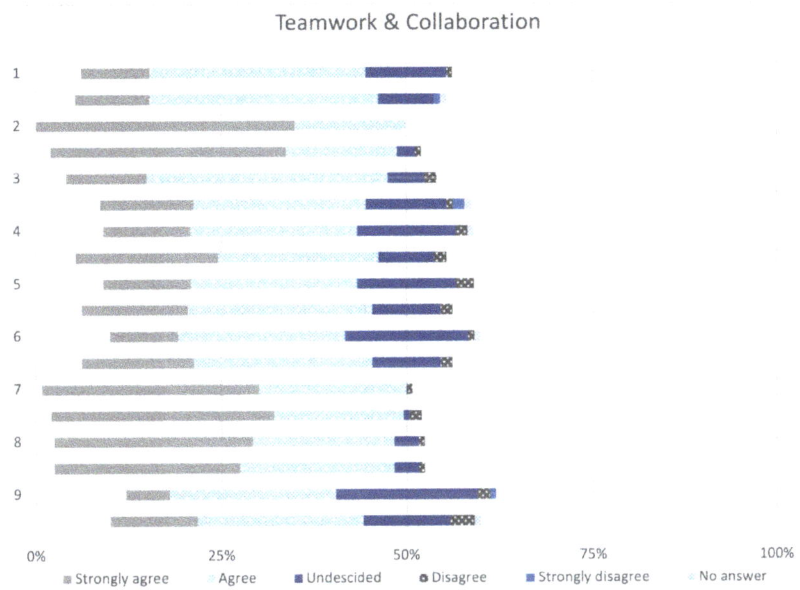

Figure 2. Answers to items 1–9 of the subscale "Teamwork & collaboration" of the pretests and post-tests of both courses (paired samples, n = 60). The items 1–9 of the subscale "Teamwork & collaboration" are shown in Table 1.

In Figure 3, items 10 to 16 of the RIPLS are presented which constitute the subscale of "Professional identity". For each statement, the pretests and post-tests from both courses were combined and compared for all paired samples. Items 10 to 12 consist of negatively formulated statements about interprofessional communication. These mainly received little to no agreement. Items 13 to 16 are positive statements, which were mainly rated positive by the participants.

The last three items of the RIPLS are presented in Figure 4. These constitute the subscale "Roles and responsibilities". Again, for each statement the pretests and post-tests from both courses were combined and compared for all paired samples. These statements were answered in a more varied manner. Concerning the item "The function of nurses and therapists is mainly to provide support for doctors", in the pretest, about half of the apprentices (53.85%, n = 7) agreed with the statement, in contrast to the percentage of students who chose "Strongly agree" and "Agree" less often ("Strongly agree": 6.38%, n = 3; "Agree": 25.53%, n = 12). In the post-test, there were similar differences between the two professions; the apprentices rated the statement more positively than the students. The item

"I'm not sure what my professional role will be" was answered with more disagreement in the post-test than in the pretest by both professions. The last statement "I have to acquire much more knowledge and skills than other health care students" was also rated with more agreement in the pretest than in the post-test.

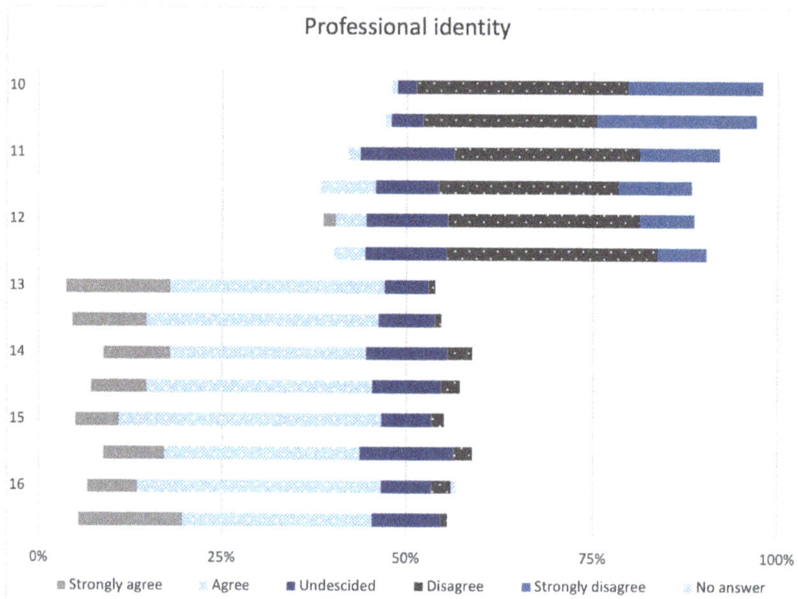

Figure 3. Answers to items 10–16 of the subscale "Professional identity" of the pretests and post-tests of both courses (paired samples, n = 60). The items 10–16 of the subscale "Professional identity" are shown in Table 1.

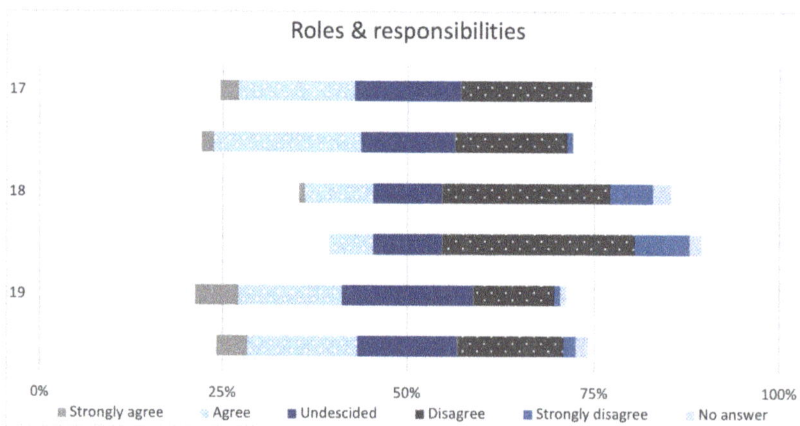

Figure 4. Answers to items 17–19 of the subscale Roles and responsibilities of the pretests and post-tests of both courses together (paired samples, n = 60). The items 17–19 of the subscale "Roles & responsibilities" are shown in Table 1.

3.2. *Interference Statistical Analysis*

In the total of all pre- and post-tests, mainly fair to moderate agreement between the answers of the pre- and the post-test of both professions was apparent using the Cohen's

(PaBaK) kappa test. Only item 12 had a slight agreement. In the analysis of the students as a separate group, the findings showed mainly fair to moderate agreement. Three items (items 6, 12 and 19) had a slight agreement and item 8 had a substantial agreement. On the other hand, the results of the apprentices mainly showed a slight to moderate agreement. Only item 12 showed no agreement at all. All results of the McNemar test are presented in Supplementary Table S1.

The statement "Shared learning will help me to think positively about other professionals" was answered highly significantly (p = 0.0098) differently by the two professions in the pretest. In the post-test, the statement "Shared learning will help to clarify the nature of patient problems" was rated also significantly (p = 0.0366) differently by the professions.

Furthermore, there were significant differences when looking at the data from both courses together: in the post-test, almost three different statements of the RIPLS were answered significantly differently by the professions. The statement "It is not necessary for undergraduate health care students to learn together" scored a highly significant p = 0.0089 in Fisher's test. "Shared learning with other health care students will help me to communicate better with patients and other professionals" was rated significantly differently (p = 0.0133) and "Shared learning will help to clarify the nature of patient problems" received a value of p = 0.0375 and showed also a significant difference. All other exact Fisher tests had a p = >0.05 and showed no significant differences in the responses of students and apprentices (Supplementary Table S2).

4. Discussion

In this study, we explored the readiness for interprofessional learning of German veterinary students and apprentices (including those who had already completed apprenticeship training). We compared the attitudes before and after an interprofessional communication course to find out whether a common event effects any change in assessment of the 19 statements of the RIPLS. Despite challenges in participant linking, significant findings emerged between the student and apprentice groups in specific areas of the RIPLS, notably in the "Professional Identity" subscale post-course. Regarding the research question, there appears to be no overall improvement in readiness for interprofessional learning following the 4-month course. Only in item 12 is there a lack of agreement between the pre- and post-tests. Notably, there are several significant differences in the assessment of the statements that differ between students and apprentices.

Both courses taken together resulted in a total of 88 evaluable pretests, 78 post-tests and 60 paired samples linked by an individual code. Only the linked samples were included in the analysis; the remaining questionnaires could not be included due to missing links caused by incorrect codes. These problems were also reported in a previous study on learning interventions [23]. The participants received instructions on how to create an individual, anonymous code based on their personal data. While the instructions for the pretest and post-tests were identical, different codes were generated in some cases. These observations should be taken into account in the future, and a simpler instruction could be a possible solution to avoid unassignable datasets. The validated RIPLS, created in 1999 [12], has filled an empirical gap and continues to be a tool for measuring the attitudes of students in health professions towards interprofessional learning. Other questionnaires like the CSAS (Communication Skills Attitude Scale) also exist to measure positive and negative attitudes towards learning communication skills [24] but without the focus on interprofessional learning. However, there are indications that the questionnaire is particularly unsuitable for before-and-after studies, as it inadequately reflects changes in attitudes [25]. This could be based on the assumption that the elements which are relevant for the stable factor values are more strongly correlated with each other than initially assumed. Based on these indications, it must be determined whether a measuring instrument for this specific case does not yet exist. Other studies describe low values of internal consistency in the Cronbach's alpha method in the subscales, although the values overall show higher reliability [15]. Furthermore, studies indicate that the psychometric integrity of various measurement instruments for interprofessional education is limited [26]. The observation that increased interprofessional contact leads to decreased ratings of the RIPLS items has already been made in Brazil [27]. This is an interesting result which could indicate that the results could be lower after an interprofessional event. However, there is also evidence that interactive communication training promotes learning success [28], which makes the assumption plausible that the attitudes change through such training. In 2021, there was already a needs assessment towards interprofessional training, in which participants of all five veterinarian institutions underlined their wish to participate in such a training [6]. That finding is supported by our result in item five of the RIPLS, namely, "Communication skills should be learned with other health care students", which was mainly positive in the pre- and post-tests. In addition, we have many different professions working together in veterinarian practice [1], which is why it is important to pay more attention to interprofessional communication. The negative formulated items 10 to 12 mainly received little to no agreement, which illustrates that the participants read the statements attentively and were not distracted due to the length of the whole questionnaire.

In our study design, we compared two different courses with varying face-to-face contact between the professions to check for a correlation between the two different types of courses and the rating of the RIPLS. It is plausible that there was no correlation between contact or shared learning of different professional groups and the assessment of the items, as in our study design, a clear increase in ratings could not be observed. It is noteworthy that during the planning phase of the first course in 2022, finding dates and times during which both participating professions were available was challenging. Providing one live online seminar during the second course was similarly problematic. It became clear that although efforts were made to create joint and interprofessional learning interventions, the current timetables and schedules of different professions do not easily allow for this. In addition, a comparison was made to determine whether different professions exhibited significantly different readiness for interprofessional learning before and after the course. In this context, differences in readiness between medical students and nursing students have already observed [29]. This observation might be applicable to veterinary medicine students and prospective veterinary medical assistants as well. In our datasets, we could also find some significant differences in the rating of some of the RIPLS items between students and the apprentices in specific questions, especially in the overall post-tests under the subscale "Professional identity". In other countries, significant differences in the response to the various subscales were observed among the different health care groups [30].

The translations of the English language RIPL scale vary, which may lead to a conceptual imbalance that affects its utility, whereas the translation from English into other languages has proved to be reliable in initial tests [31]. Nonetheless translations could lead to variations in the meaning of certain words or phrases, as different languages might not perfectly align. Changes in wording or structure could impact the scale's psychometric properties, such as internal consistency or construct validity. Comparing the results across different languages might lead to different response patterns. As a limitation of this study, we must admit that we had a relatively small sample size, which was further skewed due to the non-proportional distribution of the two surveyed professions. The sample size of this study may not appear to be particularly large at first glance, but in reality, the response rate, especially concerning the first course and the prospective veterinary medical assistants, was very high. Out of a total of 21 trainees working at the University of Veterinary Medicine, 13 signed up for the course. Compared to the first course, more participants in the second course showed interest in the learning intervention, with more registrations, thereby highlighting the relevance and readiness for interprofessional learning. To further generalise our results, comparable studies at the other four German veterinary institutions would be helpful. Generating a more proportional sample size of the different professions seems to be the biggest challenge because of the huge difference in the numbers of apprentices and students of the professions at universities. Therefore, the acquisition of veterinarian professions outside of the universities would help to balance the proportion. However, when examining the results concerning the various professions, it is important to note that even small changes in absolute numbers can reflect significant percentage changes. Also, the fact that we had various training occupations, such as biology laboratory technicians who have typically less patient and interprofessional contact as they often work in separate labs, may have influenced the needs assessment. The small sample size also leads to rare statistical findings and some tests simply are not possible with the low number of datasets. Nevertheless, the preliminary results suggest that we could have more significant findings with a larger sample size. This study also only rates the subjective perspective of the participants without having an objective measurement tool to compare with. The duration of the course (October 2022 to February 2023 and April 2023 to August 2023) may not have been sufficient for a significant change in attitudes, so a study comparing attitudes before and after the start of a degree course programme or training and after completion may yield more concrete results.

In both courses, 96.67% of the participants were female. This is slightly higher than the percentage reported by the Federal Chamber of Veterinary Surgeons (Bundestierärztekammer) concerning the student statistics of recent years [32]. These statistics show that the number of female veterinarians has increased significantly since 2002. In general, it has already been proven that women are more willing to participate in surveys [33], which can also be seen in other surveys conducted for veterinary students and veterinarians in Germany [23,34], and that female medicine and nursing students have a more positive attitude towards teamwork than male students [35,36]. The fact, that mostly females participated in our study could have had an impact on the results; referring to the mentioned studies, this impact seems to be a positive one. Also, the amount of datasets could be higher with a majority of female participants than with more male ones.

Based on our study, using the Readiness for Interprofessional Learning Scale, it becomes evident that the readiness for interprofessional learning is high. Following the initial course iteration, additional professions (e.g., animal keepers) reached out to us, expressing interest in the event. Implementing interprofessional interactions during education and training would be welcomed in further projects and curriculum adjustments and should not be limited to a few professional groups.

In conclusion, the preliminary evaluations indicate a high willingness towards interprofessional learning. The possibility of a shared communication course was well received in both university terms and was successfully completed on a voluntary basis. Regarding attitude change, initial indications are evident, which would most probably become more conclusive with a larger sample. These findings underscore the need for interprofessional learning during studies and training, as well as the desire and necessity to acquire communication skills. The results can be used to establish additional courses and programmes in this area.

Supplementary Materials: The following supporting information can be downloaded at: https://www.mdpi.com/article/10.3390/ani14020229/s1, Table S1: Chi-square and PaBaK tests of the total pretests and post-tests and specifically for the professions; Table S2: p-values of the exact fisher test showing the difference of the answers between apprentices and students (paired samples: n = 60).

Author Contributions: S.A.C.H. and C.K.: study design, data collection, data analysis, results interpretation, and writing and review of the manuscript. A.T.: study design, results interpretation and review of the manuscript. K.R.: data analysis, results interpretation and review of the manuscript. All authors have read and agreed to the published version of the manuscript.

Funding: This study was supported by the project Innovation Plus 2022/2023, No. T0049 of the Ministry of Science and Culture of Lower Saxony. This Open Access publication was funded by the Deutsche Forschungsgemeinschaft (DFG, German Research Foundation) 491094227 "Open Access Publication Funding" and the University of Veterinary Medicine Hannover, Foundation.

Institutional Review Board Statement: This study was conducted in accordance with the ethical standards of the University of Veterinary Medicine Hannover Foundation. The entire project was approved by the university's data protection officer. The voluntarily participating students consented to the processing of their data in accordance with the EU General Data Protection Regulation of 2018 (General Data Protection Regulation Art. 6 I 1 lit. e i.V.m. 89 and Lower Saxony Data Protection Act § 3 I 1 No. 1 NHG, § 13). All collected data were evaluated and processed anonymously in accordance with the data protection regulation of the university. Due to the lack of the ethics approval code the doctoral thesis committee of the university, which acts as the University's ethics committee, validated the project in accordance with ethical guidelines regarding research with human participants and approved this study. Written consent to participate in the study was obtained from all participants. The data protection officer reviewed the proposed project regarding observance of the Data Protection Law and gave permission to perform this study. All of the data obtained were processed and evaluated anonymously and in compliance with EU's General Data Protection Regulation. All data presented in this study are available on request from the corresponding author. The data are not publicly available due to ethical and privacy restrictions.

Informed Consent Statement: Informed consent was obtained from all subjects involved in this study. Consent forms were approved by the Data protection officer and the doctoral thesis committee of the University.

Data Availability Statement: All data presented in this study are available on request from the corresponding author. The data are not publicly available due to ethical and privacy restrictions.

Acknowledgments: We wish to thank all enrolled participants in the courses and evaluations. Also, special thanks go to Ellen Preussing who led one seminar session each year as the communication coach. Furthermore, we appreciate the work of our actors who professionally performed and improvised during the simulation sessions, providing thoughtful feedback to students and course facilitators.

Conflicts of Interest: The authors declare that the research was conducted in the absence of any commercial or financial relationships that could be construed as a potential conflict of interest.

References

1. Kinnison, T.; May, S.A.; Guile, D. Inter-professional practice: From veterinarian to the veterinary team. *J. Vet. Med. Educ.* **2014**, *41*, 172–178. [CrossRef]
2. Antoni, C.H. Interprofessional teamwork in health care. *Z. Evid. Fortbild. Qual. Gesundhwes.* **2010**, *104*, 18–24. [CrossRef]
3. Gruber, C.; Dilly, M.; Bahramsoltani, M.; Kleinsorgen, C.; Engelskirchen, S.; Ramspott, S.; Ehlers, J.P. Communication as teaching content of veterinary studies—A joint position paper from the DVG specialist group "communication and didactics" and the GMA veterinary medicine committee. *GMS J. Med. Educ.* **2021**, *38*, Doc84. [CrossRef]
4. Kleinsorgen, C.; Ramspott, S.; Ehlers, J.P.; Gruber, C.; Dilly, M.; Engelskirchen, S.; Bernigau, D.; Bahramsoltani, M. Kommunikative Kompetenzen im Studium der Veterinärmedizin in Deutschland—Ansätze für die Entwicklung eines Mustercurriculums. *Berl. Und Münchener Tierärztliche Wochenschr.* **2020**, *133*. [CrossRef]
5. Pohl, A.; Klass, L.G.; Kleinsorgen, C.; Bernigau, D.; Pfeiffer-Morhenn, B.; Arnhold, S.; Dilly, M.; Beitz-Radzio, C.; Wissing, S.; Vogt, L.; et al. Integration and potential of teaching communication skills in the study of veterinary medicine in Germany. *GMS J. Med. Educ.* **2021**, *38*, Doc53. [CrossRef] [PubMed]
6. Rauch, M.; Wissing, S.; Tipold, A.; Kleinsorgen, C. Interprofessional survey on communication skills in veterinary and veterinary-related education in Germany. *BMC Med. Educ.* **2021**, *21*, 516. [CrossRef] [PubMed]
7. WHO. *Framework for Action on Interprofessional Education & Collaborative Practice*; No. WHO/HRH/HPN/10.3; World Health Organization: Geneva, Switzerland, 2010.
8. Verordnung über die Berufsausbildung zum Tiermedizinischen Fachangestellten/zur Tiermedizinischen Fachangestellten. 2005. Available online: https://www.gesetze-im-internet.de/tiermedfangausbv/BJNR252200005.html (accessed on 2 January 2024).
9. Verordnung zur Approbation von Tierärztinnen und Tierärzten (TAppV) vom 27. 2016. Available online: https://www.gesetze-im-internet.de/tappv/BJNR182700006.html (accessed on 2 January 2024).
10. Hattie, J.; Biggs, J.; Purdie, N. Effects of Learning Skills Interventions on Student Learning: A Meta-Analysis. *Rev. Educ. Res.* **1996**, *66*, 99–136. [CrossRef]
11. Miller, M. Teaching and Learning in Affective Domain. *Emerg. Perspect. Learn. Teach. Technol.* **2005**, *6*, 2008.
12. Parsell, G.; Bligh, J. The development of a questionnaire to assess the readiness of health care students for interprofessional learning (RIPLS). *Med. Educ.* **1999**, *33*, 95–100. [CrossRef]
13. Reid, R.; Bruce, D.; Allstaff, K.; McLernon, D. Validating the Readiness for Interprofessional Learning Scale (RIPLS) in the postgraduate context: Are health care professionals ready for IPL? *Med. Educ.* **2006**, *40*, 415–422. [CrossRef]

4. Luderer, C.; Donat, M.; Baum, U.; Kirsten, A.; Jahn, P.; Stoevesandt, D. Measuring attitudes towards interprofessional learning. Testing two German versions of the tool "Readiness for Interprofessional Learning Scale" on interprofessional students of health and nursing sciences and of human medicine. *GMS J. Med. Educ.* **2017**, *34*, Doc33. [CrossRef] [PubMed]
5. Mahler, C.; Rochon, J.; Karstens, S.; Szecsenyi, J.; Hermann, K. Internal consistency of the readiness for interprofessional learning scale in German health care students and professionals. *BMC Med. Educ.* **2014**, *14*, 145. [CrossRef]
6. Sollami, A.; Caricati, L.; Mancini, T. Attitudes towards Interprofessional Education among Medical and Nursing Students: The Role of Professional Identification and Intergroup Contact. *Curr. Psychol.* **2017**, *37*, 905–912. [CrossRef]
17. Burford, B. Group processes in medical education: Learning from social identity theory. *Med. Educ.* **2012**, *46*, 143–152. [CrossRef]
18. Roopnarine, R.; Boeren, E. Applying the Readiness for Interprofessional Learning Scale (RIPLS) to medical, veterinary and dual degree Master of Public Health (MPH) students at a private medical institution. *PLoS ONE* **2020**, *15*, e0234462. [CrossRef] [PubMed]
19. Rauch, M. Interprofessionelle Bedarfsermittlung von Kommunikationsfähigkeiten und Evaluation von Schauspielereinsatz im Kommunikationstraining in der Tiermedizin. 2021. Available online: https://elib.tiho-hannover.de/servlets/MCRFileNodeServlet/tiho_derivate_00001121/Rauchm-ss21.pdf (accessed on 2 January 2024).
20. Interprofessional Education Collaborative. *Core Competencies for Interprofessional Collaborative Practice*; 2016 Update; IPEC: Washington, DC, USA, 2016.
21. Mahler, C.; Giesler, M.; Stock, C.; Krisam, J.; Karstens, S.; Szecsenyi, J.; Krug, K. Confirmatory factor analysis of the German Readiness for Interprofessional Learning Scale (RIPLS-D). *J. Interprof. Care* **2016**, *30*, 381–384. [CrossRef]
22. Landis, J.R.; Koch, G.G. An Application of Hierarchial Kappa-Type Statistics in the Assessment of Majority Agreement among Multiple Observers. *Biometrics* **1977**, *33*, 363–374. [CrossRef]
23. Zintl, J.; Kleinsorgen, C.; Tipold, A.; Schaper, E. Die Studieneingangsphase in der Tiermedizin—Herausforderungen, Chancen und Bedarfe. *Berl. Und Münchener Tierärztliche Wochenschr.* **2023**, *135*, 1–16. [CrossRef]
24. Rees, C.; Sheard, C.; Davies, S. The development of a scale to measure medical students' attitudes towards communication skills learning: The Communication Skills Attitude Scale (CSAS). *Med. Educ.* **2002**, *36*, 141–147. [CrossRef]
25. Schmitz, C.; Brandt, B.F. The Readiness for Interprofessional Learning Scale: To RIPLS or not to RIPLS? That is only part of the question. *J. Interprof. Care* **2015**, *29*, 525–526. [CrossRef]
26. Oates, M.; Davidson, M. A critical appraisal of instruments to measure outcomes of interprofessional education. *Med. Educ.* **2015**, *49*, 386–398. [CrossRef] [PubMed]
27. de Oliveira, V.F.; Bittencourt, M.F.; Navarro Pinto, I.F.; Lucchetti AL, G.; da Silva Ezequiel, O.; Lucchetti, G. Comparison of the Readiness for Interprofessional Learning and the rate of contact among students from nine different healthcare courses. *Nurse Educ. Today* **2018**, *63*, 64–68. [CrossRef]
28. Meehan, M.P.; Menniti, M.F. Final-year veterinary students' perceptions of their communication competencies and a communication skills training program delivered in a primary care setting and based on Kolb's Experiential Learning Theory. *J. Vet. Med. Educ.* **2014**, *41*, 371–383. [CrossRef]
29. Keshtkaran, Z.; Sharif, F.; Rambod, M. Students' readiness for and perception of inter-professional learning: A cross-sectional study. *Nurse Educ. Today* **2014**, *34*, 991–998. [CrossRef]
30. Aziz, Z.; Teck, L.C.; Yen, P.Y. The Attitudes of Medical, Nursing and Pharmacy Students to Inter-Professional Learning. *Procedia-Soc. Behav. Sci.* **2011**, *29*, 639–645. [CrossRef]
31. Pype, P.; Deveugele, M. Dutch translation and validation of the readiness for interprofessional learning scale (RIPLS) in a primary healthcare context. *Eur. J. Gen. Pract.* **2016**, *22*, 225–231. [CrossRef] [PubMed]
32. Bundestierärztekammer. Statistik 2022: Tierärzteschaft in der Bundesrepublik Deutschland. *Dtsch. Tierärzteblatt* **2023**, *71*.
33. Petermann, S. Rücklauf und systematische Verzerrungen bei postalischen Befragungen: Eine Analyse der Bürgerumfrage Halle 2003. *ZUMA Nachrichten* **2003**, *29*, 55–78.
34. Losansky, V.A.; Arnhold, S.; Aschenbach, J.R.; Göbel, T.; Fey, K.; Kleinsorgen, C.; Mülling, C.; Schaper, E.; Seeger, J.; Tipold, A.; et al. Umfrage zur Relevanz der Fächer veterinärmedizinischen Lehre und zukünftigen Studienausrichtung bei Tierärztinnen sowie Stuiderenden in Deutschland. *Berl. Und Münchener Tierärztliche Wochenschr.* **2022**, *2022*, 135. [CrossRef]
35. Visser CL, F.; Wilschut, J.A.; Isik, U.; van der Burgt SM, E.; Croiset, G.; Kusurkar, R.A. The Association of Readiness for Interprofessional Learning with empathy, motivation and professional identity development in medical students. *BMC Med. Educ.* **2018**, *18*, 125. [CrossRef]
36. Wilhelmsson, M.; Ponzer, S.; Dahlgren, L.O.; Timpka, T.; Faresjö, T. Are female students in general and nursing students more ready to teamwork and interprofessional collaboration in healthcare? *BMC Med. Educ.* **2011**, *11*, 15. [CrossRef] [PubMed]

animals

MDPI

Article

Developing Communication Competency in the Veterinary Curriculum

Ingrid van Gelderen (Mabin) * and Rosanne Taylor *

Sydney School of Veterinary Science, Faculty of Science, The University of Sydney, Camperdown 2006, Australia
* Correspondence: ingrid.vangelderen@sydney.edu.au (I.v.G.); rosanne.taylor@sydney.edu.au (R.T.)

Simple Summary: Effective communication skills are vital for successful veterinary practice and are a core component of veterinary programs. Veterinary schools design their programs to ensure that all veterinary graduates can demonstrate Day One competencies in clinical communication and provide evidence of this to accrediting bodies. The methods of teaching clinical communication in veterinary medicine have developed since this became a required part of the curriculum over two decades ago, and there is a growing evidence base for their effectiveness. However, validated 'best practices' for teaching and assessing 'real-world' communication competency are less well established. Here, we report three recent developments in communication skills training in the Doctor of Veterinary Medicine program at the University of Sydney and evaluate implications with respect to curriculum design. The developments are the following: increasing the realism of simulated communications using clinical skills laboratories, embracing a focus on primary care; including telehealth delivery in communications training; and tackling the challenge of "minding the gap" when applying theory to veterinary clinical practice. We conclude that communication in the veterinary curriculum can be more engaging and effective with student-centred design, which increases the realism and authenticity of the student experience.

Abstract: Veterinary graduates require effective clinical communication skills for a successful transition to practice. The ways of teaching and assessing veterinary communication skills have developed and are increasingly supported by research. However, some students have difficulty applying the skills learned in a simulated consultation to working with real clients, particularly in the second part of a standard consultation, where the student communicates the reasons for their clinical decision making and assists the client's treatment decisions. The authors explore three key developments in communication skills training in the Doctor of Veterinary Medicine program since 2015 at the University of Sydney: (1) Workshops were designed to include communication scenarios that were contextualised in ways that embraced a spectrum of care. These were facilitated within a clinical skills laboratory, and student surveys were used to evaluate this teaching and learning activity; (2) student and facilitator perceptions of the value of online communication skills training were evaluated using surveys; and (3) perceptions of the gap between pre-clinical training and the demonstration of communication competency in authentic clinical settings were evaluated using a survey. We conclude that the communications curriculum can be made more engaging and effective by student-centred design, which increases the realism and authenticity of the student's experience.

Keywords: veterinary communication; communication competency; simulated consultations; contextualised scenarios; clinical consultation skills; veterinary curriculum

1. Introduction

1.1. The Importance of Clinical Communication Skills in the Veterinary Curriculum

The teaching and assessment of communication competency are a necessary inclusion in veterinary school curricula. There is a robust body of evidence demonstrating that a successful and safe graduate transition to practice is associated with communication competency development in health professions, including medicine [1] and veterinary science [2,3]. Veterinary schools around the world no longer view communication competency as an optional inclusion or as a set of skills that are learned by example in the curriculum. This is because these skills are amongst the most highly valued and necessary workplace skills for new graduates [4–21], and accrediting bodies explicitly require that these competencies be demonstrated by all graduates [22–24].

In the packed modern veterinary curriculum, there is a need to explicitly and purposefully embed learning activities and the assessment of communication competency. Explicit communication curriculum frameworks developed from other disciplines such as medicine [25] are widely used as the foundation from which communication skills are taught and assessed in many veterinary curricula [8]. This includes the veterinary curriculum at the University of Sydney, where the skills curriculum has been developed and refined over two decades. With respect to clinical consultation skills (CCSs), the widely accepted framework based on the Guide to the Veterinary Consultation based on the Calgary–Cambridge Model (GVCCCM) [3,8,16] is used to teach and assess CCSs at most veterinary schools in Australia. Clinical consulting skills in a veterinary setting are those behaviours that are demonstrated when undertaking a consultation with a client and include structuring the interaction, developing a rapport and building a relationship, active listening, reflecting, explaining, responding, and concluding with spoken and written interactions. It is expected that the teaching and assessment of CCSs are integrated and sequentially developed within an education program that provides students opportunities to apply these skills in simulated and authentic clinical encounters [26–30]. This is to ensure that students are well prepared to communicate with clients during clinical placements and can demonstrate communication competency at the time of graduation. While the emphasis today is on competency-based education, a review of the medical education literature flags the important link between confidence and competence. With scaffolded experiences and feedback, competency develops over time. As such, activities that enhance students' confidence contribute to competency development, and, as described in medical education [31], this ultimately helps with a safe transition to professional practice.

1.2. Evolving Veterinary Curricula

Veterinary curricula at the University of Sydney have been adapted to address the significant impact of technology and client expectations on the role of veterinarians. This paper describes the changes made to strengthen the scaffolding of students' communication competency and to smooth their transition to practice.

In the early years of the DVM at the University of Sydney, the focus is on pre-clinical areas of study, and in these pre-clinical years, CCSs are first taught and assessed. CCS training should represent current clinical practice so that students can translate these competencies into a workplace context. This includes the use of clinical skills laboratories where students can practice their skills in safe and structured environments. The curricular revisions described in this paper have focused on strengthening the ways in which students learn CCSs through their experiences, and this was guided by an evaluation of graduate outcomes. Communication skills training plays a significant role in developing veterinarians' professional identities [32]. As such, course design needs to include resources and environments that afford students authentic opportunities to learn, practice, receive feedback, and be assessed [3,8,10,26,27,33]. Resources such as case studies or scenarios are widely used in different ways in veterinary curricula. This includes their use as a stimulus in workshop discussions, tutorials, problem-based learning activities, and communication skills training. Authentic opportunities to learn and assess CCSs can range from low-fidelity simulations such as role-plays with case scenarios facilitated in a physical classroom (in a clinical skills laboratory or virtually via videoconference) through to immersion in authentic clinical settings where students are supported and supervised whilst applying their communication skills and knowledge in ways expected for a novice veterinarian. The university's veterinary teaching services are a major site for these authentic environments, where students' communication skills are then assessed. These experiences are usually in the context of practicing "gold standard" care or a highly specialised approach to veterinary medicine.

A spectrum of care (SoC) approach has recently been recognised as an essential component of practice readiness that requires specific communication strategies [34,35]. To keep pace with industry standards and community expectations, veterinary schools must provide authentic learning activities that reflect a full range of care options, that is, where there is provision and adaptation of veterinary care that suits clients' preferences, limitations, and relationship with their pet, for example, through shelter medicine or community clinical services [34,35]. With respect to CCSs, veterinary schools are well placed to design case scenarios that reflect complex clinical presentations across a broad range of species and in situations where communication may be challenging. Situated in an environment where research drives the pursuit of new knowledge and innovative practice, highly specialised veterinary teaching hospitals are equipped to scaffold skill and knowledge development that represents a gold standard of care, including advanced diagnostic and therapeutic services. However, veterinary schools must also spend time and resources on the communications skills required for common presentations and routine cases with accreditation bodies in the UK, Australia, and New Zealand, now requiring a substantial focus on common, entry-level practice [22,24]. In practice, the goal of veterinarians is to provide valued services to meet the needs of clients and the animals in their care. So, while offering the best standard of care available to them, their clients will expect to have a range of options communicated to them and receive guidance in the selection of the treatment plan most appropriate to their needs. Clients may experience significant financial or practical constraints or simply have different priorities in what health care they are able to support for their animals [34,36,37]. As such, it is important for veterinary schools to include the teaching and assessment of communication techniques that help the veterinarian navigate this SoC approach.

Opportunities to apply clinical knowledge and skills in a spectrum of authentic professional practice environments are a critical component of veterinary education programs, and these are most effective when they build students autonomy and decision making in a supported environment. These holistic experiences afford students the opportunity to integrate communication skills with the full range of technical and non-technical competencies expected of a veterinarian. Veterinary schools achieve this in a variety of ways, including the involvement of veterinary teaching hospitals within the university in contracted practices as well as supervised practice with external partners in the industry. This presents a range of challenges, one of which is ensuring that there is vertical alignment between formal teaching and assessment activities and what is then subsequently expected of students when they apply their skills in authentic clinical encounters. Clinical placements in the final years of a veterinary program are recognised to be an effective way to link theory to practice [38]. However, research investigating work-integrated learning environments in other disciplines (health, education, psychology, and law) has shown that aligning authentic assessment activities in this complex context is challenging and problematic [39]. For example, when confronted with an actual clinical case in veterinary practice, information is often incomplete, or the veterinarian is presented with a client that has limited funds or does not have the capacity to understand or adhere to the recommended therapeutic plan. Communication with clients is impacted by the student's ability to manage time, reach probabilistic decisions, and explain these as they guide the client's treatment choices. How students experience the practice of communication skills in clinical placements and how well clinical teachers' and supervisors' assessment and feedback align with underpinning theoretical frameworks such as the GVCCCM is not well understood and remains an ongoing challenge with respect to consistency in feedback and assessment by clinical teachers and supervisors.

The challenge for veterinary schools is to make sure that curriculum review and renewal reflect industry and community expectations. Over the past 30 years, innovations in the way we communicate have been phenomenal: the general public has access to a vast amount of information via the internet, and they bring this with them to the consultation room; the widespread use of social media impacts the veterinarian–client relationship in varying ways; the role, skills, and daily work of veterinarians are much better understood due to extensive exposure through documentaries on television; telehealth is now widely practiced in human health; and the use of technology has revolutionised the way in which veterinarians record their consultations and communicate with their clients. In sum, clinical communication skills are not static competencies. This was starkly illustrated during the recent COVID-19 pandemic. As universities and veterinary schools grappled with the required shift to online teaching and learning, the same social distancing requirements led to the rapid industry uptake of telehealth consultations. That is, as the teaching and assessment of CCSs moved online, veterinarians were moving to telehealth consultations. This presented a unique opportunity to explore and review the way in which many aspects of the veterinary curriculum were taught and assessed, both in terms of educational value and industry currency.

1.3. Curriculum Progression of CCSs at the University of Sydney

Since 2015, at the University of Sydney, CCSs have been formally taught and assessed in the first and second years of the DVM program of study (DVM1 and DVM2). Opportunities to practice, demonstrate competency, and be assessed on these skills are subsequently provided in community spey-neuter clinics in the third year of the DVM (DVM3), in teaching hospitals, and in external placement rotations of final year (DVM4). The formal teaching of CCSs is first integrated into a professional practice Unit of Study (UoS), and this is followed by a series of small workshops in a module that sits within a larger, first-year Professional Skills UoS in the DVM program. Workshops are conducted throughout the first semester in DVM1 and the second semester in DVM2.

In the first year of the DVM program, the formal clinical communication curriculum involves an introductory lecture and a large-group workshop that is then followed by a series of small-group workshops (5–6 students per group). The small-group workshops are facilitated by veterinarians who have recent or current clinical experience. It is intended that the introductory lecture on clinical communication focus on understanding the generic skills required for effective communication as well as describing models for effective clinical consultations. The first large-group workshops (20–24 students per group) take place after the introductory lecture and involve several activities and group discussions. These explore elements of the clinical consultation framework and include activities that examine specific communication skills such as empathy, non-verbal communication, and the use of proxemics when communicating in a consultation. The subsequent small-group workshops involve students conducting simulated consultations as both a veterinarian and a client for a range of common companion animal health issues that include advice on desexing procedures, weight management recommendations, dental care, guidance on rabbit husbandry, and an equine health issue. Students conduct the simulated consultations for a standardised series of cases, and during the workshops, they reflect on their achievement against their own communication SMART goals, that is, goals that are Specific, Measurable, Action-oriented, Realistic, and Time-limited [40]. Students then receive structured feedback from their peers and their facilitator using the GVCCCM framework. At the end of the workshop series, students are allocated an assessment case from one of the health issues that they have been introduced to, and they conduct a simulated consultation with a professional actor taking on the role of a client. The facilitator then assesses student competency based on the core clinical consultation skills that are mapped to the GVCCCM.

In the second year of the DVM program, students' second professional practice UoS has a focus on some more challenging elements associated with clinical consultations. Students then practice their communication skills and receive feedback in a series of workshops that spotlight more challenging clinical consultations. In these workshops, the standardised cases now focus on issues such as revisit, euthanasia, emergencies, and discharge consultations for complex cases. Hospital teaching placements during Professional Skills UoS in DVM1 and DVM2, pre-clinical placements in DVM3, the community spey-neuter clinic in DVM3, and the final year placements provide students with opportunities to apply their CCSs in authentic clinical encounters that vary based on species and context.

At the University of Sydney, Units of Study with explicit learning outcomes and assessment activities associated with clinical communication skills are intentionally mapped across all stages of the DVM (Table 1). This table shows how these Units of Study are sequentially developed at the University of Sydney, with underpinning knowledge of CCS frameworks explored in the professional practice Units of Study in DVM and opportunities for the application of CCSs at the pre-novice stages in the Professional Skills Units of Study, industry, and pre-clinical placements. Context- and species-specific clinical communication learning outcomes are mapped across all DVM3 Units of Study, along with the experience of leading a community spey-neuter consultation and discharge. During the final clinical DVM4 year, learning outcomes that align with communication skills competency are articulated in all final year placements. Students are scaffolded with increasing levels of complexity and challenge as they progress through the DVM program and move from the pre-clinical to the clinical curriculum in DVM4. The authors submit that CCS training should be introduced early in the curriculum and progressively developed in challenge and complexity across the years.

Table 1. Units of Study with explicit communication learning outcomes and assessments in the DVM program at the University of Sydney.

	Professional Practice	Professional Skills	Placements
DVM1	VETS6101: The Veterinary Professional 1	VETS6102: Professional Skills 1A VETS6106: Professional Skills 1B	
			VETS6121–VETS6128: Industry Placements These placements occur at farms and other commercial animal enterprises for different animal species.
DVM2	VETS6201: The Veterinary Professional 2	VETS6202: Professional Skills 2A VETS6206: Professional Skills 2B	VETS6121–VETS6128: Industry Placements
			VETS6221–VETS6222: Preparatory Clinical Placement
DVM3	VETS6301–VETS6314: VETS6308: Veterinary Practice Management: Professional Practice Unit of Study VETS6314: Small Animal Desexing Clinic All other DVM3 units include clinical communication learning outcomes that are context- and species-specific.		VETS6221–VETS6222: Preparatory Clinical Placement
DVM4			VETS6401–VETS6404: Small Animal Clinics VETS6405–VETS6406: Large Animal Clinics VETS6408: Public, Industry or Community Placement VETS6409–VETS6412: Extra-mural Placements

This article explores the dynamic evolution of CCS education in veterinary medicine since its inception in the DVM curriculum at the University of Sydney. Three key developments are explored, and their implications are critically evaluated. These developments include:

1. Enhancing contextualisation through skills laboratories: a close examination of CCS sessions in DVM1 and DVM2, embracing the spectrum of care approach.
2. Navigating the era of online CCSs: analysing the impact of COVID-19 restrictions on CCSs, with insights into telehealth and future pedagogical implications.
3. Bridging theory and practice: an in-depth evaluation of the application of CCS training in authentic clinical environments throughout the DVM program, tackling the challenge of 'minding the gap'.

2. Materials and Methods

2.1. Utilising Skills Laboratories—Enhancing the Spectrum of Care Approach

In 2017, a pilot was conducted in which technical skills typically conducted in a consultation were incorporated into the CCS module for DVM students. DVM students engage in a series of CCS workshops in DVM1 (CCS1-6) and then DVM2 (CCS7-10). A single CCS session was dedicated to performing a "bed-side" selection of routine tasks such as calculating drug doses, blood collection, and routine diagnostics while students undertake four simulated consultations. Several skills were embedded within each simulated consultation, but they were skills that are performed by veterinarians within the time constraints of a typical consultation. The pilot focused on a single DVM2 workshop session, as students in this cohort had developed and practiced a greater range of routine technical skills at this stage of their study program. Consultation with other staff coordinating professional skills guided the CCS coordinators in aligning this session with the curriculum in DVM1 and DVM2. Facilitators were trained in a short workshop, had access to online readings and additional preparatory materials for each class, and then reflected on their experiences with the coordinator.

Groups of 5–6 students and one facilitator rotated through four "bed-side" stations within a clinical skills laboratory (CSL), also referred to as a clinical skills space at the Sydney School of Veterinary Science (and previously named the clinical skills hub). This space is a large, flat-floored teaching room equipped with benches for groups of up to 6 students per bench and a range of equipment for common veterinary procedures conducted in a routine consultation. Each station was conducted around a common clinical scenario. Students were given a brief case history, a list of tasks to perform, and the skill set that was required to manage the case. Instructions for each task were provided in the form of step-by-step procedure guides, images, and short videos where relevant. These instructions were available on the Learning Management Platform via an iPad at each station and were available in hard copy during the workshop. A series of questions and prompts were provided to facilitators to initiate discussion amongst students about the role of communication in the management of each case. Students were on their feet and were required to make decisions, perform the procedures, and role-play communication with their clients and team members as they proceeded through the cases. The time spent on the role-play was purposely limited to 10 min to encourage time management. The four cases were structured around common clinical scenarios that are routinely seen in veterinary clinical practice (Table 2).

Anonymous student feedback evaluating the value of this teaching and learning experience was gathered via an online student survey administered using Survey Monkey® (basic). This was a reflective teaching evaluation activity, and no statistical analysis was performed on the data. There were 84 responses from a cohort of 120 students.

Table 2. Pilot DVM2 communication workshops in the CSL: case scenarios and technical and communication skills.

Case	Technical Skills	Focused Communication Skills
Clinical consultation room—first-time client with new puppy	Using clinic software (Rx Works—demonstration version) to gather information when taking a history and advising on diet, training, and behaviour.	Gathering appropriate amount and type of information and managing proxemics in the consultation room.
Trauma case—hit by car	Dose calculation, placing IV catheter, calculating fluid rates, wound care, bandaging, and completing drug register for controlled drugs.	Evaluating barriers to effective communication and expressing empathy (owner was the driver and incident witnessed by children).
Revisit case—fractious cat with elderly client	Administering subcutaneous drugs, venepuncture, and performing routine blood tests (PCV, TPP), cystocentesis, and urinalysis.	Evaluating barriers to effective communication, understanding client perspective, empathy, structure of explanation and plan, and chunk-and-check techniques.
Rescue case—sick puppy presented by foster carer	Basic clinical pathology such as faecal float, heartworm test, fine-needle aspirate, and dose calculation.	Evaluating barriers to effective communication, gathering history when information is incomplete, and communicating complex therapeutic plans in situations that are complex with barriers to adherence.

2.2. Online Teaching and Assessment of Clinical Consultation Skills

In response to the COVID-19 restrictions regarding social distancing, CCS workshops for DVM1 and DVM2 students moved to online delivery (using Zoom) and assessment in 2020 and 2021. Offshore and onshore students were located across three continents and multiple time zones. Many key elements in the administration of CCS workshops remained the same. The case-scenario health issues were the same as those used for in-person delivery, and groups of 4–6 students participated in a series of workshops that were facilitated by a veterinarian with recent or current clinical experience. Once all workshops were completed, students were individually assessed by a facilitator, and the 'client' was a professional actor. Students were given feedback and assessed on the same core communication skills as those used for in-person delivery. These included preparing and initiating the consultation; exploring the patient's history; using attentive and reflective listening strategies; demonstrating effective explanation and planning; closing the consultation; providing structure to the consultation; employing effective non-verbal communication; expressing empathy; seeking and receiving constructive feedback; and structuring and providing constructive feedback for peers.

Some changes to the teaching and assessment of CCSs were required in response to the need for social distancing and the COVID-19 restrictions. Prior to the first two workshops in the COVID-19 lockdown period, students were required to submit a video of themselves conducting a simulated consultation (adhering to isolation requirements). This video was uploaded to a discussion page on the Learning Management Platform, Canvas. For the remaining CCS sessions, simulated consultations were conducted live during the Zoom workshops. Small-group, facilitator-led workshops were all conducted via Zoom and involved student goal setting, reflection on the consultations, and constructive feedback shared by peers and the facilitator. The final workshop and the assessment involved students conducting a consultation using existing cases that were modified to suit a telehealth format, and this was based on the Australian Veterinary Association telemedicine guidelines released in response to the COVID-19 restrictions. In the workshop, the role of 'client' was filled by a fellow student, and for the assessment, a professional actor was used. Constructive feedback was provided by peers and facilitators during the workshop, and for the assessment, student competency was determined by the facilitator with respect to the core communication skills that are mapped to the elemental stages in the Guide to the Veterinary Consultation based on the Calgary–Cambridge Model (GVCCCM) [8].

As reported in van Gelderen et al. [41], an online, anonymous survey evaluating the student, facilitator, and actor experience was administered at the conclusion of the program, with data collected via the secure data collection instrument Qualtrics®. The survey was administered to all DVM1 students (119) and facilitators and actors (14), with 20 completed survey responses received from students and 10 from facilitators and actors. Facilitators who were involved in collecting and analysing the data were not included. The survey questions were designed to evaluate four key areas:

Value of the learning experience
Level of confidence
Perceived ability
Emotional response

Questions had five response options using a Likert scale from 'strongly disagree' to 'strongly agree', and an optional open-text response box was available to gather additional comments for each question. Questions for the facilitators and actors were modified to reflect their perspective and to seek comparative data as this group of participants had prior experience with CCSs offered in person [41].

For each of the four key areas under investigation, the levels of agreement (strongly agree and agree) were measured for the participant groups. Data comparing the online experience to the in-person CCS experience were only collected from the facilitators and actors. Free-text responses to the open-ended questions were reviewed by all researchers, with the lead researcher initially developing key themes through keyword searches and pattern identification. Repeated discussions amongst the research group addressed biases, and a final set of themes was established based on a concordance of views from the three researchers [41] (see https://library.iated.org/view/VANGELDEREN2021FRO (accessed on 23 November 2023)).

Ethics approval for this study was granted by the University of Sydney's Human Research Ethics Committee, Project Number 2020/496.

2.3. *Evaluating the Application of CCSs in Authentic Clinical Settings*

In 2022, a survey was designed to evaluate the effect of clinical communication skills training on supporting DVM students' application of CCSs in authentic clinical encounters. The study sought to evaluate students' perceptions of their competency in communication skills, their confidence levels, and whether training supported their application in an authentic environment. Due to pandemic isolation impacts, these students had varying levels of opportunity to apply communication skills in authentic settings, so the survey included questions to establish the students' stage of learning and level of opportunity.

An online anonymous survey instrument was administered to all DVM students at the University of Sydney who had completed formal CCS training in DVM1 and DVM2, and survey questions were modelled on a study designed to track the acquisition of CCSs and student confidence following training using the GVCCCM framework [29]. This survey was anonymous and was administered after all teaching and learning and formal assessments of CCSs were complete. Qualtrics®, a secure survey data collection instrument, was used for survey administration.

General descriptive data were gathered from students regarding the stage of the degree that they were in, the number of opportunities that they had experienced to apply their communication skills, where they had applied these skills, confidence levels for different types of skills, and capability levels for different types of skills. Questions exploring students' confidence level in individual communication skills included response options on a five-point Likert scale from 'lack confidence completely' to 'completely confident.' Additional questions included a yes–no–unsure assessment of the effectiveness of clinical communication skill training and a self-assessment of the ability to build rapport, take a comprehensive history, and make a client feel valued.

Survey data were collected over 12 weeks, and 35 valid responses from the 272 students invited to participate were received. The data analysis report was downloaded from Qualtrics®, and raw data were then cleaned for analysis. The data were analysed using GenStat® using a logistic regression model with an underlying binomial distribution. This analysis sought to identify if there was a statistical association between the outcomes (building rapport, taking a history, making a client feel valued) and stage of degree and the number of opportunities the students had to apply their skills.

Ethics approval for this study was granted by the University of Sydney's Human Research Ethics Committee, Project Number 2022/058.

3. Results

3.1. Utilising Skills Laboratories—Enhancing the Spectrum of Care Approach

The informal survey evaluating the utilisation of the clinical skills space for a single session in the CCS workshop series revealed that the majority of students either strongly agreed or agreed (96%) that this session helped their learning. Most students (93%) could understand the link between the skills performed and the impact on communication during a consultation, and 96% of respondents believed that this session helped their learning of clinical communication. The areas identified for improvement were associated with logistics, namely the organisation of the stations in the space, the quality of the supporting materials for students, and the scaffolds for facilitators and students (Table 3).

Table 3. Questions and survey responses from DVM2 students evaluating a CCS workshop in the CSL (clinical skill hub), $n = 84$.

Questions	Strongly Agree	Agree	Neutral	Disagree	Strongly Disagree
Q1: Working on skills commonly encountered during a consultation in the clinical skills hub helped my learning	71%	25%	1%	1%	1%
Q2: I understood the link between the skills performed and the impact that this has on communication in a consultation	62%	31%	5%	1%	1%
Q3: The stations in the clinical skills hub were well organised	43%	51%	4%	2%	0%
Q4: I had enough time to work through the skills at each station	19%	37%	19%	20%	5%
Q5: The supporting videos and information material on the Learning Management Platform helped me to prepare for the session in the clinical skills hub	36%	44%	19%	1%	0%
Q6: The discussion questions for each scenario helped my learning	46%	43%	8%	1%	1%
Q7: Overall the CCS clinical skills hub session helped my learning of clinical communication	55%	36%	6%	2%	1%
Q8: Overall the CCS clinical skills hub session helped me to develop skills I will need for success as a veterinarian	70%	26%	1%	1%	1%

In response to the student feedback received, the module coordinator developed and incorporated a similarly designed session into the series of DVM1 CCS workshops in 2022. The DVM1 sessions in the CSL focused on simple cases and skills that aligned with this stage of the curriculum (Table 4). More emphasis was placed on facilitator prompts, guidance, just-in-time feedback, and short role-plays to promote the discussion of communication skills so that students could clearly identify the links between the performance of these 'bed-side' skills and their impact on communication skills. These were provided to facilitators to improve the consistency and organisation of activities in the clinical skills space. Additional prompts were included to highlight issues related to cultural competency.

Table 4. DVM1 communication workshops in the CSL (clinical skills hub): case scenarios and technical and communication skills.

Case	Technical Skills	Focused Communication Skills
Obese dog with osteoarthritis	Dose calculation, administration of subcutaneous injection, and interpretation of feeding instructions	Structuring an explanation and plan, achieving shared understanding, expressing empathy, and cultural competency (owner is elderly, hearing and vision impaired, and cannot read the feeding instructions on the bag of dog food)
Cat abscess and castration advice	Dose calculation, writing drug labels, interpreting in-house rapid blood tests (e.g., FIV/FeLV SNAP test), and oral tablet administration	Structuring an explanation and plan, expressing empathy, negotiating a therapeutic plan, achieving shared understanding, and cultural competency (owner is resistant to castration based on prior experiences and cultural norms)
Dog with sore ears, retained deciduous teeth, and ovariohysterectomy advice	Use of equipment (otoscope), basic ear cleaning, and use of anatomical models to demonstrate normal and pathologies, e.g., those observed in canine ears and teeth	Structuring an explanation and plan, expressing empathy, negotiating a therapeutic plan, achieving shared understanding, closing the consultation, and discussion of costs
Annual health check and prophylactic care (vaccination and internal and external parasite control)	Dose calculation, microchip scanning, vaccination card completion, review, and selection of appropriate parasiticide product	Questioning techniques, signposting techniques, reflective listening, structuring an explanation and plan, negotiating a plan with shared understanding, and closing the consultation

3.2. Online Teaching and Assessment of Clinical Consultation Skills

In evaluating online teaching and assessment of CCSs, participant responses were grouped according to four key areas (Table 5). High levels of agreement (>90%) were identified from the student and facilitator/actor groups with respect to the 'value of the learning experience' and the 'increasing ability to communicate effectively'. Facilitators and actors reported lower levels of agreement than students for 'increasing confidence to communicate in a veterinary consultation', 'dealing with clients', and 'encouraged active participation'. Students reported higher levels of 'increased ability to structure a consult based on GVCCCM' compared to facilitators and actors. Most facilitators and actors (70%) reported that online CCS teaching and assessment were not more effective than in-person delivery.

Table 5. Levels of agreement evaluating four key aspects of the online CCS teaching and learning experience for students (n = 20) and facilitators/actors (n = 10) (taken from van Gelderen et al., 2021 [41]).

	Students: Proportion Reporting Strongly Agree and Agree (%)	**Facilitators/Actors: Proportion Reporting Strongly Agree and Agree (%)**
	Value of learning experience	
Was a valuable learning experience	95	100
Effective in developing communication skills	95	100
Effective in the integration of clinical knowledge and communication skills	100	90
Was more valuable than face-to-face	N/A	10
	Confidence	
Increased confidence to communicate in a veterinary consultation	90	70
Increased confidence to deal with clients	80	60
More effective than face-to-face CCSs in developing confidence	N/A	30
	Ability	
Increased ability to communicate effectively for common scenario	95	90
Increased ability to structure consult based on GVCCM	100	80
More effective than face-to-face	N/A	20
	Emotional response	
Was a stressful experience	20	30
Encouraged active participation	95	80
More stressful than face-to-face	N/A	0

There were six themes identified from the qualitative survey data describing the participants' experiences of online CCS teaching and assessment. Consistent themes were identified in both the student (ST) and facilitator (FA) groups, with some variation in emphasis and focus within each theme. See Table 6 for themes, key points, and illustrative quotes.

3.3. Evaluating the Application of CCSs in Authentic Clinical Settings

The data obtained from the survey (response rate 13%) evaluating the students' application of CCSs in an authentic environment revealed information about the opportunities that students had to apply CCSs, the overall confidence levels in CCSs (Figure 1), the confidence levels in specific skills (Figure 2), the perceived competence in taking a comprehensive history, the building of client rapport and making a client feel valued (Figure 3), and an evaluation of whether CCS training supported the application of skills in an authentic clinical encounter (Figure 4). The respondents were at varying stages of their degree. Those at the early stage (43%) had completed their CCS training workshops in DVM1 and DVM2 and had just commenced DVM3. Most of these early-stage students (70–80%) had completed their two 2-week pre-clinical placements in university-operated or private veterinary clinics. The remaining respondents were either in the mid stage (49%), having completed DVM3; their pre-clinical placements and one or two final year rotations; or their late stage (9%), where they had completed all final year rotations in DVM4 and had just recently graduated.

Table 6. Participants' experiences of online CCSs: emergent themes and illustrative quotes from 197 comments (94 comments from 10 facilitators/actors (FAs) and 103 comments from 20 students (STs)) (taken from van Gelderen et al., 2021 [41]).

Theme	Key Points	Illustrative Quotes
1. Online teaching and learning	Benefits associated with online formats, such as more time to prepare video uploads, which reduced stress. Online had inherent limitations but was an authentic representation of the shift to telehealth	*[online] less confronting for students and promoted discussion* (FA) *[online] not a full substitute for some physical consultations, different feel* (ST)
2. Skills and knowledge	Development of non-technical skills Challenges with non-verbal communication cues Authentic and common scenarios	*setting the right mindset of how to communicate effectively with clients and gather information while building rapport with them* (ST) *many aspects of body language are lost as mainly the face is seen online* (FA) *students did learn to communicate with clients in common scenarios* (FA)
3. Feedback and reflective practice	Receiving feedback from peers and facilitators Preparation and active engagement	*receiving feedback from other students and a tutor was really helpful; improved a lot between first and last workshop* (ST) *being given different cases each week and having time to prepare allowed me to be fully invested in the class and participate as actively as possible...get the most out of the sessions* (ST)
4. Workshop structure	Facilitator-led small groups GVCCM framework	*good to have small groups where instructors can give personal comments* (ST) *I think it works as a guide but I always stress the need for flexibility* (FA)
5. Ability and confidence	Progression Prior experience	*practice increases confidence; notable progression throughout the course* (FA) *the students that came with experience as a generalisation did the best (FA)*
6. Emotional response	Stress levels	*they were not so much stressful as much as they were engaging, enjoyable and fun, especially the assessment* (ST) *they didn't seem unduly stressed. A bit of nerves, but that is good* (FA)

More than half of respondents reported having had more than 10 opportunities to apply CCSs in an authentic clinical setting, and the highest number of opportunities were undertaken during pre-clinical placements. The 'other' opportunities were all linked to external work as a veterinary nurse or technician. The majority of respondents (77%) reported that formal training in CCSs supported their skill development (Figure 4). Most respondents (66%) were confident or extremely confident in applying CCSs, 20% were neutral, and 14% were not confident or lacked confidence completely. Statistically, there was no significant association between confidence levels and the stage that respondents were up to in their degree (Table 7). However, an analysis revealed that those respondents who had more opportunities to apply their skills were more likely to report being confident or extremely confident.

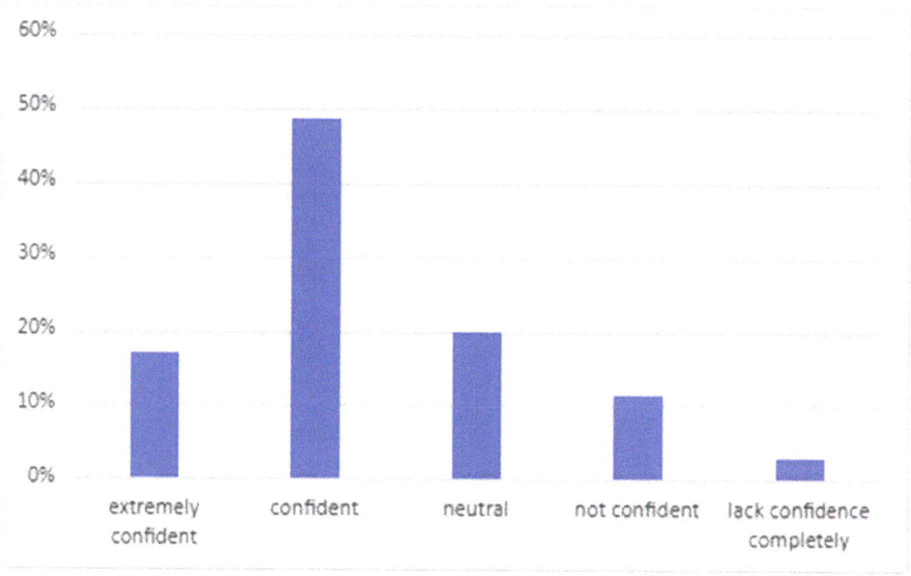

Figure 1. Students' perceptions of overall confidence in clinical consultation skills (n = 35).

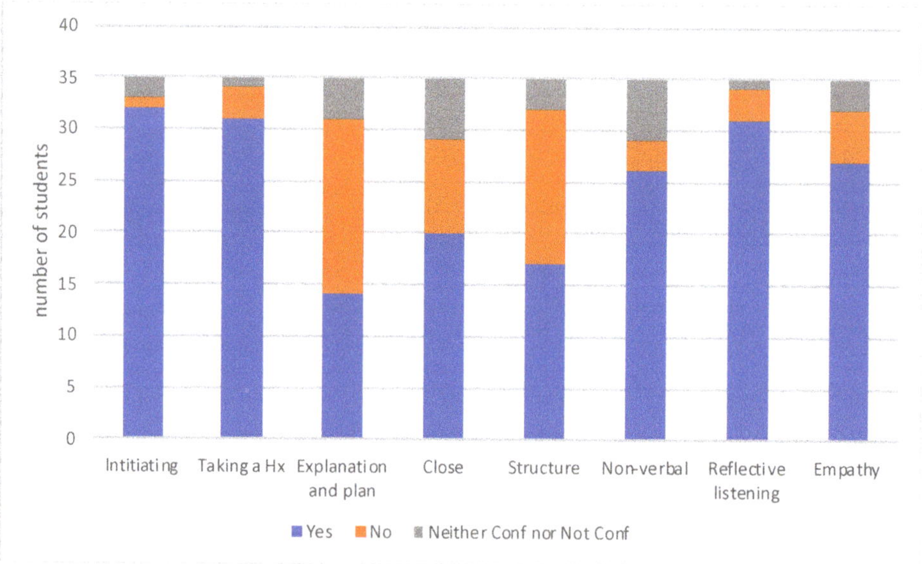

Figure 2. Students' perceptions of confidence in specific clinical consultation skills (n = 35).

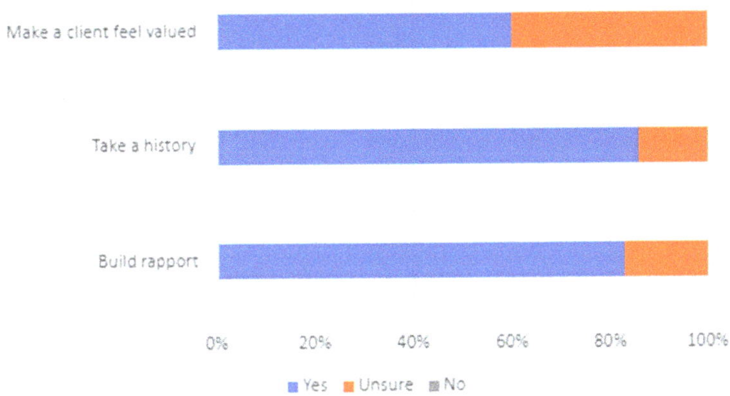

Figure 3. Students' perceptions of competency in specific clinical consultation skills (n = 35).

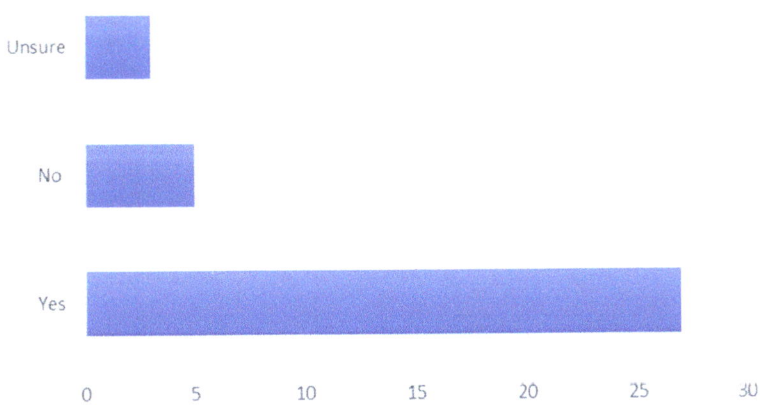

Figure 4. Students' evaluation of whether CCS training in DVM1 and DVM2 supported application in an authentic clinical encounter (x-axis is the number of students and n = 35).

Table 7. p-values measuring associations between confidence levels and the number of opportunities to apply skills and the stage of degree.

Communication Skill	Number of Opportunities p-Value	Stage of Degree p-Value
Build rapport	0.125	0.938
Patient history	0.183	0.799
Client feels valued	**0.027**	0.889

The specific CCS skills based on the GVCCCM framework where students reported the highest confidence were 'initiating a consultation', 'taking a history', and 'reflective listening' (Figure 2). Those CCS skills where students reported the lowest confidence were 'explanation and planning', 'providing a structure', and 'closing the consultation'. With respect to students' perceptions of their competence in CCSs, it was revealed that most respondents were certain that they could build rapport with a client and take a comprehensive history, but there were higher levels of uncertainty when asked about making a client feel valued (Figure 3). Statistically, there was no significant effect of the stage of degree on any of the questions relating to perceived competence, and the only significant association was related to the number of opportunities that a student had to apply their skills in an authentic clinical setting and make a client feel valued (Table 7). That is, those respondents who had more than 10 opportunities to apply their CCSs in an authentic clinical setting were nine times more likely to perceive that they were competent in making a client feel valued (95% CI 1.8–44.8) (Table 8).

Table 8. Predicted proportions for making a client feel valued based on the number of opportunities to apply skills.

	Predicted Proportion for "Yes"	Standard Error
No Opportunity	0.5	0.354
<10	0.307	0.128
>10	0.8	0.089

4. Discussion

A spectrum of care (SoC) approach is recommended in veterinary education [35–37], and there are many ways that this can be successfully achieved across a veterinary curriculum with respect to communication competence. Veterinary graduates are expected to have competence across multiple domains and be able to adapt in response to the diverse needs of their clients and society. Competency-based veterinary education (CVBE), as described by the Association of American Veterinary Colleges, describes nine domains of expected competence necessary for veterinary graduates [42]. Suggested subcompetencies within the Communication Domain explicitly address the fact that clients and society have varied needs, wants, and understandings regarding the health of animals. Clinical consultation case studies or scenarios are a widely used curriculum resource with respect to communication skills training and assessment, and these scenarios are easily adapted to demonstrate a wide range of different outcomes with respect to patient care. The capacity to tweak and modify case scenarios in real time was a key feature identified in the CCS workshops that were undertaken in the clinical skills space at the University of Sydney. Moreover, the scenarios were designed with consideration of time management with respect to making decisions on clinical information and communicating that to the client, making these simulations a valuable tool for assessment and feedback. Facilitators were able to prompt students to consider how they would need to adapt communication styles as well as diagnostic and therapeutic plans because of varied client understandings, needs, wants, and financial capacities.

Training and guidelines for facilitators and teachers are necessary to achieve the communication competency outcomes described here [6,8,25]. Facilitators of CCS workshops at the University of Sydney are practitioners who have recent or current experience in veterinary practice, and they are well placed in their understanding of common scenarios and the variation in what clients understand, need, and want with respect to the care of their animals and their capacity to support that care. It is, however, critical that facilitators are active in promoting these discussions with their students. As such, facilitator training and supporting guidelines with suggested prompts are required to support the standardised case scenarios used in CCS training and assessment. Moreover, guidance to facilitators and students on providing and receiving effective feedback is needed to reinforce, encourage, and scaffold [41].

Simulations can greatly assist in preparing students for the responsibility of case management [43]. Learning through the experience of being responsible for case management is an essential aspect of students' final rotations during veterinary school, and it is critical when they transition into clinical veterinary practice. Indeed, the transition to taking responsibility for decisions and communicating with others is a difficult transition for many students, challenging their confidence and self-perceptions of competence. This is true for both technical skills and non-technical skills, such as clinical communication. Case management involves communication that does more than inform clients about diagnostic and therapeutic plans. When communicating with clients, veterinarians guide clients in the decision-making process, and they need to help their clients understand the implications of the choices made. This includes, but is not limited to, consideration of finances, understanding cultural differences, and client constraints. Simulated consultations, embedded early in the veterinary curriculum, are effective in providing students with repeated opportunities in a safe environment to practice and finesse those communication skills that are required for effective case management. This includes experiencing the impact of client 'pushback' or negative emotions in response to veterinary advice, navigating and negotiating diagnostic and therapeutic plans, and managing time in a consultation. According to the study reported in this paper, most students reported that the formal integration of simulations was effective in supporting their development of clinical communication skill competency. Using the GVCCCM framework to interrogate this further, it is evident that CCS training supported students' confidence and competence in gathering a history, active listening, and building a rapport with their client, but there was less certainty in students' confidence for making a client feel valued. Significantly, students who had more opportunities to apply their communication skills in an authentic clinical setting reported higher confidence levels in making a client feel valued. Providing context is key to the assessment of communication skills [44], and it is not surprising that authenticity in the design of learning experiences is critical to enhancing student confidence.

Communication skills cannot simply be viewed as individual competencies. In research investigating the factors contributing to complaints and litigation in the veterinary profession [20], communication issues played a role in 80% of cases. This means that when we teach and assess communication skills, consideration must be given to organisational systems and communication within teams. As such, this must underpin the design of simulations (case studies, facilitator prompts, environment, distractions, etc.) that are used in communication skills training. For example, when using the clinical skills space for the session when communication skills were contextualised, students were time-limited when conducting the role-plays whilst performing routine skills expected during a consultation (for example, administering a tablet to a fractious cat owned by an elderly and frail client). This challenged the student to consider how they would communicate with the client and their team to ensure that the consultation was completed in a timely way whilst at the same time achieving the desired outcome, maintaining the client's trust, and maximising the chance of client adherence to the therapeutic plan.

There are aspects of clinical communication competency that are likely to present greater challenges to the veterinary student and will be more difficult to teach and assess in the veterinary curriculum. This is particularly the case in the early stages of the DVM when students have little or varied experience and their knowledge is still foundational. As such, their clinical reasoning skills and their capacity to make decisions and take responsibility for those decisions are limited. Clinical reasoning relies on the ability to prioritise problems and then take a systematic and reflective approach to investigate and take action on those plans [3,45]. Even a reliance on the risky practice of pattern recognition using a non-analytical form of reasoning will pose challenges for the novice with limited experience of common presentations. It is therefore unsurprising that students report lower levels of confidence when structuring a consultation, providing their client with an explanation and plan, and closing the consultation. That is, when they must integrate interpersonal communication with clinical decision making. This is supported by previous research that found students demonstrate lower levels of competence with organisation and sequencing [28], and in Meehan and Menniti's study [46], students found it more difficult to manage the consultation with respect to time, structure, and discussions of costs. This is likely to be amplified when problems are complex and there are higher levels of uncertainty. In real time and with a foundational knowledge base, it will be more challenging for students to prioritise information, design, and then action plans in collaboration with their clients.

In this paper, we have described an integrated approach in which students are given explicit opportunities to apply communication skills using simulations that utilise clinical skills laboratories in the pre-clinical stages of the degree and then in actual consultations in their final year placements. Clinical skills laboratories are used in many veterinary schools for the provision of self-directed learning opportunities and the formal teaching of technical skills prior to performing the skills in a live setting (see Baillie et al. [47]). This paper reports on the use of a CSL in the teaching and assessment of communication skills, and, whilst this is not a widely reported use of a CSL, it was raised in some of the survey feedback reported in Baillie et al.'s study [47]. For the use of a CSL to work in communication skills training, the authors suggest that case scenarios be carefully designed so any inclusion of "bed-side" technical skills aligns with what students would already know and would be able to perform at the stage of the curriculum when communications skills workshops take place. Time-bound simulations where students experience performing a range of routine skills, such as dose calculations for medications, whilst communicating with their client are a way to help students practice their communication skills in a safe, low-stakes environment. The role-plays conducted for the CSL pilot were limited to 10 min to encourage time management, and this feature was incorporated into the design of subsequent CSL workshops in DVM1 and DVM2. The authors recommend that the emphasis on facilitator scaffolding and feedback remain focused on communication skills, and this needs to be reinforced in facilitator training. Prompts that can be used to tweak the scenario to represent the spectrum of care options need to be provided to facilitators and reinforced with training. Small student groups are therefore essential so that students are able to practice and receive meaningful feedback. This aligns well with the core components of a competency-based veterinary education curriculum, in which learning outcomes can be progressively sequenced across the program of study [42].

When veterinary educators review a veterinary curriculum in the context of competency-based education, the teaching and assessment of communication skills can be enhanced by explicitly describing observable markers, or milestones, that define the level of skill for each competency in the Communication Domain in the pre-clinical (pre-novice) stages and then from novice to advanced beginner, competent, and proficient in the clinical rotations in the final year. In the final placement year, a way to link communication competency to application in a professional, authentic workplace may be through a defined Entrustable Professional Activity (EPA). The AAVMC CBVE has described core EPAs [42], and the authors posit that the integrated and authentic context for learning and the communication skills feedback provided by an EPA may go some way to enhancing students' confidence in the face of uncertainty and complexity that is typically faced in practice. The authors acknowledge that the small sample sizes of students participating in the surveys are a limitation for the results reported in this paper. However, we maintain that monitoring the student's experience across the program is necessary to assure the integrity of communication skill training, and this may be achieved through student and graduate surveys, focus interviews, and supervisor feedback reports.

Finally, it is worth noting that recent innovations in the way that professionals communicate in practice should be given some consideration with respect to future curriculum planning. By way of example, the impacts of the COVID-19 pandemic amplified the use of communication methods that use technology, and this was demonstrated in the widespread endorsement of online teaching and learning in higher education [41] and the increased uptake in telehealth services by veterinary practitioners [48,49]. Prior to this, veterinarians in practice had not widely embraced telehealth options [49], and, to the authors' knowledge, there is no evidence that these methods of communicating are widely embedded in communication skills training in veterinary schools. The survey reported in this paper indicates that facilitators and some students recognised the value of the online CCS training implemented during the pandemic as it aligned with what practitioners were required to embrace at the height of the pandemic restrictions [41]. As new ways of accessing and communicating information continue to develop at an astounding pace (see Aliwi et al. [50] for a review of the use of augmented and virtual reality technologies in medical communication), it is likely that the practice of veterinary telemedicine or telehealth will increase [49,51]. As such, it behoves educators to consider how this can be addressed in the teaching and assessment of communication skills in the curriculum, which is an area for future research.

5. Conclusions

Mastering effective communication skills is vital in veterinary education. Public trust, accreditation mandates, and research-backed methodologies converge to emphasise the essential role communication skills play in ensuring optimal animal welfare outcomes, making them a cornerstone of veterinary training. However, validated 'best practices' for teaching and assessing 'real-world' communication competency are not well established [12,18]. The authors of this paper present several strategies to develop communication skills training in a veterinary curriculum and also suggest areas that may be considered for future research. These strategies enhance the ways in which CCS training and assessment are contextualised. Clinical skills laboratories can provide a more authentic, enriched, and engaging learning experience and introduce students to communications with clients around selecting patient care options from the spectrum available. Students can be better prepared for telehealth consultations by incorporating these into clinical communications training. Finally, veterinary schools should monitor the cohesion and integration of the communication elements in the curriculum and understand students' experiences and graduates' perceptions of their confidence as well as competence to ensure that all veterinary program graduates are ready for a smooth transition to practice. A dynamic and ever-evolving curriculum is essential, and our proposed strategies for developing communication competency offer practical ways for veterinary schools to ensure graduates are not only well prepared for current challenges but also equipped for the evolving demands of the future.

Author Contributions: Conceptualisation, R.T. and I.v.G.; methodology, formal analysis, investigation, and writing—original draft preparation, I.v.G.; writing—review and editing, R.T. and I.v.G. All authors have read and agreed to the published version of the manuscript.

Funding: This research received no external funding.

Institutional Review Board Statement: Two of the studies reported in this paper received human ethics approval from the Human Research Ethics Committee of the University of Sydney (Project No. 2020/496, Approval Date: 25 August 2020, and Project No. 2022/058, Approval Date: 16 February 2022), and one involved the use of anonymous teaching evaluation data. Participants cannot be identified, and the surveys were all anonymous.

Informed Consent Statement: Informed consent was obtained from all subjects in this study.

Data Availability Statement: The data presented in this study are available on reasonable request from the corresponding author.

Acknowledgments: The authors acknowledge the valuable contributions from academic and technical staff in the Sydney School of Veterinary Science at the University of Sydney. These include Evelyn Hall, in the Sydney School of Veterinary Science, for the statistical analysis of the data collected to evaluate clinical communication skills training and the application of skills in an authentic clinical setting; Sanaa Zaki, Katrina Walker, Alyssa Matthews, and Amy Draper for their significant collaboration in the design, implementation, and evaluation of the pilot utilising the clinical skills space (CSL) in the teaching of clinical communication skills for DVM2 students and for the subsequent development of a similar workshop for DVM1 students; and Paul Sheehy for his significant collaboration on the review and evaluation of the online teaching and assessment of clinical communication skills during the COVID-19 pandemic.

Conflicts of Interest: The authors declare no conflict of interest.

References

1. Silverman, J.; Kurtz, S.; Draper, J. *Skills for Communicating with Patients*, 3rd ed.; CRC Press: London, UK, 2013. [CrossRef]
2. Cake, M.A.; Bell, M.A.; Williams, J.C.; Brown, F.J.L.; Dozier, M.; Rhind, S.M.; Baillie, S. Which professional (non-technica competencies are most important to the success of graduate veterinarians? A Best Evidence Medical Education (BEME) systema review: BEME Guide No. 38. *Med. Teach.* **2016**, *38*, 550–563. [CrossRef]
3. Hodgson, J.L.; Pelzer, J.M. (Eds.) *Veterinary Medical Education: A Practical Guide*; Wiley Blackwell: Hoboken, NJ, USA, 2017.
4. Adams, C.L.; Kurtz, S.M. Building on existing models from human medical education to develop a communication curriculum veterinary medicine. *J. Vet. Med. Educ.* **2006**, *33*, 28–37. [CrossRef] [PubMed]
5. Gray, C.A.; Blaxter, A.C.; Johnston, P.A.; Latham, C.E.; May, S.; Phillips, C.A.; Turnbull, N.; Yamagishi, B. Communicatic education in veterinary education in the United Kingdom and Ireland: The NUVACS project coupled to progressive individu school endeavors. *J. Vet. Med. Educ.* **2006**, *33*, 85–92. [CrossRef] [PubMed]
6. Kurtz, S. Teaching and learning communication in veterinary medicine. *J. Vet. Med. Educ.* **2006**, *33*, 11–19. [CrossRef] [PubMe
7. Mills, J.N.; Irwin, P.; Baguley, J.; Meehan, M.; Austin, H.; Fitzpatrick, L.; Parry, B.; Heath, T. Development of Veterina Communication Skills at Murdoch University and in Other Australian Veterinary Schools. *J. Vet. Med. Educ.* **2006**, *33*, 93–9 [CrossRef] [PubMed]
8. Radford, A.; Stockley, P.; Silverman, J.; Taylor, I.; Turner, R.; Gray, C.; Bush, L.; Glyde, M.; Healy, A.; Dale, V.; et al. Developmer teaching, and evaluation of a consultation structure model for use in veterinary education. *J. Vet. Med. Educ.* **2006**, *33*, 38–4 [CrossRef] [PubMed]
9. Shaw, D.H.; Ihle, S.L. Communication skills training at the Atlantic Veterinary College, University of Prince Edward Island. *J. V Med. Educ.* **2006**, *33*, 100–104. [CrossRef]
10. Chun, R.; Schaefer, S.; Lotta, C.C.; Banning, J.A.; Skochelak, S.E. Didactic and experiential training to teach communication skil The University of Wisconsin-Madison School of Veterinary Medicine collaborative experience. *J. Vet. Med. Educ.* **2009**, *36*, 196–2C [CrossRef]
11. Rhind, S.M.; Baillie, S.; Kinnison, T.; Shaw, D.J.; Bell, C.E.; Mellanby, R.J.; Hammond, J.; Hudson, N.P.H.; Whittington, R.I Donnelly, R. The transition into veterinary practice: Opinions of recent graduates and final year students. *BMC Med. Educ.* **201** *11*, 64. [CrossRef]
12. Hodgson, J.L.; Pelzer, J.M.; Inzana, K.D. Beyond NAVMEC: Competency-based veterinary education and assessment of th professional competencies. *J. Vet. Med. Educ.* **2013**, *40*, 102–118. [CrossRef]
13. McDermott, M.P.; Tischler, V.A.; Cobb, M.A.; Robbé, I.J.; Dean, R.S. Veterinarian-client communication skills: Current stat relevance, and opportunities for improvement. *J. Vet. Med. Educ.* **2015**, *42*, 305–314. [CrossRef] [PubMed]
14. Mossop, L.; Gray, C.; Blaxter, A.; Gardiner, A.; MacEachern, K.; Watson, P.; Whittlestone, K.; Robbé, I. Communication skil training: What the vet schools are doing. *Vet. Rec.* **2015**, *176*, 114–117. [CrossRef] [PubMed]
15. Adams, C.L.; Kurtz, S.M.; Bayly, W.; Mülling, C.; Suchman, A. *Skills for Communicating in Veterinary Medicine*; Otmoor Publishin Oxford, UK, 2017.
16. Adams, C.L.; Kurtz, S.M. Chapter 23, Communication. In *Veterinary Medical Education: A Practical Guide*; Hodgson, J.L., Pelze J.M., Eds.; Wiley Blackwell: Hoboken, NJ, USA, 2017; pp. 357–377.
17. Haldane, S.; Hinchcliff, K.; Mansell, P.; Baik, C. Expectations of graduate communication skills in professional veterinary practic *J. Vet. Med. Educ.* **2017**, *44*, 268–279. [CrossRef] [PubMed]
18. Shaw, J.R. Evaluation of communication skills training programs at North American veterinary medical training institution *J. Am. Vet. Med. Assoc.* **2019**, *255*, 722–733. [CrossRef]
19. Reinhard, A.R.; Hains, K.D.; Hains, B.J.; Strand, E.B. Are they ready? Trials, tribulations, and professional skills vital for ne veterinary graduate success. *Front. Vet. Sci.* **2021**, *8*, 785844. [CrossRef] [PubMed]
20. Russell, E.; Mossop, L.; Forbes, E.; Oxtoby, C. Uncovering the "messy details" of veterinary communication: An analysis c communication problems in cases of alleged professional negligence. *Vet. Rec.* **2022**, *190*, e1068. [CrossRef]
21. Bahramsoltani, M.; Bröer, S.; Langforth, S.; Eule, C.; Prior, A.; Vogt, L.; Li, T.-T.; Schirone, R.; Pohl, A.; Jensen, K.C. Outcom of communication training in veterinary studies: Influence on the perception of the relevance of veterinary competencies an self-assessment of communication skills. *Animals* **2023**, *13*, 1516. [CrossRef]
22. AVBC. AVBC Day One Competencies. Version 1: January 2024. Australasian Veterinary Boards Council. 2023. Available onlin https://avbc.asn.au/wp-content/uploads/2023/01/AVBC-Day-One-Competencies_Final_2024-v1-Jan-24.pdf (accessed o 29 September 2023).
23. AVMA. COE Accreditation Policies and Procedures: Requirements: Standard 9, Curriculum and Standard 11, Outcome Assessment. American Veterinary Medical Association. 2023. Available online: https://www.avma.org/education/center-fo veterinary-accreditation/accreditation-policies-and-procedures-avma-council-education-coe/coe-accreditation-policies-anc procedures-principles (accessed on 20 June 2023).
24. RCVS. RCVS Standards and Guidance for the Accreditation of Veterinary Degree Programmes. Royal College of Veterinary Su geons. 2023. Available online: https://www.rcvs.org.uk/document-library/rcvs-standards-and-guidance-for-the-accreditatior of-veterinary/ (accessed on 20 June 2023).
25. Kurtz, S.; Draper, J.; Silverman, J. *Teaching and Learning Communication Skills in Medicine*, 2nd ed.; CRC Press: London, UK, 201 [CrossRef]

Brandt, J.C.; Bateman, S.W. Senior Veterinary Students' Perceptions of Using role play to learn communication skills. *J. Vet. Med. Educ.* **2006**, *33*, 76–80. [CrossRef] [PubMed]

Barron, D.; Khosa, D.; Jones-Bitton, A. Experiential learning in primary care: Impact on veterinary students' communication confidence. *J. Exp. Educ.* **2017**, *40*, 349–365. [CrossRef]

Stevens, B.J.; Kedrowicz, A.A. Evaluation of fourth-year veterinary students' client communication skills: Recommendations for scaffolded instruction and practice. *J. Vet. Med. Educ.* **2018**, *45*, 85–90. [CrossRef]

Englar, R.E. Tracking veterinary students' acquisition of communication skills and clinical communication confidence by comparing student Performance in the first and twenty-seventh standardized client encounters. *J. Vet. Med. Educ.* **2019**, *46*, 235–257. [CrossRef]

McDavid, L.; San Miguel, S.F. Using a community engagement program to promote veterinary medicine while helping veterinary students improve their communication skills and increase their cultural understanding and well-being. *J. Am. Vet. Med. Assoc.* **2021**, *258*, 1322–1324. [CrossRef]

Gottlieb, M.; Chan, T.M.; Zaver, F.; Ellaway, R. Confidence-competence alignment and the role of self-confidence in medical education: A conceptual review. *Med. Educ.* **2022**, *56*, 37–47. [CrossRef] [PubMed]

Gaida, S.; Härtl, A.; Tipold, A.; Dilly, M. Communication identity in veterinary medicine: A grounded theory approach. *Vet. Rec. Open* **2018**, *5*, e000310. [CrossRef]

Hafen, M.; Drake, A.A.S.; Rush, B.R.; Nelson, S.C. Using Authentic Client Interactions in Communication Skills Training: Predictors of Proficiency. *J. Vet. Med. Educ.* **2013**, *40*, 318–326. [CrossRef] [PubMed]

Brown, C.R.; Garrett, L.D.; Gilles, W.K.; Houlihan, K.E.; McCobb, E.; Pailler, S.; Putnam, H.; Scarlett, J.L.; Treglia, L.; Watson, B.; et al. Spectrum of care: More than treatment options. *J. Am. Vet. Med. Assoc.* **2021**, *259*, 712–717. [CrossRef] [PubMed]

Fingland, R.B.; Stone, L.R.; Read, E.K.; Moore, R.M. Preparing veterinary students for excellence in general practice: Building confidence and competence by focusing on spectrum of care. *J. Am. Vet. Med. Assoc.* **2021**, *259*, 463–470. [CrossRef] [PubMed]

Stull, J.W.; Shelby, J.A.; Bonnett, B.N.; Block, G.; Budsberg, S.C.; Dean, R.S.; Dicks, M.R.; Forsgren, B.W.; Golab, G.C.; Hamil, J.A.; et al. Barriers and next Steps to Providing a Spectrum of Effective Health Care to Companion Animals. *J. Am. Vet. Med. Assoc.* **2018**, *253*, 1386–1389. [CrossRef] [PubMed]

Block, G. A new look at Ssandard of care. *J. Am. Vet. Med. Assoc.* **2018**, *252*, 1343–1344. [CrossRef]

Baguley, J. The role of final year extramural placements in the undergraduate veterinary curriculum. *Aust. Vet. J.* **2006**, *84*, 182–186. [CrossRef]

Ajjawi, R.; Tai, J.; Huu Nghia, T.L.; Boud, D.; Johnson, L.; Patrick, C.J. Aligning assessment with the needs of work-integrated learning: The challenges of authentic assessment in a complex context. *Assess. Eval. High. Educ.* **2020**, *45*, 304–316. [CrossRef]

Jevring-Bäck, C.; Bäck, E. *Managing a Veterinary Practice*, 2nd ed.; Elsevier Saunders: Edinburgh, UK, 2007.

van Gelderen, I.; Sheehy, P.; Taylor, R. From face-to-face to remote learning. Evaluating online clinical communication workshops for veterinary science students. In *INTED2021 Proceedings*; IATED: Barcelona, Spain, 2021; pp. 2867–2877.

AAVMC. Competency Based Veterinary Education: CBVE Framework, American Association of Veterinary Medical Colleges, CBVE Working Group. 2023. Available online: https://www.aavmc.org/programs/cbve/ (accessed on 3 October 2023).

Pollock, K.; Morton, C.; Spielman, S. Teaching clinical skills mastery using immersive simulation. *J. Am. Vet. Med. Assoc.* **2023**, *261*, 46. [CrossRef]

Hecker, K.G.; Adams, C.L.; Coe, J.B. Assessment of first-year veterinary students' communication skills using an objective structured clinical examination: The importance of context. *J. Vet. Med. Educ.* **2012**, *39*, 304–310. [CrossRef] [PubMed]

Maddison, J. Chapter 24, Clinical Reasoning Skills. In *Veterinary Medical Education: A Practical Guide*; Hodgson, J.L., Pelzer, J.M., Eds.; Wiley Blackwell: Hoboken, NJ, USA, 2017; pp. 380–395.

Meehan, M.P.; Menniti, M.F. Final-year veterinary students' perceptions of their communication competencies and a communication skills training program delivered in a primary care setting and based on Kolb's Experiential Learning Theory. *J. Vet. Med. Educ.* **2014**, *41*, 371–383. [CrossRef] [PubMed]

Baillie, S.; Dilly, M.; Ciappesoni, J.L.; Read, E. The Rapid and International Expansion of Veterinary Clinical Skills Laboratories: A Survey to Establish Recent Developments. *J. Vet. Med. Educ.* **2023**, e20220113. [CrossRef] [PubMed]

Dubin, R.J.; Angliss, G.; Eng, C.; Cisneros, T.; Griffon, D. Veterinarians' perceptions of COVID-19 pandemic–related influences on veterinary telehealth and on pet owners' attitudes toward cats and dogs. *J. Am. Vet. Med. Assoc.* **2021**, *259*, 1140–1147. [CrossRef]

Wells, J.; Watson, K.; Sharma, M.; Davis, R.E.; Gruszynski, K.; Robertson, S.R.; Nahar, V.K. Application of the multi-theory model to explain veterinarians' intentions to use telehealth/telemedicine. *Vet. Rec.* **2023**, *192*, e2385. [CrossRef]

Aliwi, I.; Schot, V.; Carrabba, M.; Duong, P.; Shievano, S.; Caputo, M.; Biglino, G. The role of immersive Virtual reality and augmented reality in medical communication: A scoping review. *J. Patient Exp.* **2023**, *10*, 23743735231171562. [CrossRef]

Cushing, M. What Is Telemedicine, Telehealth, and Teletriage. The Veterinary Clinics of North America. *Small Anim. Pract.* **2022**, *52*, 1069–1080. [CrossRef]

animals

Article

Conversation Analysis of Clients' Active Resistance to Veterinarians' Proposals for Long-Term Dietary Change in Companion Animal Practice in Ontario, Canada

Clare MacMartin [1,*,†], Hannah Wheat [2,†] and Jason B. Coe [3]

1 Department of Family Relations and Applied Nutrition, University of Guelph, 50 Stone Road East, Guelph, ON N1G 2W1, Canada
2 Community and Primary Care Research Group, Faculty of Health, University of Plymouth, Plymouth PL4 8AA, Devon, UK; hannah.wheat-1@plymouth.ac.uk
3 Department of Population Medicine, University of Guelph, 50 Stone Road East, Guelph, ON N1G 2W1, Canada; jcoe@uoguelph.ca
* Correspondence: cmacmart@uoguelph.ca
† These authors contributed equally to this work.

Simple Summary: Research suggests that half of all veterinary clients fail to adhere to veterinarians' dietary recommendations, which can lead to serious consequences for pet health. However, little is known about what clients' resistance to such recommendations looks like in actual talk in veterinary consultations and how veterinarians respond. The present study aimed to fill this gap by using conversation analysis to investigate clients' active resistance to veterinarians' proposals for long-term changes to cats' and dogs' diets in 23 segments from 21 videotaped appointments in Ontario, Canada. Clients responded by suggesting that the proposals themselves or the nutritional modifications were potentially unnecessary, inappropriate, or unfeasible. Justifications were most frequently based on their pets' food preferences, multi-pet feeding issues, their current use of equivalent health strategies, or their current enactment of the proposed changes. Thus, client resistance occurred when veterinarians did not first gather relevant diet- and patient-related information, solicit clients' perspectives, or educate them about the benefits of the recommended changes before proposing them. Veterinarians subsequently accommodated clients' resistance more often when barriers to adherence involved patient- or client-related issues rather than clients' lack of medical knowledge. Findings provide valuable evidence for developing effective veterinary communication training and practice guidelines in nutritional assessment and shared decision-making.

Abstract: The impact of nutrition on animal health requires effective diet-related treatment recommendations in veterinary medicine. Despite low reported rates of veterinary clients' adherence with dietary recommendations, little is known about how clients' resistance to nutritional proposals is managed in the talk of veterinary consultations. This conversation-analytic study investigated clients' active resistance to veterinarians' proposals for long-term changes to cats' and dogs' diets in 23 segments from 21 videotaped appointments in Ontario, Canada. Clients' accounts suggested the proposals themselves or nutritional modifications were unnecessary, inappropriate, or unfeasible, most often based on patients' food preferences, multi-pet feeding issues, current use of equivalent strategies, or current enactment of the proposed changes. Resistance arose when veterinarians constructed proposals without first gathering relevant diet- and patient-related information, soliciting clients' perspectives, or educating them about the benefits of recommended changes. Veterinarians subsequently accommodated clients' concerns more often when resistance involved patient- or client-related issues rather than clients' lack of medical knowledge. The design of subsequent proposals accepted by clients frequently replaced dietary changes in the initial proposals with nutritional or non-nutritional alternatives and oriented to uncertainty about adherence. This study provides evidence-based findings for developing effective communication training and practice guidelines in nutritional assessment and shared decision-making.

Keywords: adherence; communication; compliance; conversation analysis; decision-making; treatment recommendations; nutrition; qualitative analysis; veterinary education

1. Introduction

In companion animal medicine, the powerful role of nutrition in the prevention and treatment of acute and chronic diseases is well established [1–3]. Some gastrointestinal disorders and hepatopathies, along with chronic kidney disease, are diet-sensitive and hence amenable to nutrition-based treatment approaches [4]. The relationship between diet and disease is even more direct in the case of diet-induced health issues; there can be significant health problems involving contaminant ingestion, nutritional deficiencies, and the consumption of excess nutrition [4]. For example, the growing problem of overweight and obesity in cats and dogs [5–9] has been linked to early mortality and health concerns ranging from diabetes mellitus and cardiovascular diseases to osteoarthritis and hepatic lipidosis. [10,11]. It is not surprising, then, that guidelines for assessing patient nutrition in all veterinary appointments with cats and dogs have been published by the American Animal Hospital Association and the World Small Animal Veterinary Association [1,3] and that dietary management of obesity in cats and dogs has assumed a crucial role in their veterinary care [12].

Underutilization and improper utilization of therapeutic diets are longstanding, large-scale problems [13,14]. The American Animal Hospital Association published a major study [13] in 2003, reporting that, in the United States, owners of 9 million cats and 11.6 million dogs with health conditions that could benefit from therapeutic diets failed to provide such diets for their pets or did not do so for the necessary period of time. Ineffective clinician communication about nutritional recommendations in some cases and the failure to make any nutritional recommendations at all in others have been suggested as probable factors [13]. In just over half (55%) of the cases in which veterinarians recommended the use of therapeutic diets for canine and feline patients with associated health conditions, owners bought the recommended food; adherence declined further over time either because owners failed to keep purchasing the therapeutic diet or because they fed their pets additional food, thereby undermining the diet's impact [13]. Similarly, a survey study conducted in 2004 found that only 12% of cat and dog owners whose pets had been diagnosed with diseases that could be ameliorated through nutritional changes (e.g., cardiac, gastrointestinal tract/hepatic, lower urinary tract, musculoskeletal and periodontal diseases) reported feeding their pets a therapeutic diet [14]. Veterinarians need to learn to communicate more effectively with their clients about their pets' nutrition [14], primary health care practitioners play a pivotal part in assessing patient nutrition, educating clients, and supporting client adherence with sound treatment planning and decision-making in the interests of patient well-being [15–17].

Patient adherence in human medicine has been defined as "the extent to which a patient follows an agreed-on mode of treatment" ([17], p. 51). Studies of doctor–patient communication in human medicine have identified key characteristics of physicians' communicative activities that are associated with patient adherence [18–22] and positive health outcomes [23–26]. Adherence with treatment recommendations has been predicted by the quality of physicians' communication (assessed through patient and observer ratings) and training in communication skills [22]. Positive patient health outcomes have been linked with highly informative communications by physicians, the clarity of their recommendations, and a high degree of doctor–patient collaboration in treatment decision-making [24].

Although much less communication research on veterinarian–client treatment decision-making has been conducted in veterinary medicine, findings point to implications similar to those in human medicine [13,27–29]. Ineffective veterinary communication can limit client understanding of the health benefits of practitioners' treatment recommendations and can reduce clients' belief in their importance for patients [13,27,28]. Higher client adherence with medication-related treatment has been associated with the amount of time veterinarians spend with clients [28,29], written instructions and demonstrations regarding medication use [29], and follow-up calls and reminders [29].

A limitation of such research is its reliance on retrospective reporting by clients to identify the important characteristics of treatment-related communication that serve to support subsequent adherence. One study avoided this problem by studying recordings of actual veterinary communication [30]. Variables from the Roter interaction system (RIAS) adapted for the study of veterinarian–client–patient interaction were used to code videotaped interactions involving surgery and dentistry recommendations during companion animal consultations to determine which variables might predict subsequent adherence (measured by information kept in clinic medical files) and client satisfaction (captured in a post-consultation questionnaire) [30]. While overall client adherence was only 30%, it was associated with longer visits, more frequent positive statements by veterinarians toward clients, more sympathetic/empathetic and non-rushed/non-hurried communication by veterinarians, higher proportions of client-centred talk, and higher client satisfaction ratings [30]. Another factor strongly predictive of client adherence in the study was the clarity of veterinarians' treatment recommendations (as assessed by the researchers); clear recommendations for surgical and dental procedures were seven times more likely to result in client adherence than were ambiguous recommendations [30].

The RIAS study [30] is laudatory in its investigation of actual talk rather than relying on informants' retrospective reporting of prior treatment discussions. However, the generation of composite variables in the RIAS framework necessarily removed information about the possible impact of sequential context on treatment decisions. An inspection of the details that might have been implicated in later adherence (e.g., how the recommendations were specifically designed, how clients responded, and how veterinarians took up clients' responses) was not possible using this method. Hence, little is known about how treatment discussions, including those related to patient nutrition, unfold turn-by-turn as veterinarians and clients interact with each other.

But such features may be crucial. The 2009 follow-up study [28] to the 2003 American Animal Hospital compliance study [13] suggested that there had been a fundamental misunderstanding among veterinary healthcare providers in the earlier study; "doctors and staff alike confused telling clients what to do with having the client *accept* the recommendation and follow through on it" ([28], p. 16, emphasis added). Furthermore, in her discussion of adherence in veterinary medicine, Abood [17] emphasized that the mode of treatment followed must be something previously agreed upon by both the client and clinician. But how is veterinarian–client agreement or disagreement co-constructed in actual treatment discussions, including those about dietary modification? What do verbal displays of client resistance to veterinarians' nutritional recommendations look like and on what grounds do clients resist such recommendations? How do veterinarians respond to client resistance, and how do these responses and ensuing interactions between veterinarians and clients shape the ultimate trajectory of diet discussions and resulting treatment plans? Knowledge about real-life verbal interactions between veterinarians and clients, including nutrition discussions and their outcomes, can be a tool in the development of evidence-based, effective communication curricula in veterinary medical education and sound guidelines for clinical practice by current professionals.

Conversation analysis is a form of qualitative research that can answer the above questions. It has long been employed to investigate healthcare practitioner–patient interactions in human medicine [31], including treatment recommendations [32–42] and healthcare advice-giving [43–46]. For example, conversation analysis of physician–patient interactions has demonstrated a pattern of maximizing agreement and minimizing disagreement between physicians and patients in the negotiation of treatment recommendations; a patient withholding a response for two seconds after the physician's treatment proposal or a patient's weak acceptance can result in the physician immediately revising the nature of the proposal in subsequent turns to elicit patient agreement [31,47]. Nonadherence in human medicine has been studied by conversation analysts who examine the interactional phenomenon of active resistance where patients question, challenge, or otherwise reject medical recommendations [36,38,39,41,42]. Because clinicians and patients have been shown to orient closely to each other's contributions in ways that shape the emerging treatment discussion, treatment recommendations are not viewed by conversation analysts as actions attributable to physicians alone at one point in a sequence of talk but rather as joint social action, involving both physician and patient, unfolding over time in multiple turns [36,40,47]. Increasingly, conversation analysis has been applied to the study of veterinary communication in companion animal practice [48–52], most recently in the areas of dietary history-taking [51] and nutritional recommendations [52].

The present study is part of a larger project that employed conversation analysis to study veterinarian–client interactions in the negotiation of veterinarian-initiated long-term changes to cats' and dogs' diets in companion animal clinics in Ontario, Canada [52]. We adopted a broad definition of the phenomenon under study in that we investigated not only instances of clear advice on a single preferred course of action recommended by the clinician, but also proposals that discussed multiple options. In a previous publication [52], we reported on the linguistic design of the nutritional proposals initiated by veterinarians, the types of changes proposed, and the health concerns targeted, along with the phases of the visits during which the proposals were introduced.

Very few proposals (4%) took the conventional form of "I would recommend ... "; the most frequent designs (25%) involved descriptions of options, actions, or foods (e.g., "There are also special diets .... .") [52]. The prescriptiveness of the proposals was often reduced through various grammatical and lexical features such as the use of modals (e.g., "may"; "might"), qualifying adverbs (e.g., "maybe"), and verbs that were oriented to attempting a food change (e.g., "try") or to merely considering one (e.g., "One thing you may wanna consider ... ") [52]. Thus, veterinarians mitigated their own authority to impose nutritional changes on clients and patients; by reducing the certainty with which adherence with proposed changes could be presumed, veterinarians' proposals implicitly or explicitly oriented to various contingencies that could affect adherence [52]. Veterinarians mentioned multiple product options for clients when proposing nutritional changes requiring the purchase of new food, rather than promoting veterinarian-only therapeutic diets exclusively [52].

The present study builds on those findings by reporting on one strand of our analyses of clients' responses to veterinarians' initial proposals for longer-term dietary change: clients' displays of active resistance to veterinarians' proposals. Because of the potential health consequences for patients of nonadherence to veterinarians' dietary proposals, we analyzed the sequential organization and linguistic design of such responses. Specifically, we investigated how clients disaffiliated with (i.e., resisted) veterinarians' proposals, the grounds on which clients justified their potential nonadherence with proposed nutritional modifications, and what happened subsequently. That is, we also investigated veterinarians' responses to client resistance and the unfolding trajectories and outcomes of the resulting veterinarian–client discussions.

2. Materials and Methods

2.1. Data Archive

The data used in the present study were drawn from a set of 350 videotaped appointments collected in 2006 involving 20 veterinarians and their clients in clinics in 14 counties in Ontario, Canada for quantitative research on veterinarian–client–patient communication [53]. Details about the design of the original study have been previously provided [53]. Seventeen of the 20 clinicians and their clients consented to the archiving and use of their videotapes (284 consultations in total) for subsequent secondary research, approved by the University of Guelph Research Ethics Board (see Figure 1).

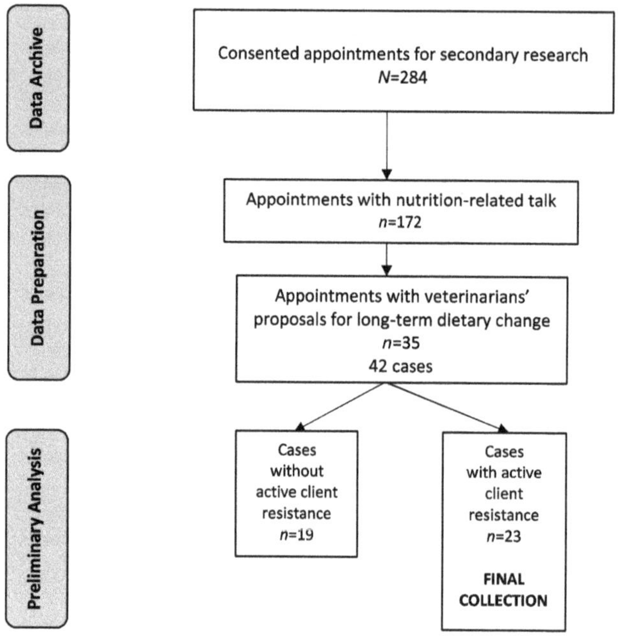

Figure 1. Data preparation, preliminary analyses and development of final collection of cases of active client resistance to veterinarians' proposals for long-term dietary change.

2.2. Data Preparation

Creation of the collection of segments containing clients' active resistance to veterinarians' proposals for long-term nutritional change began with a screening of the 284 consented visits available for secondary data analysis (Figure 1) to flag only those in which veterinarians and clients talked about patient diet. We identified 172 such appointments (Figure 1). These appointments comprised 61% of the consented archive available for analysis. Basic orthographic (i.e., word-for-word) transcription was performed on all diet-related talk. Pseudonyms for the proper names of geographic locations, people, and pets were used to anonymize the data.

Long-term nutritional modifications to patients' diets were discussed in 55 (32%) of the 172 visits containing nutritional talk (Figure 1). Long-term dietary changes were selected as the focus of analysis of client resistance because of the significant impact long-term nutritional modifications could have on patient health. Proposed changes variously involved the addition or replacement of current main foods or treats and/or the cessation of current favoured foods and treats (including cow's milk), details of which have been provided elsewhere [52].

Proposals initiated by veterinarians rather than clients were chosen for conversation analysis because of the possible challenges for clinicians in proposing such alterations and the need to initiate such recommendations to support patient health [52]. Among the 55 appointments containing long-term dietary proposals, 35 (64%) involved veterinarians initiating the proposals rather than clients (Figure 1). Transcripts of dietary discussions in the 35 appointments were used to identify 42 discrete segments in which veterinarians proposed to clients some type of long-term alteration to patients' diets (Figure 1). There were more segments than appointments because some appointments contained multiple kinds of nutritional proposals. The 42 segments included a broad spectrum of proposals. These ranged from recognizable recommendations or suggestions to adopt a singular course of action calling for client acceptance or rejection (e.g., "So she should be getting onto … "; "I would recommend definitely trying to ... "; "we could put him on ... ") to descriptions of diets or nutritional options possibly hearable by clients as merely information-sharing [52].

2.3. Characteristics of Appointments Containing Veterinarian-Proposed Long-Term Dietary Change

In the collection of 35 appointments in which veterinarians proposed long-term nutritional modifications, 15 (88%) of the original 17 practitioners in the consented archive were retained (10 women and five men). The median length of time in veterinary practice was 10 years (range, 2 to 25); 14 of the veterinarians practiced in clinics in which two or more veterinarians worked. Of the 15 clinics included in the present study, seven were in urban areas, five in suburban areas, and three in rural areas. In 18 (51%) of the 35 appointments, patients were dogs and in 17 (49%) appointments, patients were cats. Regarding the type of appointment, 25 (71%) of the 35 were wellness visits, nine (26%) were problem visits, and one (3%) was a follow-up visit. Wellness visits were regular appointments scheduled for routine and preventative care of apparently healthy patients, while problem visits involved special appointments scheduled to address injury or illness in sick patients.

2.4. Analytic Method: Conversation Analysis

Conversation analysis involves the qualitative study of audio and video recordings of naturally occurring conversations along with extremely detailed, specially notated transcripts of those recordings to identify the social actions that are being performed [54].

Language and social interaction have been shown to be deeply ordered in nature; the study of patterns of interaction between speakers across a sequence of turns taken by different speakers during a conversation is the typical focus of conversation-analytic research [55–58], including the present study.

In line with the methodological procedures of conversation analysis, for a past study [52] and the present one, we repeatedly listened to and observed the videotaped dietary proposal segments [55–58], further refining the word-for-word transcripts using special transcription notation [59,60] that captured features like overlaps during which more than one person was speaking, gaps between stretches of talk, shifts in speech volume and speed, and changes in vocal intonation. Additional information about nonverbal activities (e.g., head nods, eye gaze) was also incorporated on the transcripts as potentially consequential for the investigation of client resistance.

Conversation analysis has identified a basic sequence in interaction called an *adjacency pair* [60] whereby a first turn taken by one speaker (the *first pair part*) expects a particular sort of responsive action in the form of a second turn by another speaker (the *second pair part*) [61]. An easily recognizable type of adjacency pair involves a question–answer sequence whereby, for example, a veterinarian's question to a client about the contents of a pet's diet expects an answer to that question [51]. If an answer is not forthcoming, the smooth progression (or *progressivity*) of the conversation is threatened [61]. Similarly, a medical treatment recommendation is the first pair part in an adjacency pair sequence calling for the patient to accept or reject (the second pair part) the recommendation; if a patient fails to accept or reject the recommendation, the physician may modify the recommendation, provide justifications for it, and/or otherwise pursue acceptance from the patient [31].

A crucial concept in the analysis of adjacency pair sequences in the present study involves *preference* [62], whereby a recipient of a recommendation or proposal tends to minimize overt rejection of the proposal as demonstrated in the sequential structure and the design of their response [61,62]. It is important to note that "preference" refers not to individual internal preferences, but rather to principles that are culturally shared and observable in action by examining orderly patterns of talk in line with those principles [62]. Thus, although a recipient of a proposal can either accept or reject it, the two types of responses are non-equivalent; the preferred response to a proposal is acceptance and the dispreferred response is rejection [61]. Preferred responses tend to be delivered more rapidly than dispreferred responses and are typically shorter and less elaborated in design than are dispreferred responses, which are often delayed and accompanied by accounts [61].

Two additional important conversation-analytic concepts informing the present study are the domains of *epistemics* [63] and *deontics* [64]. "Epistemics" refers to the "distribution of rights and responsibilities regarding what participants can accountably know, how they know it, [and] whether they have rights to describe it" ([63], p. 16). "Deontics" refers to "the right to determine others' future actions" ([64], p. 297). Parallel to descriptions of human medical encounters [42], veterinarians' epistemic primacy is grounded in their expert medical knowledge, including the ability to interpret clinical signs in their patients, to diagnose, and to know what tests and treatments could be helpful; their deontic authority is based on their rights to make treatment recommendations, such as dietary modifications, and to prescribe and dispense drugs, the latter involving legal control. Clients' epistemic primacy is based on knowledge of their own preferences, of patients' preferences and experiences, including patients' illnesses, and on their own perceptions of medical aspects such as diagnoses and nutrition. Similar to the agency that parents exercise regarding their children as patients in pediatric medicine [42], veterinary clients' deontic authority is grounded in their right to make healthcare decisions on behalf of animal patients, including whether to agree to certain tests, to fill out and administer prescription drugs, and to purchase food items and feed patients. The deontic authority of clients' access to nutritional resources is thus somewhat different than that involving access to prescription medications, which are regulated and can legally be obtained only from veterinarians.

It is important to note that epistemic primacy and deontic authority are not exercised in a static manner; conversation analysts differentiate between *status*, which refers to the enduring elements of knowledge and agency participants possess, and *stance*, by which a participant's expressions of knowledge and agency in conversation can vary from moment to moment [65,66]. For example, although a veterinarian demonstrates their deontic authority in announcing a treatment recommendation, such as switching to a therapeutic diet, the way they design such a recommendation for a client may invoke a stance that downgrades their own authority to impose such a change (e.g., "You may wanna consider ... " [52].

We studied both the position [61,67] and composition [68] of veterinarians' and clients' turns at talk in those segments in which veterinarians proposed long-term changes to patients' diets. Drawing on previous conversation-analytic work on the negotiation of treatment proposals in human medicine [32–47], including research on patient resistance [34–36,38,39,41,42], we analyzed clients' responses to veterinarians' proposals in terms of the timing, grammatical design, and wording of clients' responses with a particular focus on cases of clients' active resistance towards veterinarians' dietary proposals and how veterinarians responded to client resistance. In order to determine the final outcomes of dietary decision-making, we also reviewed subsequent portions of the relevant videotaped visits and transcripts for any further veterinarian–client interactions relevant to the dietary proposals and/or alternative non-nutritional strategies.

2.5. *Identification and Categorization of Clients' Responses*

To finalize the collection of active resistance cases as the phenomenon of interest for the present study, we first needed to exhaustively identify and categorize all types of clients' responses to veterinarians' proposals. Within the 42 segments involving veterinarian-initiated proposals for long-term dietary change, varying types of client responses following the proposals were identified. Sometimes, more than one type of response occurred in the same proposal segment. Clients were variously found to accept the proposals; withhold acceptance of them in a display of passive resistance by offering acknowledgment tokens, head nods, or continuers like "Mm hm" that enact a listener stance [36,43]; remain silent/fail to take up a proposal with a nutrition-related response; and/or demonstrate active resistance to the proposals, sometimes after initially accepting or withholding acceptance of a previously uttered proposal (see [35,41]).

In order to arrive at a final collection of active resistance cases, once the various types of client responses had been identified, we dichotomized segments and appointments in terms of whether they did or did not contain active resistance by clients (Figure 1). Drawing on definitions of patients' active resistance in conversation-analytic research in human medicine, e.g., [35,36,41], active resistance in the present study was defined as lexical content introduced by a client in the form of a question or comment that implicitly or explicitly provided an account for the possible non-acceptance of the proposal. We also investigated the characteristics of those appointments containing active client resistance and compared them with the characteristics of those appointments containing no active resistance. The aim was to gather as much contextually relevant information as possible because of the important implications of active resistance for the phenomenon of nonadherence. Similarly, so as to situate active resistance in the broader context of the range of possible client responses to a veterinarian's proposal, a brief description is provided below of the preliminary analyses of clients' responses in those segments lacking active resistance.

2.5.1. Cases without Active Client Resistance

In the total set of 42 proposal segments, 19 (45%) of cases contained no instances of active resistance (Figure 1). Response types included acceptance of the proposal, passive resistance/withholding of acceptance, no response, and one ambiguous response. For instances to be classifiable as client acceptance cases, the proposals needed to have been unequivocally designed as veterinarians' recommendations or suggestions calling for client acceptance or declination (e.g., "And she should be on a large breed puppy food").

In 16 of these 19 cases, there was client acceptance of the proposals. In line with the notion of preference, acceptances were typically delivered without delay in the simple form of the response token "Okay," intoned with falling pitch; this accords with the analysis of patient acceptance of treatment recommendations in human medicine [34–36,40,47]. Among the 16 acceptance cases, 14 involved early client acceptance of the proposals, coming promptly on the heels of the veterinarians' proposal turns. In two segments, there was delayed client acceptance because of constraints imposed by the linguistic design of veterinarians' initial proposals. They were formatted as complex turns that did not provide a clear opportunity for the clients to respond and did not otherwise clearly expect initial client acceptance or declination because the proposal turns ended with only information-sharing by the veterinarian. In those two cases, the veterinarians treated client acceptance of their initial dietary proposals as due by pursuing (and ultimately receiving) client acceptance through the subsequent re-issuing of their proposals.

Three of the 19 cases lacking active resistance contained client responses other than acceptances. In one of these segments, signs of passive resistance to the dietary proposal were demonstrated by one of two clients attending a problem visit involving a dog with a cut paw. Passive resistance in conversation-analytic work in human healthcare encounters can involve silence and/or unmarked acknowledgment tokens (e.g., "Mm hm") following the clinician's health advice [43] or treatment recommendation. [36]. In another case, the client failed to respond to the veterinarian's dietary proposal which had been uttered during other medical activities involving a client's competing serious concern about the patient. The final segment was a case in which the veterinarian's complex dietary proposal was designed in such a way that the status of the client's response as acceptance was ambiguous.

2.5.2. Cases with Active Client Resistance

The collection of 42 proposal segments included 23 (55%) segments (Figure 1) containing one or more instances of active resistance by clients in the form of asking questions or making statements that explicitly suggested various grounds for potential disaffiliation with the dietary proposals. A range of response types was identified in the 23 segments, such that some of the segments containing active client resistance opened with early acceptance or passive resistance to veterinarian's dietary proposals before active resistance was displayed.

3. Results

3.1. Characteristics of Appointments with/without Active Client Resistance

In order to explore whether the prevalence of clients' active resistance varied depending on patient species and type of appointment, we drew on counts for those characteristics generated for our earlier study [52] (see Table 1). The number of appointments exceeds 35 because three appointments each contained two proposals, one of which elicited no active resistance and one of which elicited active resistance. Due to the unequal numbers of appointments associated with the presence versus absence of active resistance, prevalence figures are reported below as percentages to aid in making comparisons.

Table 1. Characteristics of appointments (patient species and type of appointment) based on presence or absence of active resistance in clients' responses to veterinarians' proposals for long-term dietary change.

	No. (%) of Appointments with and without Active Resistance		
Characteristics	**Active Resistance** n **= 21 (60%)**	**No Active Resistance** n **= 17 (49%)**	**Total** n **= 35**
Patient Species			
Cat	13 (62)	6 (35)	17 (49)
Dog	8 (38)	11 (65)	18 (51)
Appointment Type			
Wellness	14 (66.7)	14 (82.3)	25 (71)
Problem	6 (28.6)	3 (17.7)	9 (26)
Follow-Up	1 (4.8)	0 (0)	1 (3)

When we compared the proportions of appointment characteristics across the two sets of client response categories, there were some noteworthy differences (Table 1). Compared to the relatively even percentages of species in the overall collection of 35 appointments, in the 21 visits containing active resistance, cats were over-represented and dogs were under-represented. Conversely, in the 17 appointments in which clients displayed no active resistance, dogs were over-represented and cats under-represented. In terms of visit type in the overall collection of 35 appointments, frequencies were skewed, with more wellness than problem visits. When appointments containing active resistance cases were examined, the proportions between wellness and problem visits were slightly less skewed than in the overall collection and more skewed than in appointments lacking active client resistance. Cases with active client resistance tended to feature proportionally more cats and more problem visits than cases without active resistance (Table 1).

3.2. Analysis of Clients' Active Resistance

3.2.1. Key Features

Conversation analyses demonstrated that the display of clients' active resistance was a complex, subtle interactional phenomenon. None of the actively resisting responses involved strongly oppositional, blatant rejections of veterinarians' proposals. In accord with the conversation-analytic principle of preference, whereby recipients' rejections of interlocutors' proposals tend to be done as *dispreferred turn shapes* [69], clients' active resistance of veterinarians' proposals for long-term dietary modification was typically delayed and mitigated, sometimes dysfluent in its delivery, and consisted of or was often accompanied by elaborated accounts providing reasons for the possible or probable rejection of the proposals. Thus, active resistance did not position clients as uncooperative towards veterinarians' advice in a blatant fashion. Indeed, some multi-unit turns in which clients demonstrated receptivity to veterinarians' nutritional expertise (e.g., asking an advice-seeking question, accepting an offer of written information about a recommended prescription diet) were the same ones in which clients showed active resistance by orienting to possible barriers to successful adherence (e.g., Extract 5.1 below).

As mentioned previously, in non-resistance cases containing client acceptance, veterinarians' dietary proposals needed to be linguistically designed as clear recommendations or suggestions for client responses to be unequivocally classified as acceptance. In contrast, client active resistance could come after clearly recognizable recommendations (e.g., "I would recommend you get him on at least partly canned food") or more tentative utterances that were merely descriptive statements (e.g., "There are some excellent diets available for dogs ... ") or evaluations (e.g., "One thing that's really easy to do is ... actually feeding a dental diet"; Extract 2.1 below). Clients oriented to veterinarians' descriptions and evaluations as projecting future recommendations to change their pets' diets by disclosing potential or actual obstacles to acceptance of the anticipated proposals. Veterinarians could thus test client receptivity to the possibility of dietary change without having to manage the interactional consequences of client disaffiliation with a canonical recommendation [52]. This was yet another manifestation in our corpus of the conversational preference for minimizing disagreement.

As will be seen in the analysis of illustrative extracts below, client active resistance sometimes occurred after a display of initial acceptance (e.g., Extract 4.1) or passive resistance (e.g., Extract 3.1). In terms of how active resistance was demonstrated, clients asked questions or offered comments that flagged why the proposal or its adoption might be problematic in some way, proposed alternative actions that deviated from those recommended by the veterinarian, and/or shared information that provided accounts as to why the proposal was unnecessary or why the dietary change itself was irrelevant, ill-advised, or unfeasible. Because of the importance of such accounts in clinical understandings of nonadherence, we engaged in close investigation of the types and frequencies of the different grounds that clients gave for resisting veterinarians' initial proposals for long-term nutritional change and the sequential environments in which they occurred.

3.2.2. Grounds for Clients' Active Resistance

Table 2 shows the types and prevalence of different categories of active resistance and examples of client utterances for each category in relation to the nutritional changes veterinarians had proposed. Across the 23 segments in which client active resistance was identified, there were 31 discrete client mentions of different bases for resisting long-term dietary change. The frequency of displays of active resistance was greater than the number of segments because in some segments clients oriented to more than one reason for possible nonadherence (e.g., Extracts 2.1 and 3.1; Table 2, Examples 2, 11). We identified a total of 11 categories of client-identified issues to which active resistance was tied. The four most frequent bases for possible nonadherence were as follows: the patient's food preferences and/or dispreferences (7/31; 22.58%); multi-pet feeding management issues of various kinds (6/31; 19.35%); current use of an alternative strategy to address the health concern motivating the dietary proposal (5/31; 16.13%); and current utilization of the proposed diet (3/31; 9.68%) (Table 2).

Table 2. Grounds on which clients actively resisted veterinarians' proposals for long-term dietary change, including prevalence and examples of client responses.

Grounds for Resistance	No. (%)	Example	Dietary Change Proposed in Example
A. Patient food preference or dispreference re. current or proposed diet (CHANGE NOT FEASIBLE)	7 (22.58)	*1. What do you use? What are you suggesting then, something they'll eat?* *2. Cuz she's asking all the time for cookies.*	Introduce dental food Replace high fat treats with baby carrots
B. Multi-pet feeding issues (food preference or dispreference of other pets, food competition, negative health consequences for other pets) (CHANGE NOT FEASIBLE)	6 (19.35)	*3. That's why yeah it's hard when for when there's three.* *4. Well cuz she seems hungry and asks for food.*	Reduce amount of dry food, increase in canned for only certain pet in multi-pet home Switch to light formulation for only certain pets in multi-pet home
C. Current enactment of other strategies to address health concern (CHANGE NOT NECESSARY)	5 (16.13)	*5. We try ta give em like tartar control treats and stuff like that as well.*	Introduce dental food
D. Current enactment of proposed dietary change (PROPOSAL NOT NECESSARY)	3 (9.68)	*6. Yeah I know. Actually I have her on that so.*	Switch to senior formulation
E. Concern about inducing new medical problem or worsening current comorbid condition (CHANGE INAPPROPRIATE)	2 (6.45)	*7. Oh yer kidding. I thought canned food was bad.*	Introduce canned food
F. Questioning of etiological role of current food in patient medical condition (CHANGE INAPPROPRIATE)	2 (6.45)	*8. I don't think that sticks to the teeth as much, do you think?*	Eliminate canned food
G. Cost of proposed food (CHANGE NOT FEASIBLE)	2 (6.45)	*9. How about a price comparison between the {Current Brand Name} and yours?*	Switch to higher-quality diet
H. Side effects of food change in patient that would be aversive for client (CHANGE NOT FEASIBLE)	1 (3.23)	*10. When I change anything her gas is awful.*	Introduce dental food
I. Client preference for or emotional attachment to current food (CHANGE NOT FEASIBLE)	1 (3.23)	*11. So if I wanna give out cookies what I'm gonna do?*	Replace high fat treats with baby carrots
J. Client lack of familiarity with proposed food (CHANGE NOT FEASIBLE)	1 (3.23)	*12. I'm not sure what the ones that yer talking about look like.*	Introduce dental food
K. Feeding information on current food packaging in conflict with proposed food change (CHANGE INAPPROPRIATE)	1 (3.23)	*13. Okay. We'll finish this bag and she'll go on adult food.*	Switch from puppy to adult formulation
Total	31 (100%)		

The different types of warrants for nonadherence can be conceptualized broadly in terms of whether they constructed the proposal as unnecessary or the nutritional modification as unnecessary, inappropriate, or impracticable. First, clients sometimes oriented to the proposal itself as unnecessary by reporting that they were already enacting the proposed regimen (e.g., Extract 1.1; Table 2, Example 6) or using another practice to address the identified health problem (Extract 2.1; Table 2, Example 5). In such cases, clients affiliated with the premise that the patient health concern identified by the veterinarian called for action but disaffiliated with the associated inference that such a strategy was not already in place.

Second, in other cases, the client's resisting turn made available an inference that the dietary intervention was not relevant. This resistance was warranted in various ways. In two cases, clients questioned the veterinarian's stance that the current food was likely contributing to the patient's health problem (Table 2, Example 8). In Extract 3.1 below, a client challenges the veterinarian's hypothesis that a food allergy might be contributing to the patient's recurrent ear infections. In Extract 4.1 below, the client accepts that the dietary change is ultimately called for but justifies a delay in enacting the recommended food change by invoking expert information conflicting with the veterinarian's proposal.

Third, other instances of client resistance suggested that the dietary change was not appropriate due to the presence or risk of additional health problems different from those triggering the proposal. Resistance was predicated on the basis that other medical conditions could be created or current ones could be exacerbated, if the dietary change were to occur.

Sometimes the conflicting health issues were confined to a single patient and involved current comorbid medical conditions or the possible advent of a new, additional health concern if the food change targeting the identified health concern were to be adopted (Table 2, Example 7). In other instances, the competing health concern was associated with multi-pet feeding involving two or more pets (e.g., Extract 2.1). Active resistance oriented to the dangers of excess or inadequate nutrition (or both) associated with the proposed dietary modification. Such instances were situated explicitly or implicitly in the context of free feeding and/or shared feeding practices in multi-pet households. Clients' accounts sometimes referenced food competition and differential feeding behaviors across pets in a household (e.g., intermittent feeding or "grazing" in one pet and rapid ingestion of an entire serving in another).

Fourth, dietary changes were sometimes resisted through client-generated accounts as to why it may not be feasible to enact the nutritional modifications despite their medical appropriateness. Clients described potential obstacles to adherence that were patient-based, client-based, or both. Patient-based accounts variously focused on pet preference for the currently favoured (to-be-eliminated) food (e.g., Extract 5.1; Table 2, Example 2) and/or dispreference for the proposed food (e.g., Extract 2.1; Table 2, Example 1); these accounts involved patients present in the consultation (Table 2, Example 1) or absent pets not part of the current visit (e.g., Extract 2.1). Dispreference-based accounts drew on specific past experiences with the proposed food or on a more general history of pet rejection of novel food items. In cases involving the proposed elimination of a favoured food, concerns about patient deprivation were sometimes raised (Table 2, Example 4). Other cases invoked multi-pet feeding management issues in the form of "dose"-related challenges: The successful implementation of the recommended nutritional change for a particular pet was characterized as uncertain or unlikely because of the difficulty in ensuring that this pet would actually follow a proposed regimen, such as reducing intake of dry food and increasing intake of canned food to manage weight in one patient in a multi-pet household (Table 2, Example 3).

Assorted client-based barriers were described. In two cases, active resistance was conveyed through clients asking questions or making comments that oriented to the possible high cost of proposed foods (e.g., Extract 5.1; Table 2, Example 9). In another case, the client appealed to the veterinarian by projecting a loss of personal enjoyment should the hedonic feeding of a favourite treat to the patient be stopped (Table 2, Example 11). In a different case, resistance involved patient side effects described as aversive for the client (i.e., a history of patient flatulence associated with past food changes) (Table 2, Example 10). In a final case, the client told the veterinarian they lacked knowledge about the proposed food (Table 2, Example 12).

3.2.3. Example Analyses of Clients' Active Resistance

Conversation analysis and its close attention to sequential organization showed these veterinarians' proposals for long-term dietary change to be interactionally problematic. That is, the proposals were ill-fitted by definition in having produced clients' dispreferred responses and accounts justifying non-acceptance. Our analyses provided important clues as to how veterinarians' proposals might have been optimized and active client resistance potentially avoided or at least attenuated had certain topics of discussion between veterinarians and clients been introduced earlier and permitted to shape the ensuing conversation, including treatment decision-making.

In this section, examples of analyses of veterinarian–client interactions featuring cases of client active resistance are provided. Presentation of the data in the form of extracts of transcripts is included as an inherent part of the validation process in conversation analysis. As experienced conversationalists, readers are invited to verify analytic claims by inspecting relevant features of excerpted portions of transcripts in which analytic claims are inductively grounded.

For ease of reader comprehension, the number of transcription symbols displayed has been reduced. Initials at the left margin are used to identify the veterinarian (V), the client (C), and the patient (P) where appropriate. Single parentheses are placed around words that were not clearly audible and hence are best guesses as to what was said. Nonverbal activities and other information (e.g., when the patient is the recipient of a particular turn at talk) are indicated through the use of italicized words inside double parentheses. The onset of overlapping talk involving two speakers is represented by the use of square brackets. Curly brackets are used to anonymize a brand, product, or parent company name. The length of pauses or gaps in talk is captured through numerals to the tenth of a second, enclosed in single parentheses. Underlining demonstrates particular stress placed on a word or syllable, and extra letters signify the elongation of a word or syllable (sound stretching). Equal signs demonstrate latching, when there is no gap between individual words in a turn or between different turns at talk. The use of a question mark indicates rising pitch and a period following a syllable or word indicates falling intonation (final pitch). Degree signs around a word or syllable show that this talk is noticeably quieter than the surrounding talk. Bold font signals those stretches of clients' talk constituting active resistance and/or reasons given for resisting veterinarians' proposals to modify patients' diets.

In Case 1, the client resists the dietary proposal on the grounds that she is already feeding the recommended diet. Extract 1.1 shows initial passive client resistance followed by active resistance. This wellness visit involves a 13-year old female dog diagnosed with arthritis. Prior to the extract below, the client reported to the veterinarian that the patient was very stiff with arthritis. The veterinarian discussed arthritis medications and the client expressed an interest in trying an arthritis medication to see if it would help the patient's mobility. The extract begins with the veterinarian announcing the results of the weigh-in of the patient (line 1).

Extract 1.1.

```
V: Uh she's ninety-one pounds but that's [exactly
C:                                       [Okay
V: what she she's exactly what she was last year=
C: =(Yeaaaah.)
   I thought she was.  Yeaah.=
V: =And [and that's
C:      [Yeah.
V: that's good.  I mean
C: [(Yeah.)
V: [One of the problems that we do run into
   with arthritic dogs is that because they exercise less
   they tend to gain weight.
C: Mm hm=
V: =And every extra pound that they're they're weighing
   is more pressure
C: [Yeah.
V: [on those arthritic joints.
   So.
C: Yeah.
V: You know i i uh just mentally
   you should make a note of that and say you know=
C: =Mm hm.
V: Maybe she doesn't need as much food as she used to.
C: Mm hm.
V: Or maybe it's time to switch to a senior food
   or a light food
C: [Yeaah.
V: [°It probably makes° it probably is time to switch
   to a senior food
C: Yeaah.  [she is
V:         [You know if she's [thirteen years old.
C:                            [Yeah.
V: Yeah it's about time.  (Is it about time?)  ((to P))
C: Yeah I know.  I actually have her on that sooo
```

Of analytic import is the design of the veterinarian's turn on lines 1 and 3. Using the contrastive conjunction "but," the weight announcement is tied to the subsequent statement, "but she's exactly what she was last year." "But" serves to somewhat downgrade the newsworthiness of the weight announcement; it also packages "ninety-one pounds" in the reassuring context of ongoing weight maintenance rather than as new weight gain. This move is perceived as a bit of a mixed message; in presenting patient weight as requiring such reassurance, the veterinarian's comments make available an inference that the patient's weight is problematic in some way.

On line 2, the client's "Okay" response acknowledges the information about the patient's current weight as identical to last year's. The client's comment, "I thought she was," and affiliative "Yeaaaaah" (line 5) orient the information as positive and position the client as a pet owner who has been successfully monitoring and maintaining the dog's weight over the past year. That the lack of change is laudatory is indicated by the veterinarian's subsequent positive assessment ("that's good," line 8), with which the client agrees (line 9); however, the veterinarian's "I mean" (line 8) signposts a possible adjustment to this positive evaluation [70]. This comes in the form of expert information-sharing warning about the increasing risk of weight gain in arthritic dogs due to their restricted mobility (lines 10–12) and the subsequent negative effect on their diseased joints (lines 14, 15, 17). "So" (line 18) projects the veterinarian's subsequent delivery of the upshot of this health risk [71] in the form of a mitigated recommendation that the client consider reducing the patient's food intake: "You should make a note of that and say you know maybe she doesn't need as much food as she used to" (lines 21, 23).

On line 24, instead of uttering "Okay," which in this slot would perform the acceptance of the recommendation, the client responds with "Mm hm"; this constitutes passive resistance in its dual function as an acknowledgment token and continuer supporting the veterinarian's continuing possession of the conversational floor [72]. In the absence of the client's acceptance of the recommendation, the veterinarian issues a different proposal, this one involving a change in food choice to either a senior or light formulation (lines 25, 26). The "or" preface at the start of line 25 latches this multi-alternative proposal to the prior, rejected proposal, packaging all three recommendations as options. This design downgrades the prescriptiveness of the deontic stance of the veterinarian and simultaneously minimizes the appearance of client disagreement by obfuscating the client's lack of affiliation with the veterinarian's prior suggestion to reduce food intake.

Of analytic interest in this extract are the client's "Yeah" turns, uttered with final pitch (lines 16, 19, 27) as response tokens during the veterinarian's description of the health risks and associated dietary proposals. While these tokens enact the listener role of the client in acknowledging the information carried by the veterinarian's contributions and acting as continuers supporting the veterinarian's ongoing role as speaker, "Yeah" uttered with falling intonation is more oriented to the potential speakership of its user and the level of her involvement in the conversation than "Mm hm" would be in those slots [72]; the implication is that the client may well have something substantial to add to the discussion. The client's "Yeah" (line 27) overlaps with the veterinarian's proposal (the line to switch the patient to a senior formulation; lines 28, 29). The "yeah" preface on line 30 begins what is perceived as the start of the client's actively resisting utterance. It is self-aborted, dropping out after "she is" is spoken in overlap with the veterinarian's justification for changing to a senior formulation on the basis of patient age (line 31).

After the veterinarian recycles part of the proposal, seemingly while addressing the patient (line 33), the client finally produces and completes the actively resistant turn in the clear: "Yeah I know. I actually have her on it that" (line 34); "I know" treats the proposal and the reasoning accompanying it as unnecessary by underscoring the epistemic stance of the client as knowledgeable about the health risks to the patient and of the appropriate remedy; "actually" indexes the client's resisting utterance as a *counter-informing* [73] that corrects the veterinarian's preceding presupposition that the client was not feeding the patient a senior formulation. At issue here are the client's epistemic primacy regarding intimate knowledge of the current feeding practices for this pet and the veterinarian's corresponding lack of knowledge.

Extract 2.1 depicts Case 2 in which a client actively resists the dietary proposal on multiple grounds: that the patient has previously rejected the recommended food; that another pet in the home is at risk of developing health problems were the food to be re-introduced; and that the client is using an alternative strategy to address the health problem the proposed dietary change was intended to address. The client displays passive resistance and then active resistance to the veterinarian's proposal. The extract is taken from a wellness appointment with a male cat. Prior to the extract, the veterinarian informed the client after the oral examination that there was tartar on the patient's teeth, discussing dental scaling first and then the idea of training the patient to have his teeth wiped or brushed as a means of slowing down tartar build-up and delaying the need for the dental procedure. The client laughed and said "Good luck," invoking patient noncompliance to resist the veterinarian's proposal to brush the patient's teeth.

Extract 2.1.

1 V: Uh one thing that's really easy ta do
2 (0.5)
3 not as effective is is actually feeding a dental diet.
4 (0.2)
5 C: Hmm *((Nods head))*
7 V: A dental [diet's
8 C: **[I did give it to him but he um**
9 **[he**
10 V: [He didn't like it?
11 C: **He didn't really like it [much**
12 V: [(No?)
13 C: **But the-deh his sister Tidbit.**
14 V: Loved it too mu[ch? Huh ha-ha=
15 C: [Ohh God
16 V: =ha-[ha
17 C: **[Well she's now fifteen pounds**
18 **and she just turned a year.**
19 [°So.°
20 V: [Uuhkaay
(0.4)
21 C: **Eats everything in sight.**
22 V: °'Kay.°
23 There are other things that can be done.
24 [There are solutions you can=
25 C: **[But he gets I give him dental treats.**
26 V: =add to the water?

The veterinarian's proposal on lines 1 and 3 is designed as a description of an alternative strategy, "feeding a dental diet," which has embedded in it assessments that characterize this dietary approach as "really easy" but not as "effective" as tooth brushing. The assessment of a dental diet as "easy" constructs it as advice-implicative [74] and contrasts it with the difficulty of attempting to brush the cat's teeth, something the client previously indicated. The informative features of the dietary proposal (lines 1, 3) implicitly position the client as someone who has never used a dental diet and explicitly construct the diet as an easy strategy to adopt.

Both of these aspects turn out to be problematic from the client's perspective. The client responds initially with the minimal response token ("Hmm") and head nod (line 5) that together merely acknowledge receipt of this information. Because this proposal is designed to present one option among several rather than as a singularly preferred course of action, the client's response is a milder form of passive resistance than might be called for if the veterinarian had said "I would recommend you put him on a dental diet." The veterinarian starts providing more information about dental diets (line 7), at which point the client, in partial overlap with the veterinarian, begins an actively resisting turn (line 8). In contrast to the canonical form of acceptance in our data (a prompt "Okay" with falling pitch), the client's response here displays the features of a dispreferred turn shape. It is performed with hesitation and disfluency: "I did give it to him but he um he" (lines 8, 9). The "but" clearly forecasts a problem with the dietary proposal, which the client seems reluctant to share.

The hitches and perturbations in the client's talk threaten the progressivity of the discussion. The veterinarian assists on line 10 as part of a *collaborative turn sequence* [75]; the veterinarian reacts to the trouble spot in the conversation with a contribution that completes the client's turn and hence affiliates with the client's experiences. Using a yes/no type declarative question [76], the veterinarian anticipates what the client was going to say and proffers a possible candidate completion of the client's turn for the client to accept or reject: "He didn't like it?" (line 10). In posing this as a question, the veterinarian ratifies the epistemic primacy of the client's knowledge of the patient's food preferences while still being the first person in the encounter to actually suggest the specific obstacle to adherence: the patient's dislike for the recommended food. In displaying knowledge about the common challenges of cat ownership, even though lacking knowledge about this specific patient, the veterinarian bridges the earlier misalignment with the client created by the ill-fitting proposal. The client accepts the candidate completion as their own by recycling it, slightly downgrading the extent of the patient's aversion to dental food by incorporating "[not] really" and "much" (line 11). In doing so, the client reduces the degree of disaffiliation with the proposal and reasserts their superior epistemic status as the expert on their pet's food preferences. This status is upheld by the questioning "No?" on line 12, which positions the veterinarian as less knowledgeable on the matter of the patient's feeding history and preferences than the client.

The client then uses the disjunctive "but" to contrast the patient's evaluative stance toward dental food with that of a female cat in the household (line 13) not present at the appointment. This launches the start of yet another reason for resisting the proposal: the potential negative health consequences for another cat in the household. Once again, the veterinarian uses a collaborative turn sequence, offering another yes/no declarative question for client ratification in the form of a different barrier to adherence posed by the other cat overindulging in the dental diet (line 14), the implications of which are softened by trailed-off laughter (lines 14, 16). The client begins a response to the candidate completion with "Oh God" (line 15), an emotionally charged, nonconforming response. The "oh" preface here establishes that the client has greater epistemic authority than the veterinarian regarding claims about the absent Tidbit, in light of the client's primary epistemic access to information about her [63].

The client then delivers an answer to the veterinarian's question starting with a "well" preface (line 17). This feature flags that the answer will be an expanded response, not a straightforward agreement [77] with the veterinarian's suggestion that Tidbit merely loved the dental diet "too much." The client's announcement of Tidbit's current weight and young age (lines 17, 18) makes available a new inference about a risk of lifetime overweight. The low-volume "so" (line 19) leaves implicit the upshot of the prior talk about Tidbit's health issues: that a dental diet is contraindicated. The client's information-sharing about Tidbit is received with a marked acknowledgment (line 20) that shows the veterinarian to accept the veracity of the health risks to her. The severity of the risk posed to Tidbit by hypothetical reintroduction of a dental diet is further underscored by the client's description of Tidbit as a cat that "eats everything in sight" (line 21), a fact that the veterinarian quietly acknowledges (line 22). "Everything" makes this an extreme case formulation [78] that by definition is rhetorically designed to discourage the undermining or challenging of the client's active resistance by the veterinarian.

Abandoning the dental diet option, the veterinarian counters the apparent hopelessness of the situation with a generic announcement about "other things that can be done" (line 23). Partway through the veterinarian's description of solutions that can be added to the drinking water, the client actively resists this strategy by informing the veterinarian of an additional, heretofore undisclosed, strategy already adopted for addressing dental concerns: the use of dental treats (line 25).

In Case 3, a client questions the veterinarian's conjecture that the patient's health problem could be caused by the current food he is being fed. Extract 3.1 contains an instance of initial client passive resistance followed by active resistance. This is a problem visit involving a dog who has a history of ear infections since puppyhood and has recently begun repeatedly scratching one ear and whimpering. Prior to the extract, the veterinarian asked the clients what food the patient was on. They described a lamb and rice calorie-reduced formulation the patient had been eating since coming to their home from the breeder. The veterinarian justified asking about diet because of a possible link between food and recurrent infection. Information-sharing about both food allergies and a possible thyroid insufficiency, raised because of the patient's age, ensued. Right before the start of Extract 3.1, the veterinarian indicated that a thyroid problem, while possible, was less likely than food allergies.

Extract 3.1.

V:	Food issues
	(0.5)
	Possible
C1:	Yeah. Yeah.
V:	You know and one thing ummm you may wanna consider
	is trying him on a vegetarian food
C1:	Mm hm. *((C2 nods))*
V:	Um if you wanna pick it up a-at the pet store
	{Parent Company} has one *((C2 nods))*
	that seems to be very good.
C1:	Mm hm.
V:	Um the prescription hypoallergenic foods are
	(0.3) better?
C1:	Yeah
V:	From a (0.3) formulation standpoint but
C1:	Mm hm.
V:	It's something you know to think about.
	(0.3)
C1:	[Yeah
V:	[You know cuz it could certainly be related to
	(0.3) the food
V:	Hi baby *((to P))*
	(1.0)
C1:	**Or just the fact that it's such a**
	(0.9)
	dark damp mess in there

The proposal to consider trying vegetarian food (lines 5, 6) comes immediately after the veterinarian's listing of "food issues" (line 1) as a hypothetical contributor to the patient's ear infection (line 3). Instead of accepting the proposal with "Okay," Client 2 demonstrates passive resistance by responding on line 7 with the continuer "Mm hm," a stance further exemplified by Client 1's silent head nod (line 7). The veterinarian pursues more engagement from the clients, keeping the topic alive by first offering a product name and assessment of a high-quality vegetarian food available at a pet food store (lines 8–10), which Client 1 acknowledges (line 11). The veterinarian then provides an assessment of in-clinic prescription diets as better than store-bought, to which Client 1 responds with "Yeah" (line 14). The veterinarian continues the topic with a turn increment (line 15) that receives minimal acknowledgment from Client 1 (line 16).

The ending of the sequence is forecasted by the veterinarian's recycling of the proposed diet as "something you know to think about" (line 17); this receives no client acceptance in the form of an "Okay" but the more ambiguous and slightly delayed "Yeah" (line 19) in overlap with the veterinarian's conjecture that the ear infection "could certainly" be related to the patient's current diet (lines 20, 21). This conjecture is an upgrading of epistemic confidence from line 3 where a food allergy was assessed merely as a "possible" contributor to the current medical problem. The veterinarian then addresses the patient (line 22) on the examining table.

It is at this late point in the segment that Client 1 demonstrates active resistance. After a 1.0 s delay, the client's "or" preface links this resisting turn to the veterinarian's prior conjecture (lines 20, 21) by proposing an alternative explanation for the patient's ear infection, one that subtly challenges the food allergy hypothesis: "Or just the fact that it's such a (0.9) dark damp mess in there" (lines 24–26). The gap in talk points to the hesitancy with which this challenge of the veterinarian's expertise is conveyed: that the structure of the patient's ear makes it a natural site for infection. While the "or" preface, on the one hand, retains this proposal's status as a conjecture that does not trump the veterinarian's prior one, "just" on the other hand marks the client's hypothesis as the more parsimonious explanation and "fact" promotes its incontestability.

Case 4 contains an example of initial client acceptance of the veterinarian's proposal followed by active resistance. Extract 4.1 is taken from a wellness visit involving a 17-month old female Labrador retriever. Prior to the extract, the client answered the veterinarian's diet history question by indicating that the patient was on a higher-quality grocery store brand of puppy food mixed with canned food. This segment occurred partially off camera, with the veterinarian and client on the floor with the patient. On line 1, the veterinarian focuses on the age of the patient as noteworthy by issuing a yes/no type declarative question asking the client to confirm the candidate estimate of the patient's age. In asking this question in the context of not having the patient file available during the examination, the veterinarian acknowledges the client's superior epistemic status regarding knowledge of the patient's age.

Extract 4.1.

V: Now (0.4) she's like a year and a half right?
C: One year five months. The twenty [fourth.
V: [Yeah.
C: November [twenty fourth
V: [Soooo
   she should be gettin' onto adult food.
C: Okay.
   (0.2) *((Clapping sound))*
C: **We'll finish this ba[g? and she'll go on=**
V: [Yeah. Like
C: **=[adult food**
V: [switch her over to adult
C: 'Kay?=
V: =Uumm
   (0.5)
C: **Cuz it says up to two years on the bag**

A type-conforming response to the veterinarian's question would be "yes" or "no." The client's answer (lines 1, 2), structured as nonconforming and dispreferred, treats the veterinarian's question as problematic in some way [76]. The answer invokes the client's epistemic primacy, as a pet owner with greater familiarity about the pet's biography than the veterinarian, to correct the imprecision of the veterinarian's over-estimation of the patient's age. This interactional detail prefigures the nature of the active resistance that subsequently emerges. The veterinarian's "Like a year and a half" (line 1) becomes "One year five months" (line 2) in the client's answer, which is expanded to include an announcement of the specific date on which the patient turned this age (lines 2, 4). The veterinarian acknowledges the initial part of the client's response (line 3) and, in overlap with the expanded answer (line 4), delivers an elongated "so" preface [70] (line 5) that displays the upshot of the previous exchange about the patient's age: the need to switch to adult food (line 6). This proposal is carried out in a relatively prescriptive fashion using the verb of necessity "should" [52].

The client initially accepts the proposal using the canonical response token "Okay" delivered with final intonation (line 7). The client expands their acceptance turn by announcing their own counterproposal: to finish the current bag of puppy food before introducing adult food (lines 9, 11). The veterinarian responds in such a way as to treat the client's plan as a problem. The turn-initial "Yeah" (line 10) acknowledges the client's proposal but does not accept it in the way that a falling-pitch "Okay" would have; the veterinarian recycles the proposal (lines 10, 12), which focuses exclusively on the food switch and deletes any reference to the client's proposal to use up the current bag of puppy food. The client's contracted "Okay" on line 13 has rising intonation which renders it ambiguous with respect to its function as acceptance of the re-issued dietary proposal; the veterinarian comes in immediately with a sound-stretched "Um" (line 14) which appears designed to reserve the conversational floor on their own behalf while simultaneously signalling a significant delay in speakership [79] (line 15). However, half a second later, which is a fairly lengthy gap in conversation [80], the client seizes the floor, giving a justification for their proposal to delay the food switch (line 16): "Cuz" makes explicit the status of this utterance as an account for the now clearly problematic proposal to delay the food switch. Here, active resistance comes in the form of citing the feeding instructions on the bag of puppy food giving two years as the upper age limit, information that is in conflict with the recommendation of the veterinarian. Client active resistance in this example is grounded in an epistemic clash between two conflicting sources of expert knowledge: the veterinarian and the pet food company that manufactured the current food.

In Case 5, active resistance is subtle, a kind of implicature in its mention of the possible expense of the recommended food and a comment about the food preference of another cat in the household. Extract 5.1 comes from a wellness visit with a male cat recently adopted from the Humane Society. Prior to the extract, the veterinarian asked history-taking questions, including one about the type of main food in the patient's diet, and completed an oral examination. The veterinarian announced to the client that the patient had some gingivitis, tartar, and plaque on his teeth, showing the client the evidence. The veterinarian explained that the best way to avoid this is to brush the patient's teeth daily, something that can be difficult to perform with cats. The non-adoption of the tooth brushing option was normalized by the veterinarian whose own cat was "not nice enough" to permit it.

Extract 5.1.

V: The other option would be to have him on a special
um dental diet. *((C nods))*
Uh the dental diet that I recommend is the
{2 Brand-Relevant Initials} diet it's for
[tooth diet
C: [°Mm.°
V: It's made by {Pet Food Company Name} and it's special
because the kibbles are larger *((C nods))*
than other kibble? and the tooth has to go all the way
into the kibble before it shatters. So it acts like a
toothbrush brushing up on the tooth when they chew the
food.
C: °Okay.°
V: Uh the last option would be to just wait until the
teeth get bad enough and then do a dental cleaning
and with cats with a dental cleaning it's anywhere
from two hundred and fifty dollars to about
[three hundred and fifty dollars.
C: [°Hm°
V: And it is under general anesthetic so it is a big
deal.
C: Mm hm.
V: So it's kinda nice to try to avoid that if you can.=
C: =(Yeah.)
V: So if you're at all interested in the diet that I was
talking about I can definitely send you home with a
pamphlet?

```
C:  That'd be good (give us) a price range [on it=
V:                                         [Yup
C:  =(°kind of thing.°) ((C nods))
V:  And then if you decide you want it I can also send you
    home with a free bag to try just to see if he likes it
    and to see if you like it.
C:  Yeah cuz Rascal's been eatin' hard kibble=Yeah he
    likes the stuff he has.
```

On lines 1 and 2, the veterinarian uses a description-type format to propose an option in lieu of tooth brushing. This initial proposal bears some resemblance to that appearing in Extract 3.1 (lines 1, 3), though that proposal was more strongly advice-implicative because it characterized the option as "easy." In Extract 5.1, the client does not respond vocally but rather minimally displays their status as an attentive listener by nodding their head. The veterinarian continues sharing information about the name of the in-clinic product that they typically recommend (lines 3–5); this recommendation is designed as a generic one associated with typical advice-giving by the veterinarian ("that I recommend"), rather than as a recommendation targeting this client and patient specifically. This construction orients to the possibility that this product will not be appropriate for this client and/or patient. It manages possible resistance by allowing the veterinarian to "test the waters" with the client to gauge possible interest in the in-clinic dental diet. The client demonstrates very limited engagement, quietly using the weak acknowledging token, "Mm" (line 6) [81]. The veterinarian shares more information about the parent company and design of the dental kibble (lines 7–12), which the client acknowledges in a more marked but still quietly uttered way with "Okay." Although the client's responses might appear at first blush to display passive resistance, it should be noted that none of the veterinarian's contributions thus far are designed as a clear recommendation targeting the patient, but are rather packaged as information. Hence, client acceptance or rejection is not expected in the way that "I would recommend you have him on a dental diet" would have.

The veterinarian then describes the final treatment option of dental scaling (lines 14, 15), providing a price range (lines 16–18) and an assessment (lines 20, 21), underscoring the seriousness of an intervention involving general anesthesia, which the client receives with "Mm hm" (line 22). The veterinarian then produces a "so"-prefaced assessment (line 23), signalling the logic involved in adopting a dietary approach: This assessment is advice-implicative in that it implicitly re-introduces the dental diet as a means of avoiding the cost and health risks to the patient posed by dental cleaning. The client appears to affiliate with this assessment by uttering "Yeah" (line 24). The veterinarian then offers a pamphlet containing information about the in-clinic dental diet (lines 25–27); the use of the if/then clausal structure delicately manages any inferences about sales pressure by making it clear that this offer is contingent on the client's interest, the presumption of which is minimized through the use of "at all" (line 25). Thus, a decision to purchase the proposed food is deferred to an uncertain future.

After initially accepting the offer with a positive assessment on line 28, the client then displays active resistance related to the expense of the dental diet by soliciting a price range (line 28, 30), something the veterinarian immediately promises to provide (line 29). Beginning on line 31, the veterinarian then delivers a second offer of a free sample of the food to "try," constructed using "if"-prefaced clauses that orient to contingencies in the form of possible dispreference for the product on the parts of the patient (line 32) and client (line 33). The client does not accept the offer; instead of using "Okay," they use "Yeah" to affiliate with the concern the veterinarian raises about food preference as another possible obstacle to the adoption of the new food: the possible rejection of the new food by a different cat in the household not in attendance at the visit (lines 34, 35).

In sum, conversation analysis of clients' initial active resistance to veterinarians' proposals for dietary change underscored the importance and dynamics of the epistemic states, statuses, and stances of veterinarians and clients. As illustrated above, nutritional proposals were sometimes issued before veterinarians had educated the client about nutrition and/or the relevant current diagnosis or potential health problem that the proposed change was intended to address or prevent; in such cases, clients sometimes questioned or challenged the relevance of the dietary proposal because they did not understand the link between the current diet and health problems. In other cases, because veterinarians had not previously conducted a thorough nutritional assessment, including dietary history-taking, they were unaware that the patient was currently on the recommended food or that it had been tried, unsuccessfully, in the past. In the latter case, this meant that the veterinarian lacked knowledge of key client-related or patient-related obstacles to adherence. And while the proposed dietary change was sometimes situated within a larger set of treatment options, including non-nutritional strategies, analyses of our collection showed that veterinarians did not explicitly solicit clients' perspectives and possible concerns about treatment options, dietary or non-dietary, before delivering their proposals. Therefore, prior to proposing modifications, some veterinarians lacked knowledge about patient or client preferences and client worries about matters such as expense and undesirable consequences of nutritional change.

3.3. *Analysis of Veterinarians' Uptake and Interactional Outcomes*

3.3.1. Key Features

This section reports on patterns of interaction and decision-related outcomes in the wake of clients' active resistance. Analyses highlight veterinarians' uptake, the ensuing client–veterinarian interactions, and what sorts of treatment plans, if any, were agreed upon by the end of the appointment. Veterinarians' responses to clients' active resistance were complex and variable, demonstrating the dynamic epistemic and deontic territories they occupied.

In epistemic terms, veterinarians' responses often contained recommendation-relevant information-sharing, including their medical justifications for the proposals. A total of 16 of the 23 resistance cases (69.6%) involved recycling of the initial dietary proposals, often in modified form, which sometimes closed down resistance-related talk and dietary discussion more generally. Veterinarians sometimes oriented to prior displays of client resistance by downgrading the proposal to a mere consideration of the dietary change or replaced the original proposal with an alternative dietary or non-dietary strategy for addressing or preventing the health issue (e.g., Extract 2.2 below). Thus, veterinarians exemplified their deontic right to recommend actions in the service of patient health but mitigated their deontic authority in imposing particular actions on clients and patients.

Table 3 shows the final outcomes of decision-making trajectories following active client resistance. Among the 23 active resistance cases, 10 cases (43.5%) involved the client ultimately accepting an alternative strategy or strategies to manage the health concern; this occurred after the veterinarian's original dietary proposal was abandoned in the wake of client resistance. The agreed-upon strategies could be nutritional or non-nutritional, including generic, downgraded recommendations that clients simply monitor the health issue (e.g., Extract 1.2). Thus, even in cases in which veterinarians accepted the basis for client resistance, they did not necessarily do so in a manner that concomitantly downgraded the seriousness of the identified health concern. In one of these cases, the veterinarian flagged that further consideration of the proposed dietary change could happen at a subsequent appointment at which the agreed-upon alternative strategy for addressing the health issue (anal gland expression) was scheduled.

Table 3. Final outcomes of decision-making trajectories in cases with client active resistance to veterinarians' proposals for long-term dietary change.

Outcome	**No. of Cases (%)**
Acceptance of Alternative Strategy (Dietary/Non-Dietary)	10 (43.5)
Acceptance of Initial Dietary Proposal	8 (34.8)
Ratification of Modified Client Counterproposal	2 (8.7)
Postponement of Decision	2 (8.7)
Outcome Unclear	1 (4.3)
Total	23 (100%)

Eight cases (34.8%) resulted in client acceptance of the veterinarian's initial nutritional proposal (e.g., Extracts 4.2 and 5.2) (Table 3). In four of the eight acceptance cases, client acceptance was *unmarked*, consisting of a falling-pitch "Okay" response without delay or elaboration. In conversation-analytic terms, the design of these turns as minimal and immediate showed them to be canonical preferred responses to veterinarians' proposals. In the remaining four cases, client acceptance was *marked*: such accepting responses included additional lexical material suggestive of intensified client engagement. For example, in Extract 5.2 below, the client accepts the veterinarian's offer of a free sample bag of dental diet and, as a way of addressing the previously identified potential barriers to adherence, proposes mixing the new food with the less expensive, favoured current food. Of note, here is how these results compared with our preliminary analysis of the non-resistance cases. In that collection, only two of the 16 early acceptance cases contained client responses that were more expansive than "Okay."

In two cases (8.7%), the veterinarian postponed further discussion of dietary change, in one case until test results were available and in the other, as previously described, until a follow-up appointment (Table 3). In two other cases (8.7%), veterinarians accepted modified counterproposals suggested by clients. In a final case (4.3%), it was not clear by the end of the appointment as to whether clients had accepted the veterinarian's dietary proposal because the veterinarian responded to the resistance with medical information-sharing that did not expect acceptance or rejection in the way that a clearly designed recommendation would have (Table 3).

3.3.2. Example Analyses of Veterinarians' Uptake of Client Active Resistance

In this section, we present additional conversation analyses of the five cases previously featured, with particular attention on veterinarians' uptake of active client resistance and subsequent veterinarian–client interactions. For each case, we also provide a brief description of any further proposal-relevant talk occurring during the visit after the resistance segment ended.

Further analysis of Case 1 shows how the progress of a treatment conversation can become hampered when the veterinarian is unaware of what the client is currently doing to address a health problem. It also shows how the recycling of previous recommendations not well fitted to the particular client and patient can lead to further disaffiliation by the client. In this case, the veterinarian ultimately dropped the dietary proposal.

Extract 1.2 captures what unfolded after the client informed the veterinarian that the patient is already eating the senior food previously recommended (line 34).

Extract 1.2.

```
C:  **Yeah I know.  I actually have her on that sooo**
V:  Okay.
C:  Yeah.
V:  All right.
    So.
C:  (But yeah.)
V:  But just you know make a mental note that you won't
    let her get overweight.
C:  Yeah [yeah.  I thought sh-
V:       [Cuz it's it just gets
    harder and harder.
C:  Oh yeaah.  Exactly.
V:  (Yeah)
C:  I thought she was maybe about the same.
V:  [She is.
C:  [I didn't notice
    that she sort of bulked up any so
V:  No=no she's good.
    Hey sweetheart ((to P))
C:  Oh good.
```

The accountability of the veterinarian in having delivered unnecessary dietary advice is conveyed by the elongated, trail-offed "sooo" (line 34) produced by the client at the end of the resisting turn; it acts as a prompt to the veterinarian to produce a relevant next action [71]. The veterinarian accepts the client's informing with "Okay" (line 35); the client's "Yeah" with falling pitch (line 36) appears to reaffirm their own earlier claim on line 34. The veterinarian's "All right" (line 37) and stand-alone "So" (line 38) are potential change-of-activity tokens [71,82], signalling a possible shutting down of the sequence. However, the veterinarian next recycles one of their previous recommendations using the imperative form (lines 40, 41). The turn-initial "but" (line 40) marks this general advice to the client—to monitor the patient and avoid letting her gain weight in the future—as disjunctive with the client's current strategy of using a senior food as a weight-control measure.

The client begins what is projectable as yet another actively resisting turn on line 42, issuing what appears to be a reiteration of their utterance on line 5 in Extract 1.1, stating their own independent perception that the patient had not gained weight over the past year. However, the client aborts completion of this utterance, dropping out in overlap with the veterinarian who justifies the recommendation with reference to their expert knowledge of the progressive challenges in keeping elderly, arthritic dogs from gaining weight: "Cuz it's it just gets harder and harder" (lines 43, 44). "Exactly" in the client's response on line 45 demonstrates strong agreement as a pet owner with the veterinarian's assessment; in combination with its "oh" preface, this response positions the client as having independently and previously come to the same opinion as the veterinarian [83]. In claiming prior awareness of the increasing difficulties in preventing the dog's weight gain, the client implies that the veterinarian's explanation and advice are not needed.

On line 47, the client restarts and completes the utterance begun on line 42, which recycles the claim on line 5 in Extract 1.1: "I thought she was maybe about the same." This repeat emphasizes the successful monitoring of the dog's weight before attending the appointment, which suggests that the veterinarian's injunction to avoid weight gain is unnecessary. The veterinarian agrees with the client's perception of the patient's weight ("She is"; line 48) in overlap with the client's continued turn. The client's statement that they "didn't notice that she sort of bulked up" (line 50) results in the veterinarian's reassuring assessment, "No = no she's good" (line 51), which repeats the positive evaluation of the patient's weight from Extract 1.1. The client receives the veterinarian's assessment on line 53 with "Oh good." Here, "Oh" marks the veterinarian's assessment as news for the client [84]; in doing so, the client upholds the epistemic superiority of the veterinarian as the medical expert who determines what an acceptable weight for the patient would be. This subordination of the client's own epistemic status on line 53 tempers the disaffiliative character of the prior talk. Ultimately, to support the mobility of the patient and encourage more exercise, the client later requests the pain medication for the patient recommended by the veterinarian near the beginning of the visit.

Case 2 is another case in which the veterinarian abandoned the original nutritional proposal. Extract 2.2 shows the veterinarian's uptake of the first types of active resistance disclosed by the client in Extract 2.1: the patient's dislike of the recommended dental food, which the veterinarian did not know the client had already tried using, and the risk of inducing overweight in another cat in the home, if the dental food were to be re-introduced.

Extract 2.2.

```
        There are other things that can be done.
        [There are solutions you can=
    C:  [But he gets I give him dental treats.
         V:  =add to the water?
    C:  (Mm hm)
    V:  They're also helpful
        and even (0.3) not even brushing the teeth
        but just rubbing ((Demonstrates on P))
        the gums up against the teeth?  ((C nods head))
        tha-that's helpful [too at slowing down=
    C:                     [Ohh yeah?  ((C nods))
    V:  =dental tartar
    C:  That's okay honey.  He's just pokin' ya ((To P))
```

The veterinarian drops the food proposal, suggesting an alternative intervention (lines 24, 26). The client pre-emptively resists the veterinarian's new proposal by announcing an alternative current strategy of which the veterinarian appears unaware: dental treats (line 25). The veterinarian responds to this with a positive assessment (line 28), and then, after discarding the previously rejected idea of teeth brushing (line 29), offers additional information about a different strategy, rubbing the patient's gums against his teeth (lines 30–31). The "Oh yeah?" (line 33) treats this advice as new information to which the client appears receptive; however, the client's subsequent talk to the patient (line 35) orients to the cat's lack of cooperation with the veterinarian's gum-rubbing (see [49,50]) and hints at the potential lack of future success in its adoption at home. It should be noted that the veterinarian does not take up this possible issue with the client. By assessing the client's current strategy of dental treats as "also helpful" (line 28) and then appending the gum-rubbing strategy as "helpful too" (line 32), the veterinarian demonstrates support of the use of dental treats while implying that singular action (i.e., the current status quo) is not sufficient in and of itself. Thus, the veterinarian promotes a multi-pronged approach, justified in terms of delaying tartar accumulation (lines 34, 36).

In Case 3, the veterinarian dropped the proposal to switch to a vegetarian diet after the client's suggestion that the patient's recurrent ear infections had a different, non-dietary etiology. Extract 3.2 begins with the client's hypothesis that the infections are caused by moisture trapped in the patient's ears.

Extract 3.2.

```
C1: Or just the fact that it's such a
    (0.9)
    dark damp mess in there
V:  Welll I mean he does have floppy ears
    I mean it does get hot and moist
    0.5 ((V sniffs P's ear))
V:  And this is yeast
```

The veterinarian takes up the client's active resistance of the conjecture on lines 24 and 26 with an answer that constitutes neither direct agreement or disagreement; the elongated "well" preface (line 27) projects that the veterinarian's response will not be straightforward or concise. The two instances of "I mean" (lines 27, 28) signpost the veterinarian's subsequent concessions [70] to the client's theory by acknowledging that the "hot and moist" (line 28) environment engendered by the patient's "floppy ears" (line 27) facilitates the overgrowth of yeast. These admissions are then linked sequentially and logically with "and" to the veterinarian's straightforward assertion, "this is yeast" (line 30). This diagnosis is supported empirically by the veterinarian sniffing the patient's ear and presumably identifying the telltale odor as a clinically relevant sign.

The confident design and delivery of this announcement upholds the epistemic authority of the veterinarian to diagnose. The announcement contrasts with the uncertain framing of the previously contested hypothesis that a food allergy may be implicated in the recurrent nature of the infection. In the absence of client endorsement of an attempt to take a nutritional approach to the prevention of future ear infections, the veterinarian focuses exclusively on treating the current one. On the basis of the unchallenged diagnosis, after this segment ends, the veterinarian recommends combination therapy, consisting of anti-inflammatory and anti-fungal medications, which the clients accept.

In Case 4, the client eventually accepted the veterinarian's proposal to immediately switch the patient from puppy to adult food. Extract 4.2 opens with the client's justification for having suggested that they finish the current bag of puppy food before effecting the change (line 16).

Extract 4.2.

```
C:  Cuz it says up to two years on the bag
V:  Yeah I know but
    (0.4)
V:  Usually with-especially with a large dog?
    (0.4)
V:  after they're about twelve months old?
C:  Oh [okay.
V:     [they get them over to adult so
C:  [Okay.
V:  [Not a big deal?
    I mean it's not like she's heavy or any[thing?
C:                                         [Noo
V:  An' ob-obviously she's good and active?
```

The veterinarian delicately disagrees with the client's reasoning. The acknowledgment of the credibility of the client's report about feeding instructions on the dog food package ("Yeah I know," line 17) is immediately appended with the disjunctive "but"; following a 0.4 s gap (line 18), the veterinarian introduces contrasting medical norms associated with the particular health needs of large breed dogs (line 19). The *self-repair* [85] whereby "especially" replaces "usually" serves to emphasize the distinctiveness of the health risk for this category of dog and, concomitantly, this patient.

The veterinarian then mentions the recommended age cut-off for large breeds "after they're about twelve months old" (line 21) at which point the client acknowledges this information with "Oh okay" (line 22). The "oh" preface indexes the shift in the client's epistemic state; once ignorant of the special nutritional requirements for large-breed dogs like the patient, the client is now informed. The veterinarian uses the generic third-person pronoun "they" (line 23) to describe what the body of experts in veterinary care do in terms of normative practices of switching large-breed dogs to adult food (line 23). Thus, the veterinarian counters client resistance and upholds the recommendation via the consensus of veterinary medical experts. The client acknowledges this generalized recommendation (line 24) in overlap with the veterinarian who uses reassuring assessments of the situation ("not a big deal," line 25) and of the patient ("not . . . heavy or anything," line 26) to position this recommendation as preventative in nature and to defuse any possible inference that the patient is already showing signs of overweight associated with excess nutrition from having eaten puppy food until now. The client promptly agrees with this last assessment (line 27). The veterinarian's comment that the patient is "good and active" (line 28) further manages the face threat of the recommendation with a positive assessment that, by implication, constructs the client's care of their pet as beyond reproach; this comment also foreshadows the veterinarian's subsequent description of adult foods formulated for active dogs. That comes after the end of the extract and elicits a request from the client for recommended brands.

As with Case 4, Case 5 led to client acceptance of the veterinarian's proposal to change the main food. Extract 5.2 opens with the client describing the preference exhibited by Rascal, another cat in the household, for his current food (lines 34, 35).

Extract 5.2.

34	C:	Yeah cuz Rascal's been eatin' hard kibble=Yeah **he**
35		**likes the stuff he has**.
36	V:	Good.
37	C:	So.
38	V:	Okay [so
39	C:	[(Now even) a free bag (would be nice) just to
40		see if he likes it=cuz I I'll see by the price and I'll
41		(portion) [it out (and see how it is.)
42	V:	[Yeah and it's not bad too because if you
43		think um with the the prescription diets they are
44		going to be a bit more expensive=
45	C:	=Mm hm. *((C nods))*
47	V:	than a lot of the grocery foods but. you don't usually
48		have to feed as much of them just cuz they're a bit
49		higher quality so more nutrient dense?
50	C:	Hm= *((C nods))*
51	V:	=So you don't have to feed as many kib[bles?
52	C:	[Or you could
53		mix them with a low [price brand.
54	V:	[Yeah or you could mix them
55	C:	Okay
56	V:	And as well if you factor in that you're using the
57		dental diet hopefully trying to extend the time
58		between a dental cleaning then that definitely saves
59		money that way.=If you're putting (that) a bit more. So
60	C:	Okay.
61	V:	Definitely I'll give you the price so you can think
62		about it.
63	C:	Yeah ((V puts on stethoscope))
64	V:	And if we can just get him over here

The veterinarian accepts this state of affairs; the positive assessment "Good" (line 36) deftly avoids taking up the client's concern about Rascal's liking of his current food as a problem. The client's stand-alone "so" prompts further action by the veterinarian who launches a turn (line 38) and promptly drops out before turn completion when overlapped by the client who performs a marked acceptance (lines 39–41) of the previous offer of the free food sample, using a positive assessment (line 39) and incorporating as contingencies the two previously mentioned possible obstacles to adherence: the food preference of the absent pet and the cost of the proposed food (line 40).

The veterinarian then shares information about the dental diet that is designed to reduce the client's concerns about the issue of cost while simultaneously demonstrating the veterinarian's sensitivity to this as a legitimate issue (lines 42–44; 47–49). The construction of the cost-related scenario of feeding the dental diet is evaluated using a mitigated negative assessment "not bad" (line 42); the cost of the prescription food relative to grocery store foods is downgraded to "a bit more expensive" (line 44), which is acknowledged by the client (line 45). In reassuring the client that cost savings are likely given that smaller portions can be served (lines 47–49), the veterinarian appears to build on the client's previously mentioned intention to portion out the free sample in an exploratory fashion (lines 40–41).

On lines 52 and 53, the client issues a candidate option of another way of rationing the dental diet to manage barriers to adherence: mixing the dental kibbles with the currently used main food. This proposal is designed as a turn increment; it begins with "or" which constructs this turn as an add-on alternative to the veterinarian's previous turn, the negatively worded utterance on line 51 regarding necessary portion sizes. This proposal by the client represents a further instance of marked acceptance of the suggested dietary change. High engagement in the diet discussion is demonstrated by the client's own independent problem-solving regarding the obstacles to adherence. The epistemic authority of the veterinarian as the medical expert to determine the acceptability of the proposed nutrition-related practices is upheld by the veterinarian's ratification of the client's proposal ("Yeah," line 54); moreover, the veterinarian's repetition of the proposal as if it is their own (line 54), which the client accepts (line 55), demonstrates strong affiliation with the client.

The veterinarian offers further information about the cost-saving benefits of mixing the current food with the dental diet: the postponement of expensive dental cleaning (lines 57–59), which the client acknowledges with "Okay" (line 60). The veterinarian then reiterates the promise to provide the client with the price of the dental food; the clause "so you can think about it" (lines 61–62) explicitly frames the proposal to use the dental diet not as an agreed-upon treatment plan but rather as something merely under consideration by the client. After the segment ends, near the end of the appointment, the veterinarian promises to obtain the sample bag of food, to which the client responds with "Okay."

In sum, conversation analysis of veterinarians' uptake of clients' active resistance demonstrated varied orientations to the barriers to adherence raised by clients in reaction to the original dietary proposals. Veterinarians responded to the superior epistemic access of clients when their resistance involved the disclosure of new information about patients' or clients' past or current experiences and preferences. Subsequent proposals were typically modified in these cases so as to incorporate the concerns of clients while still maintaining a focus on patient health. Veterinarians would suggest other options, including non-nutritional ones, for addressing or preventing the health concerns motivating the original proposal for dietary change. In light of the uncertainty regarding patient adherence and other obstacles, veterinarians' subsequent proposals were sometimes downgraded to suggestions to merely consider nutritional modification or were designed as options in a way that retrospectively constructed the initial proposal as one choice among several, rather than as the only recommended course of action. These constructions mitigated the deontic authority of veterinarians to expect clients and patients to follow the proposed strategies.

When clients' resistance manifested as questions or comments that revealed a lack of medical knowledge about the relationship between the dietary proposal and patient health, veterinarians upheld their own epistemic authority by educating clients, explaining diagnoses where appropriate, and providing reasons for the dietary proposal and/or alternative strategies, sometimes including evaluations of the relative effectiveness of the various approaches. Veterinarians did not explicitly inquire about clients' interest in addressing the patient's health issue or in a diet-related remedy. Clients deferred to the superior epistemic status of veterinarians by accepting their diagnoses, clinical interpretations, and assessments of possible treatment options. While the previously presented Case 3 might appear to be an exception, it is important to note that the veterinarian in that case epistemically downgraded the causal link between the patient's health issue and the current diet to a mere possibility when suggesting a dietary change; in contrast, the diagnosis of a yeast infection in the patient, treatable with prescription medications, was presented as a clinical certainty.

4. Discussion

Conversation analysis has shown that institutional talk like veterinary dietary discussions is built on the bedrock of ordinary conversation; this is because people in professional settings draw on the same interactional resources used for everyday communication [86]. As we have seen in the present study, those resources may help minimize disagreements and facilitate the smooth progression of the conversation, but they are not always optimal for the specialized activities and goals of veterinary appointments. The present research on clients' active resistance to long-term dietary change is one of a series of investigations of real-life veterinary–client interactions [51,52,87] aimed at informing practice guidelines for the nutritional assessment and weight management of dogs and cats [3] and, hopefully, clinical communication training in veterinary education. The implications of the present study for veterinary clinical practice become clear when the results are situated in the context of extant research and the best-practices literature on veterinary communication in the area of pet nutrition.

4.1. The Prevalence of Active Client Resistance

In our corpus of data, there were slightly more cases of initial active client resistance (n = 23) to veterinarians' proposals for long-term nutritional modification than cases of acceptance and passive resistance (n = 19). This is not necessarily surprising, given the findings of the landmark study previously cited [13]. An article promoting effective strategies for talking with clients about dog and cat nutrition normalized the potential for client resistance to dietary recommendations by suggesting that such resistance could very well arise at several decision points in every pet's lifespan: what puppy or kitten food to use, when to switch a pet to adult food and senior food, and what foods to select at those transition times [88]. Given the importance of sound nutrition for animal health, of concern is a recent survey in which 41.5% of veterinary clinicians reported that client resistance to changing their brand of pet food deterred clinicians from initiating nutrition discussions in wellness appointments [89]. That finding seems bound up with the intrinsically face-threatening nature of the topic: "Few subjects are as emotionally loaded and full of personal opinions as what and how people feed their pets" ([90], p. 907). Adding to the complexity is other survey research indicating that clients view their veterinary healthcare team as the most crucial source of information when making decisions about changing their pets' diet [91] and purchasing pet food [92].

But client resistance to dietary recommendations need not be a foregone conclusion. A conversation-analytic study in human medicine found that primary care physicians' recommendations for new drug treatments produced fewer instances of patient active resistance in cases in which physicians first requested information about prior medication use than in cases in which such preliminary inquiries did not occur [93]. Patient information gathered before delivering the recommendations permitted physicians to tailor their communications to the particular patient and avoid resistance on the following bases: patients currently taking the recommended drug; patients having previously tried the drug and found it to be ineffective; patients' aversion to taking the drug; patients' concerns about harmful drug effects; and affordability [93]. Such findings resonate with many of the barriers to adherence disclosed by clients in the present study. Thus, the prevalence of active client resistance in our study might have been reduced had veterinarians engaged in preliminary information-sharing and information-gathering with clients before proposing dietary changes.

4.2. The Importance of Nutritional History-Taking

Nutritional assessments, including thorough nutritional histories [3,52], should be conducted with clients so that veterinarians have the necessary information to customize their treatment recommendations to the particular client and patient, and reduce the likelihood of resistance. In certain cases in our study, veterinarians were unaware of the patient's current diet, such that they recommended foods that clients were already feeding their pets. In other cases, veterinarians did not know about competing health concerns in the patient, a history of gastrointestinal difficulties associated with dietary changes, or if the patient had previously rejected the specific food that was recommended. In this regard, the finding that there were proportionally more cats than dogs in the active resistance collection was partly due to species-specific difficulties switching cats to a different dry food or introducing canned food: feline neophobia [94]. In other cases, veterinarians lacked important information about feeding management in relation to the patient's environment [3] (e.g., differential food preferences among multiple pets and/or risks to the health of the patient or other pets in the household due to food competition and shared feeding scenarios). Such information can be helpful to veterinarians in developing individualized feeding plans for patients that could overcome potential obstacles to adherence [3].

Of note in our study is that veterinarians typically accommodated clients when their resistance was based on particular past or present experiences of the patient, such as dispreference for the recommended food, potentially conflicting health concerns, and possible side effects. This finding is similar to one reported in a conversation-analytic study about parents' resistance to clinicians' treatment recommendations for their children diagnosed with epilepsy in which clinicians accommodated parents (by backing down, giving concessions, and providing options) when parental resistance was based on the past experiences of their child, rather than on an anti-medication position [42].

4.3. The Importance of Educating Clients

Veterinarians need to educate clients about patient health issues before making recommendations to address them [52]. In support of this, clients surveyed at wellness appointments for one study indicated that veterinarians' statements about their pet's health would be the type of communication that would most influence them to change their pet's diet [91]. Some clients in the present study made comments or asked questions suggesting that the dietary proposals were irrelevant because they either believed that current food targeted by the proposals did not have a deleterious effect on pet well-being or they were afraid that the new food intended to support pet health would inadvertently cause other health problems. Resistance thus arose because clients lacked knowledge about nutrient-sensitive or diet-induced health disorders that could be prevented or ameliorated with nutritional modification [2,3]; other clients implied that the recommended changes were unnecessary because they were using equivalent food items or alternative practices to address the health concern, approaches that veterinarians subsequently deemed to be problematic or less effective forms of treatment than the proposed change.

In accord with their epistemic superiority regarding expert knowledge about animal health, as compared with other grounds for resistance, veterinarians were less likely in these cases to abandon or revise their initial dietary proposals; clients were more likely to ultimately accept them when their resistance was tied to a lack of medical knowledge about the benefits of the food change. Following resistance, veterinarians typically justified the prior proposal by informing the client about the health concern and/or about why the proposed dietary modification was the most effective strategy for addressing the concern. This dovetails with results of a systematic review [95] of conversation-analytic studies of primary care doctor–patient talk about health behaviour in which the physician's linking of a proposed behaviour change to a health issue that was salient for the patient was an effective tool for managing client resistance [95].

4.4. The Importance of Providing Multiple Treatment Options

When it is appropriate to do so, veterinarians should situate dietary recommendations within a list of treatment options and provide information about their benefits and drawbacks, including their relative effectiveness [3,52]. In the present study, veterinarians often accommodated clients by proposing alternative strategies in the aftermath of resistance to the dietary proposals. That the provision of multiple treatment options is important in addressing patient health is highlighted by our finding that in over 40% of the active resistance cases clients wound up accepting an alternative strategy, sometimes non-dietary, to support pet wellbeing. However, these strategies tended to be proposed in the wake of client resistance to the dietary proposals, often delivered in a series of single proposals for clients to consider individually, one by one in sequence, rather than as a range of choices to be evaluated as a set. In this sense, in the present study, there was more option-*chaining* (with client resistance to one option occasioning the mention of another one) than comprehensive option-listing. Clients most often accepted a single alternative strategy with "Okay," rather than articulating a choice among strategies. As previously noted, the sequential presentation of proposals by some veterinarians camouflaged client disagreement by recasting the previously rejected dietary proposal, not as a singular recommendation, but as one of a series of possibilities.

Of relevance is conversation-analytic research in human medicine about neurologists' recommending and option-listing approaches to treatment discussions with outpatients [95]. Results indicated that option-listing oriented strongly to patients' right to choose and also structurally expected patients to explicitly select from the list of options [96].

4.5. The Importance of Soliciting Clients' Perspectives

In order to reduce the likelihood of client resistance and to ensure that treatment recommendations are tailored to the individual client and patient, veterinarians should solicit clients' perspectives, including whether they are open to discussing their pets' nutrition [3,52]. This is critical in a medical context in which veterinary clients, as compared with patients in human medicine, have many more options available to them, including the decision to eschew treatment [48]. Information can be gathered about the client's interest in addressing their pet's health problem, their perceptions about the relevant health issue, their concerns about and commitment to nutritional change and, if appropriate, their interest in hearing about a specific, recommended food [3,52]. This solicitation begins with nutritional history-taking and proceeds through the various stages of dietary discussion in an iterative fashion [3,52].

It is noteworthy that, in our corpus, veterinarians did not explicitly invite clients' perspectives. Either these were presumed to align with those of the veterinarian as implied by clients' acceptance of veterinarians' dietary proposals, were withheld in instances of passive resistance, or "leaked out" as active resistance in the aftermath of veterinarians' dietary proposals. In line with the conversation-analytic principle of minimizing disagreement, soliciting a client's perspective may seem risky in potentially inviting their disaffiliation with the veterinarian's medical opinion, should differences in perspective be exposed. However, also in accord with the principle of minimizing disagreement, some discussions in our collection were seemingly protracted because veterinarians kept obliquely pursuing client engagement (that was not forthcoming), providing multiple pieces of nutrition-related information instead of inviting clients directly to share questions, ideas, and concerns.

Asking about possible sources of resistance normalizes their existence. Moreover, and unlike patients and parents in studies in human medicine involving prescription drug recommendations [33–40,42,93], veterinary clients exercise considerable deontic authority in being able to access a plethora of over-the-counter food choices for their pets outside of clinic-only diets.

The issue of potential patient noncompliance with a dietary switch, and the stresses associated with the change for the client, loom large in the veterinary context. Conversation-analytic studies have shown how veterinarians and clients manage interactions with animals as non-cooperative patients [49,50]. In this regard, the results of our previous study [52] and the present one that investigated veterinarians' responses to client resistance may more closely resemble conversation-analytic work on physicians' advice to patients about lifestyle changes [97] rather than physicians' drug recommendations. In the latter scenario, doctors alone have the prerogative to prescribe [42] and patients and patients' parents sometimes pursue prescriptions even when contraindicated [34–36,38,42]. In one study on lifestyle modifications, physicians advising patients about changing their behaviour avoided the use of directives, employing conditional "if" statements, information-sharing, and option-sharing to uphold the agency and autonomy of the patient in deciding to change their behaviour [97]. In a different study, physicians similarly employed conditionals when offering support to patients on smoking cessation, the design of which oriented to doctors' limited agency in shaping patient behaviour [98]; patients' perspectives on, and future intentions about, smoking cessation following such offers were frequently unclear [98].

In the present study, in spite of—and in other cases because of—veterinarians having gained important information from clients through their displays of active resistance, the design of the final proposals often oriented to possible nonadherence. Veterinarians acknowledged many contingencies, including client and patient preferences, that made the adoption of dietary modification or alternative strategies uncertain (except when the alternative strategy involved prescribed medication). Such formats included epistemically downgraded proposals to consider dietary change in the future, information-sharing about options, and generic advice (e.g., to merely keep patients' teeth clean or to keep the patient from gaining weight). Research in veterinary and human medical communication suggests that unclear, vague recommendations can reduce adherence [30,95]. Recent practice guidelines contain step-by-step communication practices that can shape clear nutritional recommendations specific to the particular client and patient [3].

Veterinarians' accommodation of relevant potential obstacles to adherence and the mitigated design of the final proposals were likely critical to the outcomes in our study whereby 78% of clients either ended up accepting the veterinarian's original dietary proposals or an alternative strategy the veterinarian proposed to address or prevent patient health problems. Clients usually responded to these proposals with a final-intonation "Okay" and no further elaboration. This is in line with conversation-analytic research demonstrating that patient acceptance of typically designed medical recommendations takes the form of a preferred turn shape, usually "Okay" [96]. While such a response to a recommendation furthers the smooth unfolding of the appointment, this sort of adjacency pair does not facilitate active patient participation in medical decision-making the way that option-listing does, whereby patients are invited to choose between treatment strategies. In contrast, "recommending turns do not *invite* patients to do more than simply accept a decision" ([96], p. 881). Interestingly, the four cases in our study in which clients demonstrated a more elaborate acceptance of veterinarians' recycled dietary proposals following active resistance involved veterinarians inviting clients to take free samples of the recommended food or to choose between two different treatment options in the wake of resistance. This finding shows that, despite some of the interactional challenges posed by initial active resistance, it does not necessarily forecast ultimate client disaffiliation with nutritional modification. Active resistance cases often included more client engagement, including client counterproposals accepted by veterinarians, than were involved in non-resistance cases.

4.6. A Collaborative Approach to Dietary Decision-Making

As described in our companion study [52] and as suggested above, a veterinarian can create the foundations for collaboration with the client in treatment decision-making by taking the necessary time to engage the client actively, and cyclically, as a partner during the dietary discussion (see also [3]). Information-sharing by both the client and the veterinarian, who have their own domains of expertise, is crucial. As we have mentioned, thorough history-taking with the client is essential so that the veterinarian avoids suggesting treatment strategies that are ill-suited to the patient and/or the client or other pets in the home. The veterinarian then needs to educate the client about the patient's health problem and ask the client explicitly about their level of interest in ameliorating or preventing the problem [52]. A range of treatment options should be described, with the veterinarian seeking the client's perspective on the options and inviting their questions and concerns [52]. In this way, potential client resistance is surfaced early and as a topic of discussion valued by the veterinarian rather than as an impediment. Should the veterinarian's treatment recommendation involve the introduction of a new food, at this juncture, the veterinarian can make a clear recommendation at a level of generality higher than a particular product name or brand [52] (e.g., a dental diet or a vegetarian diet). The veterinarian should again invite the client's perspective on the recommendation, including any concerns they may have [52]. If the client seems receptive, the veterinarian can then provide various product options, discussing the pros and cons of each, and again solicit the client's perspective on the product choices [52]. Depending on the client's response, the veterinarian can recommend a particular product, making sure to check in again with the client and to jointly create an action plan [52]; this would include steps for introducing the new food and for following up with the client to assess the success of the plan and possible need for modification [52].

4.7. Strengths and Limitations

One strength of the present study is that it provides evidence-based findings from the analysis of real-life interactions between veterinarians and clients to inform clinical practice and communication training in veterinary education regarding the nutritional assessment of dogs and cats and effective treatment recommendations. Another strength is that we examined not only the design, sequential organization, and grounds of clients' demonstrations of active resistance to veterinarians' initial long-term dietary proposals; we also studied veterinarians' uptake of client resistance and the final outcomes of nutritional decision-making so that the consequentiality of client resistance and the implications for adherence to nutritional recommendations could be better understood.

Nevertheless, certain limitations regarding our research data require mention. Unfortunately, the study did not include independent follow-up measures of adherence with agreed-upon treatment strategies. Other limitations are associated with our sample. Successful conversation analysis is frequently based on small samples, in part due to the labour-intensiveness of the methodology. However, it would be beneficial to expand the current data set by collecting additional cases from different clinics with which to compare the interactional regularities and variations identified in our study. Samples from multiple jurisdictions would also help, given the small geographic area of eastern Ontario, Canada, from which our sample was taken. Conversation analysis of large samples from England and the United States of patient resistance to treatment recommendations in primary health-care encounters demonstrated key cross-national differences in the resistant stances that patients took toward the recommendations [41].

The time frame of 2006 in which our data were collected is another possible limitation. Widespread changes since then include the following: the rise of online purchasing in the pet food industry, particularly since the inception of the recent pandemic [99]; the ever-expanding number of choices available in commercial pet foods [99]; premiumization and the increasing focus of pet owners on the healthiness of their pets' diets [99]; the associated humanization of pet food products, reflecting social trends in human dietary changes [99,100]; alternative diets [101], including organic and natural products [99,101]; grain-free options [100]; home-prepared diets [3]; plant-based diets [88]; and raw food diets [3,88]. There is also emerging medical information about diet-associated health risks (e.g., canine dilated cardiomyopathy, [101]) and guidelines for weight management [102]. With respect to feeding management, technological advances mean that clients can buy increasingly sophisticated automated feeders employing microchips or collars to restrict access of a food to one pet in multi-pet households [103].

Since the time our data were collected, these developments may well be reflected in shifts in the content of some patients' diets, the kinds of preferences clients express for particular foods, the nature of the expert information veterinarians share with clients to promote dietary change (including the risks and benefits of current pet food trends), and the increased availability of non-nutritional strategies to overcome obstacles to dietary modification. Nevertheless, the results of recent conversation-analytic studies [42,92] in human medicine on parents' and patients' resistance to doctors' treatment recommendations indicate that many of their findings, including grounds given for resisting recommendations, resonate with the results of our own study. This suggests the stability and ubiquity of the phenomenon of client resistance to dietary recommendations identified in the present study and the ongoing relevance and applicability of its findings.

5. Conclusions

The powerful impact of nutrition on animal health requires effective diet-related communication in veterinary medicine. Published work documenting veterinary clients' nonadherence to nutritional recommendations and its likely outcomes has relied on the use of client and clinician surveys (e.g., [13,89,91]) such that little has been known about how client resistance to veterinarians' dietary treatment recommendations is constructed in the language of actual appointments or how clinicians typically respond to nonadherence. The present study attempted to overcome these limitations using the qualitative research methodology of conversation analysis. Because it focuses on patterns of turn-taking and the wording of individual turns, conversation analysis can pinpoint trouble spots in interactions between veterinarians and clients, the significant features of the preceding conversational actions that shaped them, and the interactional consequences for how these trouble spots were subsequently managed. It is hoped that the results of this study demonstrate the value of this method in supporting effective veterinary communication training and professional practice guidelines, including those related to nutritional assessment and shared decision-making.

Author Contributions: Funding acquisition, J.B.C.; conceptualization, H.W.; data collection and archive management, J.B.C.; data preparation, H.W.; methodology, C.M. and H.W.; analysis, C.M., H.W. and J.B.C.; writing—original draft preparation, C.M.; writing—review and editing, H.W. and J.B.C. All authors have read and agreed to the published version of the manuscript.

Funding: This research project, entitled "Obesity Communication within Veterinary Practices," was funded by a grant from Royal Canin (Project No. 29640; Sponsor Code 43270).

Institutional Review Board Statement: This study, which involved human participants, was approved by the Research Ethics Board of the University of Guelph, Guelph ON Canada (Ethics Protocol #09JN026).

Informed Consent Statement: Informed consent was obtained from all human participants in the study who agreed to the use of their data for secondary analysis.

Data Availability Statement: Because informed consent for public posting of their videotaped data was not provided by the research participants at the time of data collection, and to protect their privacy as required by approved ethics procedures, public access to the data is not available. Excerpts of anonymized written transcripts are included in this publication as part of the standard validation practices in conversation-analytic research.

Acknowledgments: The authors wish to thank Royal Canin for their funding of the present study.

Conflicts of Interest: The authors declare no conflict of interest. Royal Canin's financial support provided for the salary of H.W. but the funder was not involved in the study design, analysis, writing, or decision to publish. J.B.C. regularly receives research funding, consults for, and receives honoraria from various veterinary organizations and commercial companies, including Royal Canin, Nestle Purina, the Purina Institute, and Hill's. J.B.C. currently holds the VCA Canada Chair in Relationship-Centred Veterinary Medicine at the Ontario Veterinary College, University of Guelph.

References

1. Baldwin, K.; Bartges, J.; Buffington, T.; Freeman, L.M.; Grabow, M.; Legred, J.; Ostwald, D., Jr. AAHA nutritional assessmen guidelines for dogs and cats. *J. Am. Anim. Hosp. Assoc.* **2010**, *46*, 285–296. [CrossRef]
2. Freeman, L.; Becvarova, I.; Cave, N.; MacKay, C.; Nguyen, P.; Rama, B.; Takashima, G.; Tiffin, R.; Tsjimoto, H.; van Beukelen, I WSAVA nutritional assessment guidelines. *J. Small Anim. Pract.* **2011**, *52*, 385–396. [CrossRef]
3. Cline, M.G.; Burns, K.M.; Coe, J.B.; Downing, R.; Durze, T.; Murphy, M.; Parker, V. AAHA nutrition and weight managemen guidelines for dogs and cats. *J. Am. Anim. Hosp. Assoc.* **2021**, *57*, 153–178. [CrossRef] [PubMed]
4. Chandler, M.L.; Takashima, G. Nutritional concepts for the veterinary practitioner. *Vet. Clin. N. Am. Small Anim. Pract.* **2014**, *44* 645–666. [CrossRef]
5. Lund, E.M.; Armstrong, P.J.; Kirk, C.A.; Klausner, J.S. Prevalence and risk factors for obesity in adult cats from private US veterinary practices. *Int. J. Appl. Res. Vet. Med.* **2005**, *3*, 88–96. Available online: http://www.jarvm.com/articles/Vol3Iss2/LUND.pdf (accessed on 19 May 2023).
6. Lund, E.M.; Armstrong, P.J.; Kirk, C.A.; Klausner, J.S. Prevalence and risk factors for obesity in adult dogs from private US veterinary practices. *Int. J. Appl. Res. Vet. Med.* **2006**, *4*, 177–186. Available online: http://jarvm.com/articles/Vol4Iss2/Lund.pdf (accessed on 19 May 2023).
7. German, A.J. The growing problem of obesity in dogs and cats. *J. Nutr.* **2006**, *136*, 1940S–1946S. [CrossRef] [PubMed]
8. Courcier, E.A.; Thomson, R.M.; Mellor, D.J.; Yam, P.S. An epidemiological study of environmental factors associated with canine obesity. *J. Small Anim. Pract.* **2010**, *51*, 362–367. [CrossRef] [PubMed]
9. Cave, N.J.; Allan, F.J.; Schokkenbroek, S.L.; Metekohy, C.A.M.; Pfeiffer, D.U. A cross-sectional study to compare changes in the prevalence and risk factors for feline obesity between 1993 and 2007 in New Zealand. *Prev. Vet. Med.* **2012**, *107*, 121–133. [CrossRef]
10. Laflamme, D.P. Understanding and managing obesity in dogs and cats. *Vet. Clin. N. Am. Small Anim. Pract.* **2006**, *36*, 1283–1295. [CrossRef]
11. Laflamme, D.P. Companion Animals Symposium: Obesity in dogs and cats: What is wrong with being fat? *J. Anim. Sci.* **2012**, *90* 1653–1662. [CrossRef] [PubMed]
12. Cline, M.G.; Murphy, M. Nutritional management of obesity. In *Obesity in the Dog and Cat*; Cline, M.G., Murphy, M., Eds.; CRC Press: Boca Raton, FL, USA, 2019; pp. 83–105. Available online: https://books.google.ca/books?hl=en&lr=&id=DTD3DwAAQBAJ&oi=fnd&pg=PP1&dq=obesity+in+the+dog+and+cat&ots=eoM-QLFhjP&sig=fAPHgwYKLG1GeegyasehMD4qwNg&redir_esc=y#v=onepage&q=obesity%20in%20the%20dog%20and%20cat&f=false (accessed on 19 May 2023).
13. American Animal Hospital Association. *The Path to High-Quality Care: Practical Tips for Improving Compliance*; American Animal Hospital Association: Lakewood, CO, USA, 2003; Available online: https://www.google.ca/books/edition/The_Path_to_High_Quality_Care/2jkMAAAACAAJ?hl=en (accessed on 19 May 2023).
14. Freeman, L.M.; Abood, S.K.; Fascetti, A.J.; Fleeman, L.M.; Michel, K.E.; Laflamme, D.P.; Bauer, C.; Kemp, B.L.E.; Van Doren, J.R. Willoughby, K.N. Disease prevalence among dogs and cats in the United States and Australia and proportions of dogs and cats that receive therapeutic diets or dietary supplements. *J. Am. Vet. Med. Assoc.* **2006**, *229*, 531–534. [CrossRef] [PubMed]
15. Michel, K.E.; Willoughby, K.N.; Abood, S.K.; Fascetti, A.J.; Fleeman, L.M.; Freeman, L.M.; Laflamme, D.P.; Bauer, C.; Kemp, B.L.E. Van Doren, J.R. Attitudes of pet owners toward pet foods and feeding management of cats and dogs. *J. Am. Vet. Med. Assoc.* **2008**, *233*, 1699–1703. [CrossRef] [PubMed]
16. Michel, K.E. Using a diet history to improve adherence to dietary recommendations. *Compend. Contin. Educ. Vet.* **2009**, *31*, 22–24. Available online: https://archive.org/details/sim_compendium-continuing-education-for-veterinarians_2009-01_31_1 (accessed on 19 May 2023).
17. Abood, S.K. Effectively communicating with your clients. *Top Companion Anim. Med.* **2008**, *23*, 143–147. [CrossRef]
18. Brown, M.T.; Bussell, J.K. Medication adherence: WHO cares? *Mayo Clin. Proc.* **2011**, *86*, 304–314. [CrossRef]
19. Bartlett, E.E.; Grayson, M.; Barker, R.; Levine, D.M.; Golden, A.; Libber, S. The effects of physician communication skills on patient satisfaction; Recall, and adherence. *J. Chronic Dis.* **1984**, *37*, 755–764. [CrossRef]
20. DiMatteo, M.R.; Sherbourne, C.D.; Hays, R.D.; Ordway, L.; Kravitz, R.L.; McGlynn, E.A.; Kaplan, S.; Rogers, W.H. Physicians' characteristics influence patients' adherence to medical treatment: Results from the Medical Outcomes Study. *Health Psychol.* **1993**, *12*, 93–102. Available online: https://psycnet.apa.org/search/display?id=20561508-4db6-71c4-4e59-6688d5c30505&recordId=1&tab=PA&page=1&display=25&sort=PublicationYearMSSort%20desc,AuthorSort%20asc&sr=1 (accessed on 19 May 2023). [CrossRef]
21. Bultman, D.C.; Svarstad, B.L. Effects of physician communication style on client medication beliefs and adherence with antidepressant treatment. *Patient Educ. Couns.* **2000**, *40*, 173–185. [CrossRef]

- Zolnierek, K.B.H.; Dimatteo, M.R. Physician communication and patient adherence to treatment: A meta-analysis. *Med. Care* **2009**, *47*, 826–834. [CrossRef]
- Kaplan, S.H.; Greenfield, S.; Ware, J.E., Jr. Assessing the effects of physician-patient interactions on the outcomes of chronic disease. *Med. Care* **1989**, *27*, S110–S127. [CrossRef] [PubMed]
- Stewart, M.A. Effective physician-patient communication and health outcomes: A review. *Can. Med. Assoc. J.* **1995**, *152*, 1432–1433. Available online: https://www.ncbi.nlm.nih.gov/pmc/articles/PMC1337906/ (accessed on 19 May 2023).
- Stewart, M.; Brown, J.B.; Boon, H.; Galajda, J.; Meredith, L.; Sangster, M. Evidence on patient-doctor communication. *Cancer Prev. Control* **1999**, *3*, 25–30. Available online: https://pubmed.ncbi.nlm.nih.gov/10474749/ (accessed on 19 May 2023). [CrossRef]
- Roter, D. The enduring and evolving nature of the patient-physician relationship. *Patient Educ. Couns.* **2000**, *39*, 5–15. [CrossRef]
- Lue, T.W.; Pantenberg, D.P.; Crawford, P.M. Impact of the owner-pet and client-veterinarian bond on the care that pets receive. *J. Am. Vet. Med. Assoc.* **2008**, *232*, 531–540. [CrossRef]
- American Animal Hospital Association. *Compliance: Taking Quality Care to the Next Level: A Report of the 2009 AAHA Compliance Follow-Up Study*; American Animal Hospital Association: Lakewood, CO, USA, 2009; Available online: https://www.google.ca/books/edition/Compliance/vFivPwAACAAJ?hl=en (accessed on 19 May 2023).
- Grave, K.; Tanem, H. Compliance with short-term oral antibacterial drug treatment in dogs. *J. Small Anim. Pract.* **1999**, *40*, 158–162. [CrossRef] [PubMed]
- Kanji, N.; Coe, J.B.; Adams, C.L.; Shaw, J.R. Effect of veterinarian-client-patient interactions on client adherence to dentistry and surgery recommendations in companion-animal practice. *J. Am. Vet. Med. Assoc.* **2012**, *240*, 427–436. [CrossRef] [PubMed]
- Gill, V.T.; Roberts, F. Conversation analysis in medicine. In *The Handbook of Conversation Analysis*; Sidnell, J., Stivers, T., Eds.; Wiley-Blackwell: Malden, UK, 2013; pp. 575–592. Available online: https://onlinelibrary.wiley.com/doi/10.1002/9781118325001.ch28 (accessed on 19 May 2023).
- Roberts, F. *Talking about Treatment: Recommendations for Breast Cancer Adjuvant Therapy*; Oxford University Press: New York, NY, USA, 1999; Available online: https://www.google.ca/books/edition/Talking_about_Treatment/LlvnCwAAQBAJ?hl=en&gbpv=1&dq=talking+about+treatment:+Recommendations+for+breast+cancer+adjuvant+therapy&printsec=frontcover (accessed on 19 May 2023).
- Robinson, J.D. Asymmetry in action: Sequential resources in the negotiation of a prescription request. *Text Talk* **2001**, *21*, 19–54. [CrossRef]
- Stivers, T. Participating in decisions about treatment: Overt parent pressure for antibiotic medication in pediatric encounters. *Soc. Sci. Med.* **2002**, *54*, 1111–1130. [CrossRef]
- Stivers, T. Non-antibiotic treatment recommendations: Delivery formats and implications for parent resistance. *Soc. Sci. Med.* **2005**, *60*, 949–964. [CrossRef]
- Stivers, T. Parent resistance to physicians' treatment recommendations: One resource for initiating a negotiation of the treatment decision. *Health Commun.* **2005**, *18*, 41–74. [CrossRef]
- Stivers, T. Treatment decisions: Negotiations between doctors and patients in acute care encounters. In *Communication in Medical Care: Interactions between Primary Care Physicians and Patients*; Heritage, J., Maynard, D., Eds.; Cambridge University Press: New York, NY, USA, 2006; pp. 279–312. Available online: https://www.cambridge.org/core/books/abs/communication-in-medical-care/treatment-decisions-negotiations-between-doctors-and-patients-in-acute-care-encounters/70882445A62D5CE019F7ACA0E254EC19 (accessed on 19 May 2023).
- Stivers, T. *Prescribing under Pressure: Parent-Physician Conversations and Antibiotics*; Oxford University Press: New York, NY, USA, 2007; Available online: https://www.google.ca/books/edition/Prescribing_Under_Pressure/Vn88DwAAQBAJ?hl=en&gbpv=1&dq=prescribing+under+pressure:+Parent-Physician+Conversations+and+antibiotics&printsec=frontcover (accessed on 19 May 2023).
- Koenig, C.J. Patient resistance as agency in treatment decisions. *Soc. Sci. Med.* **2011**, *72*, 1105–1114. [CrossRef]
- Stivers, T.; Heritage, J.; Barnes, R.K.; McCabe, R.; Thompson, L.; Toerien, M. Treatment recommendations as actions. *Health Commun.* **2018**, *33*, 1335–1344. [CrossRef]
- Bergen, C.; Stivers, T.; Barnes, R.K.; Heritage, J.; McCabe, R.; Thompson, L.; Toerien, M. Closing the deal: A cross-cultural comparison of treatment resistance. *Health Commun.* **2018**, *33*, 1377–1388. [CrossRef] [PubMed]
- Stivers, T.; Timmermans, S. Authority under siege: How clinicians transform patient resistance into acceptance. *J. Health Soc. Behav.* **2020**, *61*, 60–78. [CrossRef] [PubMed]
- Heritage, J.; Sefi, S. Dilemmas of advice: Aspects of the delivery and reception of advice in interactions between health visitors and first time mothers. In *Talk at Work: Interaction in Institutional Settings*; Drew, P., Heritage, J., Eds.; Cambridge University Press: Cambridge, UK, 1992; pp. 359–417. Available online: https://www.cambridge.org/ca/academic/subjects/languages-linguistics/sociolinguistics/talk-work-interaction-institutional-settings?format=PB&isbn=9780521376334 (accessed on 19 May 2023).
- Kinnell, A.M.; Maynard, D.W. The delivery and receipt of safer sex advice in pretest counseling sessions for HIV and AIDS. *J. Contemp. Ethnogr.* **1996**, *24*, 405–437. [CrossRef]
- Silverman, D. *Discourses of Counselling: HIV Counselling as Social Interaction*; Sage: London, UK, 1997; Available online: https://www.google.ca/books/edition/Discourses_of_Counselling/55QfnwEACAAJ?hl=en (accessed on 19 May 2023).
- Heritage, J.; Lindström, A. Motherhood, medicine and morality: Scenes from a medical encounter. *Res. Lang. Soc. Interact.* **1998**, *31*, 397–438. [CrossRef]

47. Costello, B.A.; Roberts, F. Medical recommendations as joint social practice. *Health Commun.* **2001**, *13*, 241–260. [CrossRef]
48. Stivers, T. Prediagnostic commentary in veterinarian-client interaction. *Res. Lang. Soc. Interact.* **1998**, *31*, 241–277. [CrossRef]
49. Roberts, F. Speaking to and for animals in a veterinary clinic: A practice for managing interpersonal interaction. *Res. Lang. S Interact.* **2004**, *37*, 421–446. [CrossRef]
50. MacMartin, C.; Coe, J.B.; Adams, C.L. Treating distressed animals as participants: *I know* responses in veterinarians' pet-direct talk. *Res. Lang. Soc. Interact.* **2014**, *47*, 151–174. [CrossRef]
51. MacMartin, C.; Wheat, H.C.; Coe, J.B.; Adams, C.L. Effect of question design on dietary information solicited during veterinaria client interactions in companion animal practice in Ontario, Canada. *J. Am. Vet. Med. Assoc.* **2015**, *246*, 1203–1214. [CrossRef]
52. MacMartin, C.; Wheat, H.C.; Coe, J.B.; Adams, C.L. Conversation analysis of veterinarians' proposals for long-term dieta change in companion animal practice in Ontario, Canada. *J. Vet. Med. Educ.* **2018**, *45*, 514–533. [CrossRef]
53. Coe, J.B.; Adams, C.L.; Bonnett, B.N. Prevalence and nature of cost discussions during clinical appointments in companion anim practice. *J. Am. Vet. Med. Assoc.* **2009**, *234*, 1418–1424. [CrossRef]
54. Stivers, T.; Sidnell, J. Introduction. In *The Handbook of Conversation Analysis*; Sidnell, J., Stivers, T., Eds.; Wiley-Blackwell: Malde UK, 2013; pp. 1–8. Available online: https://onlinelibrary.wiley.com/doi/epdf/10.1002/9781118325001.ch1 (accessed on 23 M 2023).
55. Hutchby, I.; Wooffitt, R. *Conversation Analysis: Principles, Practices and Applications*; Polity Press: Oxford, UK, 2000; Availab online: https://books.google.ca/books/about/Conversation_Analysis.html?id=_YJjAAAAMAAJ&redir_esc=y (accessed on May 2023).
56. Heritage, J.; Maynard, D.W. Introduction: Analyzing interaction between doctors and patients in primary care settings. *Communication in Medical Care: Interaction between Primary Care Physicians and Patients*; Heritage, J., Maynard, D.W., Ed Cambridge University Press: Cambridge, UK, 2006; pp. 1–21. Available online: https://www.cambridge.org/core/books/abs ommunication-in-medical-care/introduction-analyzing-interaction-between-doctors-and-patients-in-primary-care-encount s/7DD792E92FD5879ACF21CCFA5F9D80C0#access-block (accessed on 23 May 2023).
57. Paul, T.H. *Doing Conversation Analysis: A Practical Guide*, 3rd ed.; Sage: London, UK, 2007; Available online: https://www.g ogle.ca/books/edition/Doing_Conversation_Analysis/hew9cKFnCnQC?hl=en&gbpv=1&dq=doing+conversation+analys +a+practical+guide&printsec=frontcover (accessed on 23 May 2023).
58. Sidnell, J. *Conversation Analysis: An Introduction*; Cambridge University Press: Malden, UK, 2010; Available onlin https://www.google.ca/books/edition/Conversation_Analysis/-Wfx_uM-bmQC?hl=en&gbpv=1&dq=conversation+analys +an+introduction&printsec=frontcover (accessed on 23 May 2023).
59. Jefferson, G. Glossary of transcript symbols with an introduction. In *Conversation Analysis: Studies from the First Generation*; Lern G.H., Ed.; John Benjamins: Philadelphia, PA, USA, 2004; pp. 13–31. [CrossRef]
60. Hepburn, A.; Bolden, G.B. The Conversation Analytic Approach to Transcription. In *The Handbook of Conversation Analysis*; Sidne J., Stivers, T., Eds.; Wiley-Blackwell: Malden, UK, 2013; pp. 57–76. Available online: https://onlinelibrary.wiley.com/doi/epdf 0.1002/9781118325001.ch4 (accessed on 23 May 2023).
61. Schegloff, E.A. *Sequence Organization in Interaction: A Primer in Conversation Analysis I*; Cambridge University Press: Cambridg UK, 2007; Available online: https://books.google.ca/books/about/Sequence_Organization_in_Interaction_Vol.html?id=pJVhi FV5wC&redir_esc=y (accessed on 23 May 2023).
62. Pomerantz, A.; Heritage, J. Preference. In *The Handbook of Conversation Analysis*; Sidnell, J., Stivers, T., Eds.; Wiley-Blackwe Malden, UK, 2013; pp. 210–228. Available online: https://onlinelibrary.wiley.com/doi/epdf/10.1002/9781118325001.ch (accessed on 23 May 2023).
63. Heritage, J.; Raymond, G. The terms of agreement: Indexing epistemic authority and subordination in talk-in-interaction. *Sc Psychol. Quart.* **2005**, *68*, 15–38. Available online: https://journals.sagepub.com/doi/abs/10.1177/019027250506800103 (accesse on 23 May 2023). [CrossRef]
64. Stevanovic, M.; Peräkylä, A. Deontic authority in interaction: The right to announce, propose, and decide. *Res. Lang. Soc. Interac* **2012**, *45*, 297–321. Available online: https://www.tandfonline.com/doi/epdf/10.1080/08351813.2012.699260 (accessed on 2 May 2023). [CrossRef]
65. Heritage, J. The epistemic engine: Sequence organization and territories of knowledge. *Res. Lang. Soc. Interact.* **2012**, *45*, 30–5 Available online: https://www.tandfonline.com/doi/epdf/10.1080/08351813.2012.646685 (accessed on 23 May 2023). [CrossRe
66. Stevanovic, M.; Peräkylä, A. Three orders in the organization of human action: On the interface between knowledge, power, an emotion in interaction and social relations. *Lang. Soc.* **2014**, *43*, 185–207. [CrossRef]
67. Stivers, T. Sequence organization. In *The Handbook of Conversation Analysis*; Sidnell, J., Stivers, T., Eds.; Wiley-Blackwell: Malde UK, 2013; pp. 191–209. Available online: https://onlinelibrary.wiley.com/doi/epdf/10.1002/9781118325001.ch10 (accessed on 2 May 2023).
68. Drew, P. Turn design. In *The Handbook of Conversation Analysis*; Sidnell, J., Stivers, T., Eds.; Wiley-Blackwell: Malden, UK, 2013; p 131–149. Available online: https://onlinelibrary.wiley.com/doi/epdf/10.1002/9781118325001.ch7 (accessed on 23 May 2023).

69. Pomerantz, A. Agreeing and disagreeing with assessments: Some features of preferred/dispreferred turn shapes. In *Structures of Social Action: Studies in Conversation Analysis*; Atkinson, J.M., Heritage, J., Eds.; Cambridge University Press: Cambridge, UK, 1985; pp. 57–101. Available online: https://www.cambridge.org/core/books/abs/structures-of-social-action/agreeing-and-disagreeing-with-assessments-some-features-of-preferreddispreferred-turn-shapes/650C48185B3180764990246B9D3D7822 (accessed on 23 May 2023).
70. Beeching, K. *Pragmatic Markers in British English*; Cambridge University Press: Cambridge, UK, 2016; Available online: https://www.google.ca/books/edition/Pragmatic_Markers_in_British_English/wXjBwwEACAAJ?hl=en (accessed on 23 May 2023).
71. Raymond, G. Prompting action: The stand-alone "So" in ordinary conversation. *Res. Lang. Soc. Interact.* **2004**, *37*, 185–218. [CrossRef]
72. Gardner, R. *When Listeners Talk: Response Tokens and Listener Stance*; John Benjamins: Amsterdam, The Netherlands, 2001; Available online: https://www.google.ca/books/edition/When_Listeners_Talk/3O2wcv6bVvwC?hl=en&gbpv=1&dq=when+listeners+talk:+Response+tokens+and+listener+stance&printsec=frontcover (accessed on 23 May 2023).
73. Clift, R. Meaning in interaction: The case of actually. *Language* **2001**, *77*, 245–291. [CrossRef]
74. Shaw, C.; Potter, J.; Hepburn, A. Advice-implicative actions: Using interrogatives and assessments to deliver advice in mundane conversations. *Discourse Stud.* **2015**, *17*, 317–342. [CrossRef]
75. Lerner, G.H. Collaborative turn sequences. In *Conversation Analysis: Studies from the First Generation*; Lerner, G.H., Ed.; John Benjamins: Amsterdam, The Netherlands, 2004; pp. 225–256. [CrossRef]
76. Raymond, G. Grammar and social organization: Yes/no interrogatives and the structure of responding. *Am. Soc. Rev.* **2003**, *68*, 939–967. [CrossRef]
77. Heritage, J. Well-prefaced turns in English conversation: A conversation analytic perspective. *J. Pragmat.* **2015**, *88*, 88–104. [CrossRef]
78. Pomerantz, A. Extreme case formulations: A way of legitimizing claims. *Hum. Stud.* **1986**, *9*, 219–229. [CrossRef]
79. Clark, H.H.; Fox Tree, J.E. Using *uh* and *um* in spontaneous speaking. *Cognition* **2002**, *84*, 73–111. [CrossRef]
80. Jefferson, G. Preliminary notes on a possible metric which provides for a "standard maximum" silence of approximately one second in conversation. In *Conversation: An Interdisciplinary Perspective*; Roger, D., Bull, P., Eds.; Multilingual Matters: Clevedon, UK, 1989; pp. 166–196. Available online: https://books.google.ca/books?id=k8F24A1jC-gC&pg=PA166&lpg=PA166&dq=gail+jefferson+preliminary+notes+on+a+possible+metric+which+provides+for&source=bl&ots=LUVZGbr2tA&sig=ACfU3U0au3L2yJMTZFwss3eeNUFTozYuXw&hl=en&sa=X&ved=2ahUKEwjIsOWE5ov_AhVukokEHT0lDKsQ6AF6BAgXEAM#v=onepage&q=gail%20jefferson%20preliminary%20notes%20on%20a%20possible%20metric%20which%20provides%20for&f=false (accessed on 23 May 2023).
81. Gardner, R. The conversational object *mm*: A weak and variable acknowledging token. *Res. Lang. Soc. Interact.* **1997**, *30*, 131–156. [CrossRef]
82. Beach, W.A. Transitional regularities for 'casual' "Okay" usages. *J. Pragmat.* **1993**, *19*, 325–352. [CrossRef]
83. Heritage, J. "Oh"-prefaced responses to assessments: A method of modifying agreement/disagreement. In *The Language of Turn and Sequence*; Ford, C.E., Fox, B.A., Thompson, S.A., Eds.; Oxford University Press: Oxford, UK, 2002; pp. 196–224. Available online: https://www.google.com/books/edition/The_Language_of_Turn_and_Sequence/m2TcTircelwC?kptab=editions&sa=X&ved=2ahUKEwikwPDci4z_AhVJkIkEHZrQA1IQmBZ6BAgIEAc (accessed on 23 May 2023).
84. Heritage, J. A change-of-state token and aspects of its sequential placement. In *Structures of Social Action: Studies in Conversation Analysis*; Atkinson, J.M., Heritage, J., Eds.; Cambridge University Press: Cambridge, UK, 1985; pp. 28–52. Available online: https://www.cambridge.org/core/books/abs/structures-of-social-action/changeofstate-token-and-aspects-of-its-sequential-placement/8AACF1699E4A7AE1B19D8248B6613405 (accessed on 23 May 2023).
85. Kitzinger, C. Repair. In *The Handbook of Conversation Analysis*; Sidnell, J., Stivers, T., Eds.; Wiley-Blackwell: Malden, UK, 2013; pp. 229–255. Available online: https://onlinelibrary.wiley.com/doi/epdf/10.1002/9781118325001.ch12 (accessed on 23 May 2023).
86. Heritage, J. Conversation analysis and institutional talk. In *The Handbook of Language and Social Interaction*; Saunders, R., Fitch, K., Eds.; Erlbaum: Mawah, NJ, USA, 2005; pp. 103–147. Available online: https://books.google.ca/books/about/Handbook_of_Language_and_Social_Interact.html?id=zg8-0DKsG8IC&redir_esc=y (accessed on 23 May 2023).
87. Coe, J.B.; O'Connor, R.; MacMartin, C.; Verbrugghe, A.; Janke, K.A. Effects of three diet history questions on the amount of information gained from a sample of pet owners in Ontario, Canada. *J. Am. Vet. Med. Assoc.* **2020**, *256*, 469–478. [CrossRef]
88. Abood, S.K.; Verton-Shaw, S. Talking about dog and cat nutrition with clients. *Vet. Clin. N. Am. Small. Anim. Pract.* **2021**, *51*, 517–528. [CrossRef]
89. Alvarez, E.A.; Schultz, K.K.; Floerchinger, A.M.; Hull, J.L. Small animal general practitioners discuss nutrition infrequently despite assertion of indication, citing barriers. *J. Am. Vet. Med. Assoc.* **2022**, *260*, 469–478. [CrossRef]
90. Churchill, J.; Ward, E. Communication with pet owners about obesity: Roles of the veterinary health care team. *Vet. Clin. N. Am. Small. Anim. Pract.* **2016**, *46*, 899–911. [CrossRef] [PubMed]
91. Alvarez, E.A.; Schultz, K.K. Effect of personal, food manufacturer, and pet health statements made by a veterinarian during a pet wellness appointment on a dog or cat owner's decision to consider changing their pet's diet. *J. Am. Vet. Med. Assoc.* **2021**, *259*, 644–650. [CrossRef] [PubMed]
92. Schleicher, M.; Cash, S.B.; Freeman, L.M. Determinants of pet food purchasing decisions. *Can. Vet. J.* **2019**, *60*, 644–650. Available online: https://www.ncbi.nlm.nih.gov/pmc/articles/PMC6515811/?report=classic (accessed on 23 May 2023).

93. Barnes, R.K. Preliminaries to treatment recommendations in UK primary care: A vehicle for shared decision-making? *Health Commun.* **2018**, *33*, 1366–1376. [CrossRef] [PubMed]
94. Delgado, M.; Dantas, L.M.S. Feeding cats for optimal mental and behavioral well-being. *Vet. Clin. N. Am. Small. Anim. Pract.* **2020**, *5*, 939–953. [CrossRef]
95. Albury, C.; Hall, A.; Ziebland, S.; Stokoe, E.; Roberts, N.; Webb, H.; Aveyard, P. Communication practices for delivering health behaviour change conversations in primary care: A systematic review and thematic synthesis. *BMC Fam. Pract.* **2019**, *20*, 111. [CrossRef]
96. Toerien, M.; Shaw, R.; Reuber, M. Initiating decision-making in neurology consultations: "Recommending" versus "option-listing" and the implications for medical authority. *Sociol. Health Illn.* **2013**, *35*, 873–890. [CrossRef] [PubMed]
97. Connabeer, K. Lifestyle advice in UK primary consultations: Doctors' use of conditional forms of advice. *Patient Educ. Couns.* **2021**, *104*, 2706–2715. [CrossRef]
98. Wheat, H.; Barnes, R.K.; Aveyard, P.; Stevenson, F.; Begh, R. Brief opportunistic interventions by general practitioners to promote smoking cessation: A conversation analytic study. *Soc. Sci. Med.* **2022**, *314*, 115463. [CrossRef]
99. Wall, T.; PetFood Industry. 5 Trends Shape the Global Pet Food Industry. 2022. Available online: https://www.petfoodindustry.com/articles/11368-5-trends-shape-the-global-pet-food-industry-in-2022 (accessed on 23 May 2023).
100. Sprinkle, D.; PetFood Industry. Beyond Pet Food Humanization and Premiumization. 2018. Available online: https://www.petfoodindustry.com/articles/7635-beyond-pet-food-humanization-and-premiumization?v=preview (accessed on 23 May 2023).
101. Prata, J.C. Survey of pet owner attitudes on diet choices and feeding practices for their pets in Portugal. *Animals* **2022**, *12*, 2775. [CrossRef]
102. Brooks, D.; Churchill, J.; Fein, K.; Linder, D.; Michel, K.E.; Tudor, K.; Ward, E.; Witzel, A. 2014 AAHA weight management guidelines for dogs and cats. *J. Am. Anim. Hosp. Assoc.* **2014**, *50*, 1–11. [CrossRef] [PubMed]
103. Witzel-Rollins, A.; Murphy, M.; Springer, C.M.; Moyers, T.D.; Albright, J.D. Evaluation of a pet-separating automatic feeder and high-frequency meal feeding for weight loss in multi-cat households. *J. Feline Med. Surg.* **2022**, *24*, e281–e288. [CrossRef] [PubMed]

animals

MDPI

ticle

pplication of Blended Learning to Veterinary Gross Anatomy ractical Sessions: Students' Perceptions of Their Learning xperience and Academic Outcomes

lga Gómez †, Maria García-Manzanares †, Deborah Chicharro, Miriam Juárez, Clara Llamazares-Martín, rique Soriano and José Terrado *

Department of Animal Medicine and Surgery, Facultad de Veterinaria, Universidad CEU Cardenal Herrera, CEU Universities, C/Tirant lo Blanch, 7, Alfara del Patriarca, 46115 Valencia, Spain; olgoro@uchceu.es (O.G.); maria.garcia8@uchceu.es (M.G.-M.); debora.chicharro@uchceu.es (D.C.); miriam.juarez@uchceu.es (M.J.); clara.llamazares@ucv.es (C.L.-M.); e.soriano@vetmedia.es (E.S.)

* Correspondence: jterrado@uchceu.es

† These authors contributed equally to this work.

Simple Summary: Blended learning strategies are becoming more popular in health sciences teaching, including veterinary medicine. However, the use of these methods in practical classes is less commonly described. This paper outlines a blended learning approach using flipped classrooms, collaborative learning, and gamification in gross anatomy practicals for first-year veterinary students. The practicals were restructured to include video pre-viewing, quizzes, collaborative group work, and a card game. Results showed a small but significant improvement in practical anatomy exam scores for the locomotor apparatus, with no significant difference in organic systems exams. Student satisfaction was high, with positive feedback regarding motivation, stimulation, and learning with peers. This study demonstrates that blended learning in anatomy practicals, including a flipped classroom and gamification, can enhance the student learning experience and optimize the limited time available for practicals.

Abstract: The use of blended learning strategies is increasingly common in health sciences, including veterinary medicine; however, there are very few descriptions of these methods being applied to practicals. We describe here the application of blended learning based on the implementation of flipped classrooms with collaborative learning and gamification to the 2020–2021 veterinary medicine gross anatomy practicals at CEU Cardenal Herrera University (Spain). Students prepared for the sessions by pre-viewing videos and taking a quiz before the start. The sessions were conducted in small groups where students learned through collaborative work and reviewed their learning with a card game. A small but significant increase was observed when comparing the scores of practical exams of the locomotor apparatus with those of 2018–2019 (6.79 ± 2.22 vs. 6.38 ± 2.24, $p < 0.05$), while the scores were similar (7.76 ± 1.99 vs. 7.64 ± 1.92) for the organ system exams. Students' responses in a satisfaction survey were mostly positive (>80%) regarding the motivating and learning-facilitating effect of this educational method. Our work shows that the application of blended learning in anatomy practicals based on a flipped classroom and with elements of gamification and collaborative work can be an effective way to improve the learning experience of students.

Keywords: anatomy; flipped classroom; blended learning; dissection; prosection; team-work

1. Introduction

Higher education in health sciences disciplines is constantly evolving. Advances in technology and the application of new pedagogical approaches are modifying university teaching. In recent years, the emergence of COVID-19 has led to a rethinking of the ways of teaching and to the development of new pedagogical approaches seeking to facilitate the improvement of students' learning, giving rise to experiences that could then be applied in the post-COVID era [1]. In this context, blended learning (BL) has emerged as a strategy that uses different pedagogical approaches with the aim of modifying some aspects of how students learn to improve their learning experience [2–5]. The use of combined strategies in anatomy teaching has increased in recent years, with some studies showing the positive effects of using different methodologies [6]. This use of a diversity of e-learning resources, such as quizzes, anatomical demonstrations, computational 3D models, medical imaging, and dissection activities, has been shown to be effective in consolidating anatomical knowledge [7].

It is generally accepted that student-centered approaches and dynamic teaching methods facilitate learning. The flipped classroom (FC), collaborative learning, and gamification have emerged as three methodologies based on these principles, which facilitate active learning and student engagement and ultimately improve student learning [8].

In the FC, the ordinary roles in the learning process are reversed: the teacher acts only as a guide, and the student is the main actor. Flipped teaching is a student-centered approach where information is introduced outside the classroom, allowing more time during class to process the information and practice the content with a variety of active learning strategies [9,10]. The FC provides an opportunity for students to watch and study the course materials on their own time prior to the actual class; once they arrive, they are ready to apply the new knowledge [2,11].

In addition to the FC, peer-assisted or collaborative learning, in which students help each other and learn by teaching, has proven effective in undergraduate medical programmes [12]. More specifically, in anatomy courses, collaborative learning promotes engagement and improves the study and group-working skills of students, moving them from passive consumers to active participants [13].

Gamification experiences, or the use of game design elements in non-game environments to enhance academic performance, have also been used in different health sciences disciplines, reporting generally positive results and improving learning behaviours and learning outcomes [14].

Different BL approaches have been used in anatomy courses, and there is considerable debate about to what extent and how these new methods should be applied and can help to improve students' learning [7,15,16]. A recent systematic review concludes that the FC is often perceived positively by students and has some advantages, such as increased self-confidence, academic performance, interest, learning activity, interaction, satisfaction, and overall performance in the anatomy curriculum [17]. In relation to collaborative learning, several team learning approaches have been proposed for teaching anatomy [18], and different types of gamification experiences have also been described [19]. In our own experience, the development of a simple card game as a means to consolidate content has been well received by students, who valued the game as enjoyable, challenging, useful for improving their knowledge and understanding of clinical anatomy, and effective for anatomy exam preparation [20].

In this work, we describe a BL teaching experience that combines FC, collaborative learning, and gamification applied to practical sessions of gross anatomy for veterinary students. Similar to in the medical sciences, the use of active learning methods is increasing in veterinary education. A recent international study involving universities in the USA, United Kingdom, and Australia showed that 95% of participants were familiar with the FC technique, although fewer (64%) used it in their teaching [21]. Several studies have published different models of active or BL in veterinary medicine, most of them focusing on clinical or preclinical subjects and generally reporting positive results [22,23]; however, little has been reported in relation to practicals in veterinary anatomy.

With this background, our hypothesis was that introducing elements of flipped learning (so that students had to prepare the content of the practice beforehand), collaborative learning (so that the development of the sessions was cooperative), and gamification (applying a card game that would allow them to review the fundamental aspects of the sessions) to the practicals of veterinary gross anatomy would have positive effects on the learning experience of the students.

2. Materials and Methods

2.1. Anatomy in the Veterinary Medicine Curriculum

The teaching of anatomy subjects at the CEU Cardenal Herrera University (Valencia, Spain) is divided into three modules, called Structure and Function I, II, and III, during the first three semesters of the Veterinary Degree. The students involved in this study are those enrolled in Structure and Function (SF) I (locomotor apparatus) and II (organ systems), both in the first academic year. The practical sessions of gross anatomy in SF I in the 2020–2021 academic year included 4 sessions of comparative osteology of domestic mammals and 3 sessions of prosections on dog cadavers to study the locomotor apparatus. In SF II, 2 sessions of prosections on dog cadavers (one for the organs of the thoracic cavity and one for the abdominal and pelvic cavities) and 3 sessions of comparative anatomy of organs were carried out. The duration of each session was 2 h for both subjects. A practical exam consisting of identifying a series of anatomical structures was held at the end of each course of SF I (in December) and II (in May).

2.2. Participants and Procedure

Students enrolled in the 1st year of veterinary medicine during the academic year 2020/2021 were included in this study. There were 348 students in SF I and 325 in SF II. The students were divided into permanent and stable groups of 12–14 people for each practical. Exclusion criteria: students who did not take the practical examination were excluded from this study.

The study was approved by the Vice-Rectorate for Academic Organisation and Teaching Staff of the CEU Cardenal Herrera University, Ref: PI40A-VV-20.

2.3. Videos

Videos showing the anatomical structures to be studied in each session were recorded by the instructors and made available to the students as a basis for preparing the practicals. The videos ranged in length from 3 min to 12′ 30″. They included a description of the main anatomical details in the case of bones and viscera and explained the regional anatomy of the dog on prosections from previously dissected animals. The number of videos included in each practical was variable (between 2 and 5) depending on the content to be covered in each session. Videos were provided for all SF I and SEF II practicals. Students were encouraged to watch the videos prior to the practical as part of their learning process.

2.4. Pre-Practical Test

Twelve self-assessment tests were designed (one for each practical session, i.e., seven for SF I and five for SF II). The pre-practical tests were in multiple choice question format (with 4 possible answers, only 1 correct) and contained 5 questions on pictures of the structures explained in the videos (see supplementary material S1 as an example). They were provided via the Internet approximately one week before each practical. Students answered the questionnaire before doing the practical, and they had feedback on their answers immediately after taking the test. Access to the practical was also allowed if the student had not carried out the activity or watched the video.

2.5. Anatomy Cards Game

At the end of the practice, the students used a card game with different questions about the practical. Basically, the game consisted of answering questions related to the day's practical. These questions were organised in 4 groups and appeared on a series of previously prepared cards [20].

2.6. Teaching and Learning Approach

2.6.1. Before the Practical

At least one week in advance of each practical, the guide and the videos related to the structures to be identified were made available to the students via the Internet. Students had to study the guide and watch the videos, and then, they had to complete a five-question test via the Internet before the start of the practical. Prior to the implementation of this methodology in 2020–2021, students were provided, as support material, with the guide and a collection of videos that only partially covered the practical content, and no pre-practical quizzes were made available to them. The completion of these tests was taken into account as a component in the assessment of participation in the proposed activities (10% of the total value in SFI and 5% in SF2). The students were allowed to enter the practical regardless of whether or not they had carried out the activity and watched the videos.

2.6.2. During the Practical

In each practical, the students of each stable group (consisting of 12–14 students) were freely subgrouped into small groups of 3–4 students per dissection table to carry out the session (identification and recognition in situ of the corresponding structures). Each session lasted 2 h. Before the application of this methodology in 2020–2021, the teacher explained the structures to be identified for approximately 1 h, and the students used the remaining hour to work on the cadaver or on the models (bone pieces, viscera). In this new approach, students work on the cadaver or models from the beginning, using approximately 1 h 30 min to identify the structures and 30 min to play the self-assessment and knowledge consolidation card game. If the students were not able to identify the structures or had any doubts, an instructor was available to answer their questions. From time to time, this instructor also asked questions directly to the students to verify that the learning was being carried out correctly.

2.7. Practical Examination

At the end of each SF I (in December) and II (in May), an oral practical examination was held to assess the knowledge acquired. In the examination session, which was invigilated, the student had to identify 15 anatomical structures. There were 15 sample exams which were randomly distributed among the students at the time of the test. The student, having identified the structure, showed it to the examiner. They had a maximum time of 15 min to complete the test. The exams were similar in the academic years analyzed (2020–2021 and 2018–2019) and carried out by the same examiners in both years.

2.8. Questionnaire

At the end of the academic year, a satisfaction survey was presented to the students to find out their level of satisfaction with this teaching system. The purpose of the survey was explained to the students, and they were informed that the data would be used for academic and research purposes only. Participants were also informed that answering the questionnaire was voluntary and that responses were collected anonymously. The main objective of the survey was to determine the overall impact of this methodology on the attitude and learning experience of the students. The questions were designed in such a way that students could assess the effectiveness of the organisation of this course in their learning process. Students were asked about the effectiveness of the pre-recorded videos, the help of other students, the effectiveness in preparing for the practical exam, and about the general consideration of anatomy. For each question, students could choose their level of satisfaction between "strongly agree", "agree", "indifferent", "disagree", and "strongly disagree". Students were also given the possibility to express their opinion in qualitative responses. No demographic data were collected. This questionnaire has a Cronbach's α of 0.77.

The instructors (n = 7) also completed a questionnaire asking about the effect of this methodology on improving students' accountability, the appropriateness of following up on students' previous work, improving students' learning, the importance of videos, and the effect on student–teacher interaction. This questionnaire has a Cronbach's α of 0.60.

2.9. Outcomes Comparison

The results of the practical exams obtained by the students were compared with those obtained in the same examinations by students in the 2018/19 academic year to analyse the academic outcomes of this experience. Teaching and examinations were conducted by the same instructors in 2018–2019 and 2020–2021. The academic year 2019/20 was not considered as it was affected by the special measures for COVID 19.

2.10. Statistics

Analysis of data included variable scale parameters as mean and standard deviation. Data followed a normal distribution as calculated by Kolmogorov–Smirnov and Shapiro–Wilk normality tests and were compared using Student's *t*-test. Pearson's correlation coefficient was calculated to determine the statistical relationship between variables. $p < 0.05$ was considered statistically significant. All analyses were performed using R statistical software, version 4.2.3 for Windows (R Core Team, 2023).

3. Results

3.1. Students' Engagement and Academic Results in Locomotor Apparatus Practicals

When analysing the students' completion of quizzes prior to the practical, results showed that almost all students completed the questionnaires. In total, 74% of the 1803 proposed quizzes were completed. The number of students who completed the questionnaires, which was fairly constant (between 75% and 80%) for the first ones, decreased slightly towards the middle of the course and markedly in the last quiz proposed, which was completed by 61% of them (Figure 1).

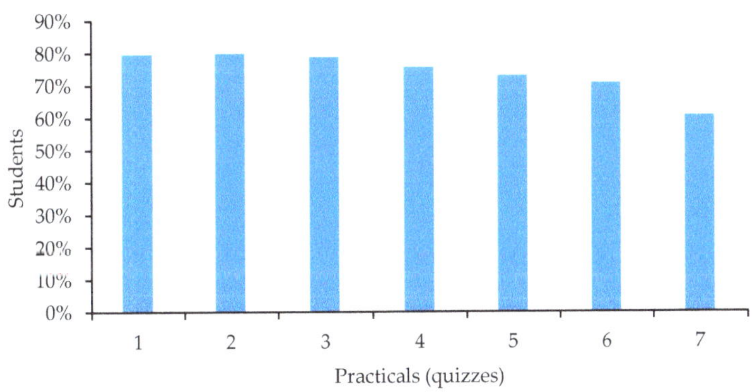

Figure 1. Percentage of students who took the quizzes corresponding to each locomotor apparatus practical.

Almost half ($n = 163$, 47%) of the students took all the quizzes and 20% ($n = 68$) only left one undone. On the opposite side, 48 students (14%) did none (Table 1).

Table 1. Number of quizzes completed by students in the locomotor apparatus study.

Number of Quizzes Completed	0	1	2	3	4	5	6	7
Number of students (%)	48 (14%)	8 (2%)	7 (2%)	11 (3%)	16 (5%)	27 (8%)	68 (20%)	163 (47%)

We then examined the correlation between having completed the quizzes and the practical exam marks. The students' final score in the anatomy practical exam was 6.79 ± 2.22

out of 10. We found a direct and discreet relationship (0.29, $p < 0.001$) between the number of quizzes completed by the students and their marks in the practical exam. We then analysed whether the opposite groups of students, i.e., those who had completed all the quizzes and those who had completed none of them, differed in their marks in the practical exam. Students who had completed all seven quizzes obtained a mean score of 7.67 ± 1.98 compared to those who had completed none, who scored 5.98 ± 1.98. This difference was very highly significant ($p < 0.001$).

Comparing these results with those obtained in the academic year 2018–2019 (the 2019–2020 academic year was not considered due to the special conditions of its teaching by the appearance of COVID-19), we found that academic results in 2020–2021 (6.79 ± 2.22) were slightly but significantly higher than in 2018–2019 (6.38 ± 2.24; $n = 353$, $p < 0.05$).

3.2. Students' Engagement and Academic Results in Organ System Practicals

In total, 78% of the 1273 questionnaires related to organ systems were completed by students. The first two questionnaires were completed by more than 80% of the students, and thereafter there was a very slight but steady decline in the number of students taking the tests (Figure 2).

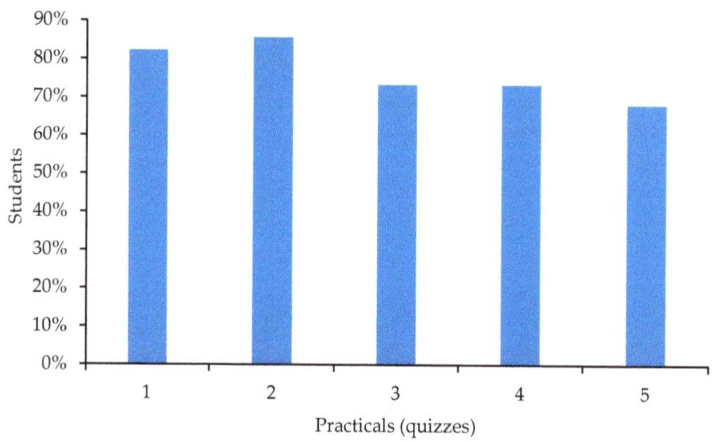

Figure 2. Percentage of students who took the quizzes corresponding to each organ systems practical.

The number of students completing the questionnaires in the organ systems practicals was slightly higher than in the locomotor system practicals, with more than half of the students ($n = 178$, 55%) completing all the questionnaires and only 23 (7%) not completing any (Table 2).

Table 2. Number of quizzes completed by students in the organ systems practicals.

Number of Quizzes Completed	0	1	2	3	4	5
Number of students (%)	23 (7%)	15 (5%)	18 (6%)	32 (10%)	59 (18%)	178 (55%)

The students' score in the final organ systems practical examination was 7.76 ± 1.99. A positive correlation (0.33, $p < 0.001$) was observed between the number of quizzes completed by the students and their marks in the practical exam. Comparing the scores of students who had completed all quizzes (8.31 ± 1.81) with those who had completed none of them (6.23 ± 2.04), a very highly significant difference was again found ($p < 0.001$). However, no difference was found, in this case, when comparing the marks for the organ systems practical exam in the year of this study (7.76 ± 1.99) and in 2018–2019, wherein students obtained 7.64 ± 1.92 ($n = 372$).

We next compared the percentage of students with low performance (those obtaining less than 5 out of 10 in the practical exam) in both SF I and SF II. The percentage of students with low performance was reduced in SF I (19% in 2020–2021 vs. 29% in 2018–2019), while in SF II, there was no change (10% in 2020–2021 vs. 8% in 2018–2019).

3.3. Students' and Instructors' Satisfaction Survey

A satisfaction survey was provided to the students at the end of the course, which was completed by 167 students. The majority of students answered positively to the proposed questions, as more than 80% of respondents agree or strongly agree with most of the proposed questions, with "*My anatomy interest has increased after practical sessions*" being the highest percentage (95%) and "*Videos helped improving my anatomy learning and knowledge*" the lowest (72%) (Figure 3).

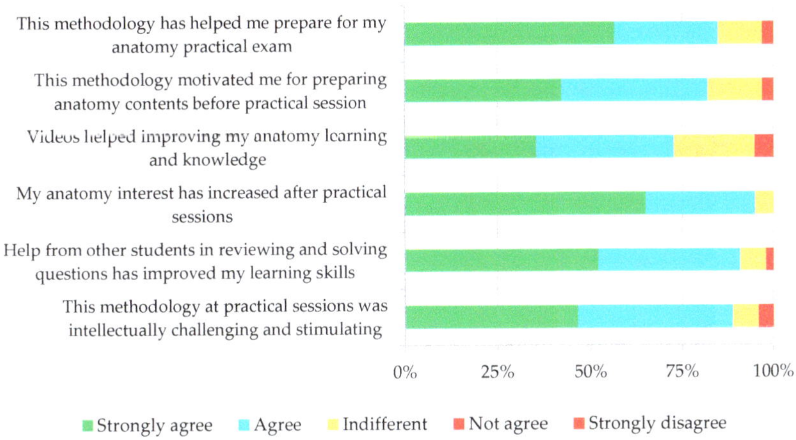

Figure 3. Results of the global satisfaction survey carried out by the students.

The students also had the opportunity to give their opinion, and 78 of them expressed their qualitative comments on the system. Most of them were positive, but in some cases, they suggested modifications in the method or in the quality of the materials provided. Some examples of the students' opinions are as follows:

> *"It would be nice to have access to the videos and tests from the beginning of the course and have the ability to do the tests multiple times".*

> *"I think videos are great bonus tools, as well as doing a test before each practical. But i prefer very much to be taught by anatomy teachers during the practical itself. So basically, watch vids, do the quizzes and then be taught by the teachers during practicals to avoid confusion. Even though they've always been available in case of doubts;)".*

> *"I would like to say that without the videos, I would never have obtained the grade I had at the anatomy practical exam. I really appreciate the videos but I can say that some of them didn't really follow the guide. The cards are really good to train ourselves during anatomy sessions. It would be great that they last longer and students helping us during the practicals is also very useful."*

Additionally, a questionnaire was also completed by the teaching staff (n = 7). The results indicate that, in the opinion of the staff, this methodology is particularly positive for improving the personal responsibility of the students and also highlights the convenience of checking the students' previous work with questionnaires before doing the practicals. On the other hand, although mostly positive, there was a diversity of opinions as to whether the videos can replace the direct explanation of the content by the teacher and whether the system increases teacher–student interaction (Figure 4).

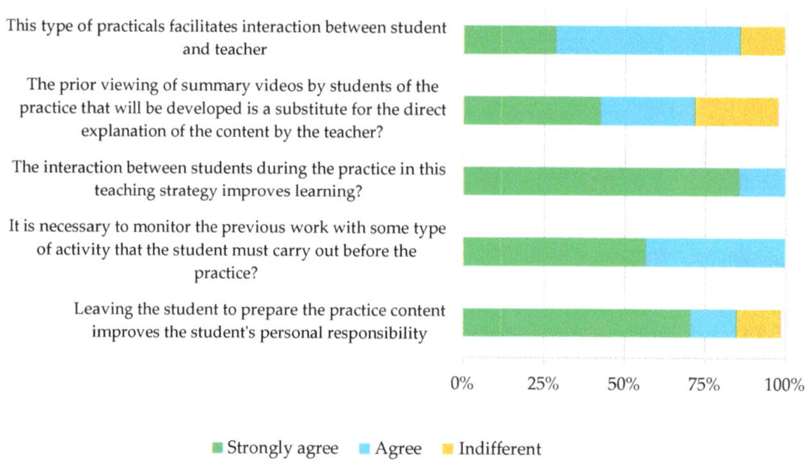

Figure 4. Results of the global satisfaction survey carried out by the teaching staff.

4. Discussion

4.1. The Usefulness of Blended Learning in the Teaching of Anatomy and the Academic Outcomes of the Students

Many different approaches are used to teach anatomy, and no single teaching tool has been found that meets all curriculum requirements [24–26]. In this regard, the application of new teaching methodologies has been described for both medical and veterinary anatomy, and ultimately, all the different changes that have occurred in recent years, including those resulting from the emergence of COVID-19, have promoted the need for adaptation and the development of new learning models [27–30].

Among the multiple forms of training, some authors consider that the best way to teach anatomy is by combining multiple pedagogical resources that complement each other, maximising interactive learning, and using time-saving materials that help students learn gross anatomy effectively and efficiently [29–31].

We describe here the transformation of traditional hands-on teaching into a BL approach in veterinary anatomy practicals. This change basically consisted of transforming sessions where a large part of the time was occupied by teacher explanation into active learning sessions, integrating flipped teaching, collaborative learning, and gamification. The results indicate that this switch was highly appreciated by the students and had some beneficial effect on academic results.

Different methods can make up a BL experience in anatomy. In our study, the FC is the central element, which is closely linked to students' cooperative work throughout the sessions and to a gamification element consisting of a card game designed to self-assess and reinforce knowledge [20]. Our results are in line with those of other authors who have reported the beneficial effects of BL in human anatomy teaching and show that active learning strategies are appreciated by students. Medical students preferred the hybrid, interactive, and student-centred learning method for practicals as a more effective system for understanding anatomy than face-to-face or online methods [32]. In another work, students appreciated the pre-class activities of this kind of learning, as they facilitated their engagement and concentration during class, thus increasing their academic performance and engagement [33]. In this regard, it has also been shown that veterinary anatomy students also favour active learning classes compared to traditional classes [34].

4.2. The Implementation and Usefulness of Flipped Classroom

Pre-class work is essential in FC pedagogies. Preparing courses by studying the material provided allows for better use of class time, creating time for integrative group activities during the session [35]. In this model, students have more responsibility for each laboratory experience, which can lead to more effort, but also to more satisfaction and confidence. While most FC approaches are applied to lecture-based courses, our results show that FC could also be applied to practicals. In our study, most of the students adequately prepared for the practicals before attending the sessions. In the preparation of the sessions, the use of videos is very important. Video as a support material for anatomy lectures is considered a very useful resource in a condensed curriculum scenario [36,37], and we have shown that their use can help decrease anxiety and enhance students' learning experience [38]. In our study, students considered these videos as important elements in the preparation of the practicals, although, in some cases, students requested more detailed documents. This would explain why the degree of satisfaction was not as high as in other questions of the survey. Although we do not have data on the video visualizations, the fact that many students completed the quizzes before the practicals suggests that most of the students prepared themselves thoroughly before attending the practicals. The number of completed quizzes exceeded 75% in the first sessions, but there was a 15–20% reduction in the number of tests completed towards the end of the semester. This decrease is consistent with Greene's [37] study, which showed a significant drop over the year in the total viewing of videos provided to review structures identified in lab sessions throughout an organ systems course. Likely, the decrease in completion of the quizzes was due to the feeling that time was not sufficient at the end of each semester, as reported in other studies [36,37,39]. At the end of the semester, there is generally a greater workload for the student; obviously, this depends on the organisation of the curriculum, but it is common for these dates to coincide with imminent exams, the preparation of which requires extra time and creates stress for students that can cause them to drop some activities. It is interesting to note that there is a correlation, though not very high, between having carried out these activities and academic outcomes. However, if we compare the results obtained by the students who completed all the tests with those who did not do any, the differences are highly significant in both topics, indicating the effectiveness of active involvement in this type of teaching.

Different results have been published on the effect of FC on academic scores in several disciplines of health sciences. Most of the studies report a slight improvement in test scores, while others show neutral results. Tune et al. [40] stated improvements of around 11–12% in the results of cardiovascular, respiratory, and renal physiology tests. Street and colleagues (2015) described a slight improvement, at the limits of the statistical significance, in a preclinical physiology course [41]. Better results after the implementation of FC have also been reported in practical examinations of dental students [42], in a pharmacotherapy course for pharmacy students [43], in an advanced physiology course for pharmacy students [44], and in physiology courses for health sciences students [45].

In other cases, the development of FC did not produce improvements in the performance of the students. No differences in grades or level of satisfaction were shown in an FC for neuroanatomy [46], and learning gains were not significantly different between a flipped biochemistry course and a traditional lecture [47]. However, in this last report, student perception of learning gains did differ and indicated a higher level of satisfaction with the flipped lecture format [47]. Indeed, students' perceptions about the effectiveness of FC are not necessarily accompanied by improvement in academic performance. This was also shown in a study performed in an introductory epidemiology class on masters-level graduate students [2].

A partial improvement has also been reported. Pharmacy students' performance in a flipped teaching pilot on cardiac arrhythmias improved in two of the three classes [48], and in a preclinical course (foundations on animal health) of veterinary medicine, FC cohorts performed well in the final exam but not in multiple-choice tests [23].

Similar results have been reported in studies specifically related to anatomy. A recent review shows that most FC experiences in anatomy report better exam scores than traditional courses, although there is also some work reporting a neutral effect [17]. Elzainy and Sadik [49] reported that FC medical students scored higher than traditional classroom students in anatomy theory classes and had lower absenteeism. Moreover, a small but significant improvement has been demonstrated in the histology exam scores of FC students compared to the control group [50], and nursing students instructed with the FC method on anatomy and physiology of the respiratory system scored higher on the final exam than the control group [51]. Finally, results reported by Yang and colleagues [52] and Elzainy and Sadik [49] on different human anatomy experiences for medical students pointed in the same direction.

As noted above, some anatomy-specific studies also describe partial improvements or neutral results from the application of FC. Fleagle et al. reported that there was no change in mean scores on the first and second lab exams, but higher scores on the final lab exam for dental gross anatomy students [35], and in another study, FC students also performed better than lecture hall students on analysis items, but there was no difference in performance between students in the two groups for knowledge [53]. Our results are close to the latter works, as the students in the experience we present here obtained a slight but statistically significant improvement in the practical examination of the anatomy of the locomotor system, while there was no effect in the examination of the anatomy of organ systems and body cavities.

4.3. The Role of Collaborative Learning and Gamification in a Model of FC

FC and peer learning are closely related since FC provides more opportunities for students to interact effectively and learn from their peers [2]. It has been shown that cooperative learning deepens student understanding but also offers them an opportunity to practice the generic skills in veterinary anatomy dissection courses, enhancing students' comprehension of the subject matter and encouraging them to share responsibility for their learning [54]. Peer-assisted learning also had positive results in a study on medical students, which appreciated most aspects of this method and obtained higher scores in osteology [55]. In this sense, it has been shown that combining flipped teaching and team-based learning results in positive outcomes in a physiology course [44]. On the basis of a different experimental design, Laakkonen and Muukkonnen [56] also pointed out the importance of collaboration between students to support mutual learning in gross anatomy courses of veterinary medicine. Among the diversity of peer-assisted learning methods, our model is based on collaborative work between students, where, organised into small groups, they received help from other students who solved their doubts in the first instance and in reviewing the content. In fact, this feature was one of the most valued aspects by the students, emphasizing the importance of collaborative work in this type of teaching. Interestingly, a positive outcome has been reported when students work cooperatively rather than when peer interaction was absent [9]; it has also been shown that the combination of e-learning, peer teaching, and FC significantly improved the average score in a physiology laboratory course for nursing students [57].

The development of the card game that ends each practical session in our model was also carried out in a collaborative environment [20] in a manner wherein everyone learns, regardless of the outcome of the game. In this sense, positive student outcomes have been reported in different gamification experiences in anatomy and related disciplines [58,59], reinforcing the positive effects of cooperative learning. Similar to other active approaches, the use of game-based methods is increasing in anatomy, and although the research concerning game-based anatomy learning is relatively limited, gamification seems to have a positive impact on different aspects of students' learning [16].

4.4. The Students and Staff Perceptions of Active Learning

Beyond the academic results, one of the advantages of the different BL models is that they are appreciated by the students as they improve their learning experience. In our work, as previously indicated, students rated the interaction with other students very positively and found the system motivating and challenging, and it increased their interest in anatomy. In the flipped model, students have more responsibility, which can increase effort but also satisfaction and confidence [35]. Active learning in anatomy demonstrations has been shown to be a preferred method by students [32], and perception surveys revealed students' enthusiasm for pre-class activities, leading to better performance in class with increased engagement with peers and teachers [60]. The positive perception of students toward active learning has been highlighted in numerous works ([60] and references therein). These results are also consistent with those shown in a systematic review showing that FC is generally perceived positively by students, increasing self-confidence, academic performance, interest, learning activity, interaction, satisfaction, and overall performance in the anatomy curriculum [17]. It is possible that this new system would entail a little more workload. This aspect was not explored, but the overall high degree of student satisfaction suggests that it was not an excessive effort.

Regarding the opinion of the staff, most of them were positive about the benefits of this method, since they all considered that it improves personal responsibility and ultimately student learning, but it is also important to point out the convenience of monitoring the work as a means of control of the preparation of the practical. This type of opinion is not always generalizable, and it has been described that, sometimes, teachers are more reluctant to implement this type of teaching than students. In this regard, it has been described that teachers sometimes consider that students do not prefer FC to traditional teaching and are not sure of the students' response to FC, in contrast to the positive views about this method in the student satisfaction survey [33].

4.5. Limitations of the Study

This teaching system was installed in the anatomy practicals for all students as a consensual teaching decision accepted by the University, so there is no control group in the same year. For this reason, the comparisons in the academic results have been made with those of the 2018–2019 academic year, the last one in which the presence of COVID-19 did not alter the teaching strategy.

On the other hand, the organisation of the teaching did not make it possible to follow the viewing of the videos.

Finally, a demographic study was not carried out, so it is not possible to know whether such factors influenced the results.

5. Conclusions

Our study shows that the development of an FC system in veterinary anatomy practices can have a beneficial effect on academic results. Moreover, it is well appreciated by students who positively value cooperation with other students to solve problems and consider this a highly motivating methodology. While most FC experiences are applied to lectures, our approach is aimed at practical gross anatomy classes. According to our experience, the application of this type of teaching organisation allows for better use of time, which is increasingly reduced in many anatomy curricula, and provides a good teaching experience for students and staff. Learning based on FC with a strong cooperative component among the students and completed with some gaming element, such as the work that we present here, can be applied, with the necessary adaptations, in a general way, both in veterinary medicine as well as in the different disciplines of health sciences that involve the practice of veterinary and human anatomy.

Supplementary Materials: The following supporting information can be downloaded at: https://www.mdpi.com/article/10.3390/ani13101666/s1, S1: Example of a question in a pre-practical quiz.

Author Contributions: Conceptualization, O.G. and J.T.; methodology, O.G., M.G.-M., D.C., M.J., C.L.-M., E.S. and J.T.; validation, O.G., M.G.-M. and J.T.; formal Analysis, O.G., M.G.-M. and J.T.; investigation, O.G., M.G.-M., D.C., M.J., C.L.-M., E.S. and J.T.; resources, O.G., M.G.-M., D.C., M.J., C.L.-M., E.S. and J.T.; data Curation, O.G., M.G.-M. and J.T.; writing—original draft preparation, J.T.; writing—review and editing, M.G.-M. and J.T.; visualization, M.G.-M. and J.T.; supervision, O.G. and J.T.; project administration, O.G. All authors have read and agreed to the published version of the manuscript.

Funding: This research received no external funding.

Institutional Review Board Statement: This study was approved by the Office of the Vice-Rector for Academic Organisation and Teaching Staff of the CEU Cardenal Herrera University (PI40A-VV-20).

Informed Consent Statement: Participants were informed of the use of the data for teaching and research purposes. The express informed consent of the participants was waived because of the analysis used anonymous data.

Data Availability Statement: The data presented in this study are available on request from the corresponding author.

Acknowledgments: The authors would like to express their gratitude to the first-year veterinary students during the 2018–2019 and 2020–2021 academic years for their participation.

Conflicts of Interest: The authors declare no conflict of interest.

References

1. Dicke, A.K.; Pilatz, A.; Wyrwoll, M.J.; Punab, M.; Ruckert, C.; Nagirnaja, L.; Aston, K.I.; Conrad, D.F.; Di Persio, S.; Neuhaus, N.; et al DDX3Y is likely the key spermatogenic factor in the AZFa region that contributes to human non-obstructive azoospermia *Commun. Biol.* **2023**, *6*, 350. [CrossRef]
2. Moraros, J.; Islam, A.; Yu, S.; Banow, R.; Schindelka, B. Flipping for success: Evaluating the effectiveness of a novel teaching approach in a graduate level setting. *BMC Med. Educ.* **2015**, *15*, 27. [CrossRef]
3. Stone, D.; Longhurst, G.J.; Dulohery, K.; Campbell, T.; Richards, A.; O'Brien, D.; Franchi, T.; Hall, S.; Border, S. A Multicentre Analysis of Approaches to Learning and Student Experiences of Learning Anatomy Online. *Med. Sci. Educ.* **2022**, *32*, 1117–1130. [CrossRef] [PubMed]
4. Atwa, H.; Shehata, M.H.; Al-Ansari, A.; Kumar, A.; Jaradat, A.; Ahmed, J.; Deifalla, A. Online, Face-to-Face, or Blended Learning? Faculty and Medical Students' Perceptions During the COVID-19 Pandemic: A Mixed-Method Study. *Front. Med.* **2022**, *9*, 791352. [CrossRef] [PubMed]
5. Xiao, J.; Evans, D.J.R. Anatomy education beyond the COVID-19 pandemic: A changing pedagogy. *Anat. Sci. Educ.* **2022**, *15*, 1138–1144. [CrossRef] [PubMed]
6. Yoo, H.; Kim, D.; Lee, Y.M.; Rhyu, I.J. Adaptations in Anatomy Education during COVID-19. *J. Korean Med. Sci.* **2021**, *36*, e13. [CrossRef] [PubMed]
7. Schulte, H.; Schmiedl, A.; Muhlfeld, C.; Knudsen, L. Teaching gross anatomy during the COVID-19 pandemic: Effects on medical students' gain of knowledge, confidence levels and pandemic-related concerns. *Ann. Anat. Anat. Anz* **2022**, *244*, 151986. [CrossRef] [PubMed]
8. Freeman, S.; Eddy, S.L.; McDonough, M.; Smith, M.K.; Okoroafor, N.; Jordt, H.; Wenderoth, M.P. Active learning increases student performance in science, engineering, and mathematics. *Proc. Natl. Acad. Sci. USA* **2014**, *111*, 8410–8415. [CrossRef]
9. Foldnes, N. The flipped classroom and cooperative learning: Evidence from a randomised experiment. *Act. Learn. High. Educ.* **2016**, *17*, 39–49. [CrossRef]
10. Morton, D.A. The flipped classroom: Starting with the end in mind. In *Teaching Anatomy. A Practical Guide*, 2nd ed.; Chan, L.K., Pawlina, W., Eds.; Springer Nature Switzerland: Cham, Switzerland, 2020; pp. 97–105.
11. Chowdhury, T.A.; Khan, H.; Druce, M.R.; Drake, W.M.; Rajakariar, R.; Thuraisingham, R.; Dobbie, H.; Parvanta, L.; Chinegwundoh, F.; Almushatat, A.; et al. Flipped learning: Turning medical education upside down. *Future Healthc. J.* **2019**, *6*, 192–195. [CrossRef]
12. Yu, T.C.; Wilson, N.C.; Singh, P.P.; Lemanu, D.P.; Hawken, S.J.; Hill, A.G. Medical students-as-teachers: A systematic review of peer-assisted teaching during medical school. *Adv. Med. Educ. Pract.* **2011**, *2*, 157–172. [CrossRef] [PubMed]
13. Scott, S.M.; Schifferdecker, K.E.; Anthony, D.; Chao, J.; Chessman, A.W.; Margo, K.; Seagrave, M.; Leong, S.L. Contemporary teaching strategies of exemplary community preceptors–is technology helping? *Fam. Med.* **2014**, *46*, 776–782. [PubMed]
14. Van Gaalen, A.E.J.; Brouwer, J.; Schonrock-Adema, J.; Bouwkamp-Timmer, T.; Jaarsma, A.D.C.; Georgiadis, J.R. Gamification of health professions education: A systematic review. *Adv. Health Sci. Educ. Theory Pract.* **2021**, *26*, 683–711. [CrossRef] [PubMed]
15. Evans, D.J.R.; Pawlina, W. The future of anatomy education: Learning from COVID-19 disruption. *Anat. Sci. Educ.* **2022**, *15*, 643–649. [CrossRef] [PubMed]
16. Chytas, D.; Noussios, G.; Paraskevas, G.; Demesticha, T.; Protogerou, V.; Salmas, M. Incorporation of team-based learning in the cadaveric anatomy laboratory: An overview. *Morphol. Bull. L'association Anat.* **2022**, *107*, 176–181. [CrossRef]
17. Kazeminia, M.; Salehi, L.; Khosravipour, M.; Rajati, F. Investigation flipped classroom effectiveness in teaching anatomy: A systematic review. *J. Prof. Nurs. Off. J. Am. Assoc. Coll. Nurs.* **2022**, *42*, 15–25. [CrossRef] [PubMed]
18. Melovitz-Vasan, C.; Huff, S.; Vasan, N.S. Teaching anatomy: Effective use of modified team-based learning strategy. In *Teaching Anatomy. A Practical Guide*; Chan, L.K., Pawlina, W., Eds.; Springer Nature Switzerland: Cham, Switzerland, 2020; pp. 161–172.
19. See, C.R. Gamification in anatomy education. In *Teaching Anatomy. A Practical Guide*, 2nd ed.; Chan, L.K., Pawlina, W., Eds.; Springer Nature Switzerland: Cham, Switzerland, 2020; pp. 63–71.

0. Chicharro, D.; Garcia-Manzanares, M.; Gomez, O.; Juarez, M.; Llamazares-Martin, C.; Soriano, E.; Terrado, J. Learning veterinary anatomy playing cards. *Adv. Physiol. Educ.* **2022**, *46*, 647–650. [CrossRef]
1. Matthew, S.M.; Schoenfeld-Tacher, R.M.; Danielson, J.A.; Warman, S.M. Flipped Classroom Use in Veterinary Education: A Multinational Survey of Faculty Experiences. *J. Vet. Med. Educ.* **2019**, *46*, 97–107. [CrossRef]
2. Kelly, R.F.; Mihm-Carmichael, M.; Hammond, J.A. Students' Engagement in and Perceptions of Blended Learning in a Clinical Module in a Veterinary Degree Program. *J. Vet. Med. Educ.* **2021**, *48*, 181–195. [CrossRef]
3. Dooley, L.M.; Frankland, S.; Boller, E.; Tudor, E. Implementing the Flipped Classroom in a Veterinary Pre-clinical Science Course: Student Engagement, Performance, and Satisfaction. *J. Vet. Med. Educ.* **2018**, *45*, 195–203. [CrossRef]
4. Ghosh, S.K. Cadaveric dissection as an educational tool for anatomical sciences in the 21st century. *Anat. Sci. Educ.* **2017**, *10*, 286–299. [CrossRef] [PubMed]
5. Varner, C.; Dixon, L.; Simons, M.C. The Past, Present, and Future: A Discussion of Cadaver Use in Medical and Veterinary Education. *Front. Vet. Sci.* **2021**, *8*, 720740. [CrossRef] [PubMed]
6. Hafez, S.A. Design for assessment of dissection in anatomy laboratory based on group identification of structures and peer evaluation. *Anat. Sci. Educ.* **2022**, *15*, 1045–1059. [CrossRef] [PubMed]
7. Kapoor, K.; Singh, A. Veterinary anatomy teaching from real to virtual reality: An unprecedented shift during COVID-19 in socially distant era. *Anat. Histol. Embryol.* **2022**, *51*, 163–169. [CrossRef] [PubMed]
8. Taylor, L.; Dyer, T.; Al-Azzawi, M.; Smith, C.; Nzeako, O.; Shah, Z. Extended reality anatomy undergraduate teaching: A literature review on an alternative method of learning. *Ann. Anat. Anat. Anz.* **2022**, *239*, 151817. [CrossRef] [PubMed]
9. Lin, D.C.; Bunch, B.; De Souza, R.Z.D.; Chen, D.; Zhou, J.; Zumwalt, A.C.; Wisco, J.J. Effectiveness of Pedagogical Tools for Teaching Medical Gross Anatomy During the COVID-19 Pandemic. *Med. Sci. Educ.* **2022**, *32*, 411–422. [CrossRef] [PubMed]
0. Shin, M.; Prasad, A.; Sabo, G.; Macnow, A.S.R.; Sheth, N.P.; Cross, M.B.; Premkumar, A. Anatomy education in US Medical Schools: Before, during, and beyond COVID-19. *BMC Med. Educ.* **2022**, *22*, 103. [CrossRef]
1. Estai, M.; Bunt, S. Best teaching practices in anatomy education: A critical review. *Ann. Anat. Anat. Anz.* **2016**, *208*, 151–157. [CrossRef]
2. Nasr El-Din, W.A.; Atwa, H.; Potu, B.K.; Deifalla, A.; Fadel, R.A. Checklist-based active learning in anatomy demonstration sessions during the COVID-19 pandemic: Perception of medical students. *Morphol. Bull. L'association Anat.* **2022**, *107*, 219–227. [CrossRef]
3. El Sadik, A.; Al Abdulmonem, W. Improvement in Student Performance and Perceptions through a Flipped Anatomy Classroom: Shifting from Passive Traditional to Active Blended Learning. *Anat. Sci. Educ.* **2021**, *14*, 482–490. [CrossRef]
4. Borroni, C.; Pimentel-Avila, A.; Stoore, C.; Hidalgo, C.; Diamond, K.; Vasquez-Carrillo, C.; Landerer, E.; Paredes, R. A Unique Approach to Project-Based Learning (PjBL) in a Veterinary Anatomy Course. *Med. Sci. Educ.* **2021**, *31*, 511–517. [CrossRef] [PubMed]
5. Fleagle, T.R.; Borcherding, N.C.; Harris, J.; Hoffmann, D.S. Application of flipped classroom pedagogy to the human gross anatomy laboratory: Student preferences and learning outcomes. *Anat. Sci. Educ.* **2018**, *11*, 385–396. [CrossRef] [PubMed]
6. Topping, D.B. Gross anatomy videos: Student satisfaction, usage, and effect on student performance in a condensed curriculum. *Anat. Sci. Educ.* **2014**, *7*, 273–279. [CrossRef] [PubMed]
7. Greene, S.J. The Use of Anatomical Dissection Videos in Medical Education. *Anat. Sci. Educ.* **2020**, *13*, 48–58. [CrossRef]
8. Terrado, J.; Gomez, O.; Chicharro, D.; Garcia-Manzanares, M.; Juarez, M.; Romo-Barrientos, C.; Mohedano-Moriano, A.; Criado-Alvarez, J.J. Anxiety, emotions, and thoughts of veterinary medicine students during their first visit to the dissection room. *Anat. Sci. Educ.* **2023**, *16*, 547–556. [CrossRef]
9. McNulty, J.A.; Sonntag, B.; Sinacore, J.M. Evaluation of computer-aided instruction in a gross anatomy course: A six-year study. *Anat. Sci. Educ.* **2009**, *2*, 2–8. [CrossRef]
0. Tune, J.D.; Sturek, M.; Basile, D.P. Flipped classroom model improves graduate student performance in cardiovascular, respiratory, and renal physiology. *Adv. Physiol. Educ.* **2013**, *37*, 316–320. [CrossRef]
1. Street, S.E.; Gilliland, K.; McNeil, C.; Royal, K. The flipped classroom improved medical student performance and satisfaction in a pre-clinical physiology course. *Med. Sci. Educ.* **2015**, *25*, 35–43. [CrossRef]
2. Bakr, M.M.; Thompson, C.M.; Massadiq, M. Anatomical sciences: A foundation for a solid learning experience in dental technology and dental prosthetics. *Anat. Sci. Educ.* **2017**, *10*, 395–404. [CrossRef]
3. Koo, C.L.; Demps, E.L.; Farris, C.; Bowman, J.D.; Panahi, L.; Boyle, P. Impact of Flipped Classroom Design on Student Performance and Perceptions in a Pharmacotherapy Course. *Am. J. Pharm. Educ.* **2016**, *80*, 33. [CrossRef]
4. Gopalan, C.; Klann, M.C. The effect of flipped teaching combined with modified team-based learning on student performance in physiology. *Adv. Physiol. Educ.* **2017**, *41*, 363–367. [CrossRef] [PubMed]
5. Megaw, P.L.; Zimanyi, M.A. Redesigning first year anatomy and physiology subjects for allied health students: Introducing active learning experiences for physiology in a first semester subject. *Int. J. Innovat. Sci. Math. Educ.* **2019**, *27*, 26–35. [CrossRef]
6. Whillier, S.; Lystad, R.P. No differences in grades or level of satisfaction in a flipped classroom for neuroanatomy. *J. Chiropr. Educ.* **2015**, *29*, 127–133. [CrossRef]
7. Ojennus, D.D. Assessment of learning gains in a flipped biochemistry classroom. *Biochem. Mol. Biol. Educ.* **2016**, *44*, 20–27. [CrossRef] [PubMed]

48. Wong, T.H.; Ip, E.J.; Lopes, I.; Rajagopalan, V. Pharmacy students' performance and perceptions in a flipped teaching pilot c cardiac arrhythmias. *Am. J. Pharm. Educ.* **2014**, *78*, 185. [CrossRef]
49. Elzainy, A.; Sadik, A.E. The impact of flipped classroom: Evaluation of cognitive level and attitude of undergraduate medic students. *Ann. Anat. Anat. Anz.* **2022**, *243*, 151952. [CrossRef]
50. Cheng, X.; Ka Ho Lee, K.; Chang, E.Y.; Yang, X. The "flipped classroom" approach: Stimulating positive learning attitudes ar improving mastery of histology among medical students. *Anat. Sci. Educ.* **2017**, *10*, 317–327. [CrossRef]
51. Joseph, M.A.; Roach, E.J.; Natarajan, J.; Karkada, S.; Cayaban, A.R.R. Flipped classroom improves Omani nursing studen performance and satisfaction in anatomy and physiology. *BMC Nurs.* **2021**, *20*, 1. [CrossRef]
52. Yang, C.; Yang, X.; Yang, H.; Fan, Y. Flipped classroom combined with human anatomy web-based learning system show promising effects in anatomy education. *Medicine* **2020**, *99*, e23096. [CrossRef]
53. Morton, D.A.; Colbert-Getz, J.M. Measuring the impact of the flipped anatomy classroom: The importance of categorizing a assessment by Bloom's taxonomy. *Anat. Sci. Educ.* **2017**, *10*, 170–175. [CrossRef]
54. Salomaki, T.; Laakkonen, J.; Ruohoniemi, M. Students as teachers in an anatomy dissection course. *J. Vet. Med. Educ.* **201** *41*, 60–67. [CrossRef]
55. Anantharaman, L.T.; Ravindranath, Y.; Dayal, S.; Shankar, N. Peer-assisted learning versus didactic teaching in osteology fo first-year Indian undergraduate medical students: A quasi-experimental study. *Surg. Radiol. Anat. SRA* **2019**, *41*, 1163–117 [CrossRef] [PubMed]
56. Laakkonen, J.; Muukkonen, H. Fostering Students' Collaborative Learning Competencies and Professional Conduct in the Conte of Two Gross Anatomy Courses in Veterinary Medicine. *Anat. Sci. Educ.* **2019**, *12*, 154–163. [CrossRef] [PubMed]
57. Meng, X.H.; Xu, X.Y.; Chen, H.L.; Zhang, L. The effectiveness of combining e-learning, peer teaching, and flipped classroom fo delivering a physiology laboratory course to nursing students. *Adv. Physiol. Educ.* **2022**, *46*, 21–26. [CrossRef]
58. Anyanwu, E.G. Anatomy adventure: A board game for enhancing understanding of anatomy. *Anat. Sci. Educ.* **2014**, *7*, 153–16 [CrossRef]
59. Donkin, R.; Rasmussen, R. Student Perception and the Effectiveness of Kahoot!: A Scoping Review in Histology, Anatomy, an Medical Education. *Anat. Sci. Educ.* **2021**, *14*, 572–585. [CrossRef]
60. Elzainy, A.; El Sadik, A.; Al Abdulmonem, W. Experience of e-learning and online assessment during the COVID-19 pandemic a the College of Medicine, Qassim University. *J. Taibah Univ. Med. Sci.* **2020**, *15*, 456–462. [CrossRef] [PubMed]

animals

MDPI

Article

The Application of 3D Anatomy for Teaching Veterinary Clinical Neurology

Lidia Blázquez-Llorca [1], Lubna Morales de Paz [1], Rosario Martín-Orti [1], Inmaculada Santos-Álvarez [1], María E. Fernández-Valle [2], David Castejón [2], María I. García-Real [3], Raquel Salgüero-Fernández [3,4], Pilar Pérez-Lloret [1], Nerea Moreno [5], Sara Jiménez [5], María J. Herrero-Fernández [6] and Juncal González-Soriano [1,*]

1 Departamento de Anatomía y Embriología, Sección Departamental de Anatomía y Embriología (Veterinaria), Facultad de Veterinaria, Universidad Complutense de Madrid, Avenida Puerta de Hierro s/n, 28040 Madrid, Spain; lidiblaz@ucm.es (L.B.-L.); lubnamor@ucm.es (L.M.d.P.); rosamart@ucm.es (R.M.-O.); inmasant@ucm.es (I.S.-Á.); pilper01@ucm.es (P.P.-L.)

2 ICTS Bioimagen Complutense, Universidad Complutense de Madrid, Paseo de Juan XXIII 1, 28040 Madrid, Spain; evalle@ucm.es (M.E.F.-V.); dcastejon@ucm.es (D.C.)

3 Departamento de Medicina y Cirugía, Facultad de Veterinaria, Universidad Complutense de Madrid, Avenida Puerta de Hierro s/n, 28040 Madrid, Spain; isagreal@vet.ucm.es (M.I.G.-R.); rsalgu01@ucm.es (R.S.-F.)

4 Hospital Veterinario Veterios, Calle Arrastaria, 23, 28022 Madrid, Spain

5 Departamento de Biología Celular, Facultad de Biología, Universidad Complutense de Madrid, Avenida José Antonio Novais 12, 28040 Madrid, Spain; nerea@bio.ucm.es (N.M.); sajime01@ucm.es (S.J.)

6 Departamento de Mineralogía y Petrología, Facultad de Geología, Universidad Complutense, Avenida José Antonio Novais 12, 28040 Madrid, Spain; mjherrer@ucm.es

* Correspondence: juncalgs@vet.ucm.es

Simple Summary: Anatomy is regarded as a key element in medical and veterinary education all over the world. It is a subject of voluminous and sometimes complex content, which normally causes students' different difficulties. These difficulties increase dramatically when it comes to the study of neuroanatomy. Hence, there have been continued efforts in developing new methods of teaching, learning and assessment that are aimed at the long-term retention of anatomical and neuroanatomical knowledge. Additionally, clinical neurology can be difficult for veterinary students to comprehend, and there is no doubt that part of its understanding is directly related to the knowledge of neuroanatomy. Therefore, the aim of this present work is to be a teaching tool oriented towards clinical neurology and clinical practice, through 3D reconstructions of magnetic resonance images of normal brains and clinical neurological cases.

Abstract: Neuroanatomy is always a challenging topic for veterinary students. It is widely accepted that understanding the anatomy of the central nervous system (CNS) is essential to explain many of the pathological processes that affect the brain. Although its study has varied over time to achieve this goal, in human and veterinary medicine it is difficult to find a teaching method that associates normal anatomy with pathological alterations of the brain. For the first time, we have created an educational tool that combines neuroanatomy and neuropathology, using different magnetic resonance (MR) images as a basis and EspINA software as analyzer, to obtain segmented structures and 3D reconstructions of the dog brain. We demonstrate that this combination is an optimal tool to help anatomists to understand the encephalon, and additionally to help clinicians to recognize illness including a multitude of neurological problems. In addition, we have tried to see whether photogrammetry, which is a common technique in other sciences, for example geology, could be useful to teach veterinary neuroanatomy. Although we still need further investigations, we have been able to generate 3D reconstructions of the whole brain, with very promising results to date.

Keywords: anatomy; neuroanatomy; teaching; magnetic resonance imaging; segmentation

1. Introduction

Anatomy is a science concerned with the identification and description of the body structures of living things [1]. It focuses on the description of form, or how body structures at different levels look, including the cells, tissues and organs and how they are organized. Consequently, veterinary anatomy is a science of which the main target is the study of animals' structure and organization.

Neuroanatomy is a very challenging topic for veterinary students, as the main goal is to associate gross anatomy with neurologic functions and, as a second step, to be able to localize neural lesions in the case of neurologic disease [2,3]. In this sense, the teaching of anatomy has evolved to the point of using different innovative methods oriented towards clinical practice [4,5]. In this present paper, we focus on the study of the central nervous system, taking the dog as a model.

Cadaver dissection started in 300 BC, and by the 15th century, it was considered the main tool for studying the structural details of the different bodily organs, including the brain [6,7]. Now, although veterinary professionals, surgeons, anatomy teachers and researchers in the anatomical field cannot completely avoid its use, anatomists often use additional methods [8,9]. In the case of the SNC, the use of different techniques for vascular casting [10] or the plastination of brain specimens is common [11]. Thus, the teaching of the CNS anatomy has evolved to introduce the use of other applied technologies. Among them, imaging techniques, X-rays, computed tomography (also called a CAT scan) or magnetic resonance imaging (MRI), stand out without a doubt. Of course, their use implies that educators must first understand how students mentally manipulate anatomical images [12–14]. At this point, it is interesting to remark that the use of three-dimensional reconstructions (3D reconstructions) is an additional and important aid to help veterinary students to study the brain, its morphology and function [2,3,15–17]. In fact, 3D reconstructions are commonly used as a teaching tool in other sciences, even those unrelated to veterinary medicine or anatomy, such as geology, for example. Between these methods, photogrammetry is very popular between earth sciences degrees, as it is able to facilitate the characterization of geological materials by the generation of 3D models [18,19]. Unfortunately, there is no previous information on the use of photogrammetry or other similar techniques in biological or medical sciences.

MRI is considered the gold standard for the diagnosis of neural pathology in medical and veterinary neurology [13]. Hence, a thorough understanding of MRI brain anatomy is essential for clinicians and surgeons. In this present paper, we analyzed different normal and pathological MR images of dog brains, by the means of EspINA Interactive Neuron Software 2.8.2 (https://cajalbbp.es/espina/, accessed on 2 May 2023). It is important to remark that EspINA allows the visualization and segmentation of large image stacks datasets, from either electron microscopy or confocal laser microscopy. Thus, the main goal of this present paper is to ascertain, for the first time, whether EspINA 3D reconstructions, proceeding from different quality MR images, could be a useful tool not only for anatomy students, but also to help clinicians recognize illness including a multitude of neurological problems. In addition, we have investigated whether photogrammetry could also be useful to produce 3D reconstructions of the brain, either from biological specimens or from brain sections or MR images.

2. Materials and Methods

2.1. Material

No dogs were sacrificed to carry out this present study. For the ex vivo experiments, we used four fixed brains, selected from the collection of specimens that are normally used to teach Neuroanatomy in the Department of Anatomy and Embryology (Veterinary Faculty, Complutense University of Madrid). In this case, the MRIs were performed at the Bioimaging Center of the Complutense University of Madrid using a Biospec BMT 47/40 system (Bruker Biospin GmbH, Ettligen, Germany) operating at 4.7 T and equipped with a 12 cm gradient system.

The in vivo MR images were performed with different equipment: a close high field MRI system (Vantage Elan 1.5 T, Canon Medical System, Otawara, Japan) from Hospital Veterios in Madrid and an open C-shape low field MRI system (Panorama 0,23 T Philips Medical Systems, Amsterdam, The Netherlands) located in the Complutense University Veterinary Teaching Hospital. The animals were 4 in total, with 2 in each system: a 9 year old female French bulldog (dog 1) and a 6 year old, neutered female (dog 2), in the first case and a middle-aged female crossbreed dog (dog 3) and a 5 year old French bulldog (dog 4), in the second. The crossbreed animals had a normal neurological examination and no signs of neural disease, whereas the other two (both French bulldogs) showed neurological symptoms.

All images were analyzed and segmented by means of the EspINA software (EspINA Interactive Neuron Analyzer, 2.8.2; https://cajalbbp.es/espina/, accessed on 2 May 2023). The 3D Viewer plugin of Image J (ImageJ 1.53, NIH, Bethesda, MD, USA) was used to generate the 3D view of the surface of the brain from the MRI stack of images of the fixed dog brain.

2.2. Methods

Two of the fixed brains were thick-sectioned (2–3 mm) by using a scalpel or simply a knife. After this, the slices were labelled by means of the Mulligan's staining [20], mainly to identify the cerebral grey matter.

The ex vivo dog brains were drained, immersed in a proton-free susceptibility-matching fluid, Fluorinert FC-40 (Sigma-Aldrich, Saint Louis, MO, USA) and placed inside a 7 cm volume radiofrequency coil. The 3D MRI experiment consisted of a T2-weighted (T2W) Fast spin echo (FSE) sequence with the following parameters: repetition time (TR) = 2500 ms; effective echo time (TE) = 35 ms; number of averaged experiments (NAQ) = 8; field of view (FOV) = 90 $\times$ 55 $\times$ 55 mm^3; acquisition matrix size = 448 $\times$ 192 $\times$ 192. The acquired data were zero-filled to obtain a reconstructed matrix size of 512 $\times$ 256 $\times$ 256; thus, the spatial resolution was 0.176 $\times$ 0.215 $\times$ 0.215 mm^3.

Concerning the in vivo experiments in the 1.5 T MRI system, a 16-channel flex medium coil, flexible 24 $\times$ 40 wrap, was used in both dogs (dog 1 and dog 2). A complete brain study was performed; however, the sequence used for this present study was a T2W FSE in a transverse plane, and the technical parameters included the following: TR = 16,569 ms and 14,052 ms, and TE = 105 ms; flip angle 90°/120°; NAQ = 2.0; FOV = 14 $\times$ 13 cm; matrix size = 256 $\times$ 272; slice thickness = 0.5 mm $\times$ 0.5 mm, with a pixel size of 1 mm.

In respect to the low field (0.23 T), an extremity coil was used for the examination of the 2 patients (dog 3 and dog 4). The sequence selected for segmentation in the case of dog 3 was a T2*-weighted (T2*W) fast field echo (FFE) 3D sequence in the transverse plane. The parameters selected for this dog were as follows: TR = 60 ms; TE = 16 ms; NAQ = 1; FOV = 330 $\times$ 200 mm; acquisition matrix size = 300 $\times$ 200. The slice thickness = 3.5 mm. The spacing between slices = 2.3 mm. The sequence used for the segmentation of dog 4 was a T2W turbo spin echo sequence in the transverse plane, and the parameters selected for this patient were as follows: TR = 4500 ms; TE = 96 ms; NAQ = 6; FOV = 343 $\times$ 200 mm; acquisition matrix size = 216 $\times$ 172. The slice thickness = 3.0 mm. The spacing between slices = 3.3 mm. In both cases, a complete brain MRI was performed. All in vivo experiments were performed under general anesthesia, and patients were positioned in sternal recumbency.

The segmentation with EspINA was manual as, to date, there are no automatic algorithms to adequately represent the structures of interest. Thus, we segmented all MRI stacks of images on a slice-by-slice basis, sometimes altering the MRI dataset contrast to help the visual identification of structures. The stacks of images of the MRI were analyzed using the EspINA software (Espina Interactive Neuron Analyzer, 2.9.15; Madrid, Spain; https://cajalbbp.es/espina/, accessed on 2 May 2023). Since EspINA allows navigation through the stack of images, it was possible to manually segment the selected brain structures in each single section where they were present. The user can create color-coded categories. The segmentations of a specific brain structure can be included in each category.

In addition, the EspINA software has a tool that allows the visualization in 3-dimensions of the reconstructed brain structures. In this present paper, we segmented and 3D reconstructed the following structures from MR images: the caudate nucleus, the cerebellum, the cerebral peduncles, the colliculi, the hippocampus, the lateral ventricles, the pyramids, the mesencephalon, the neocortex, the periaqueductal grey matter, the thalamus and the third ventricle,

Photogrammetry is the science of collecting information from 2D photos. By combining enough overlapping images of the same features, it is possible to generate realistic 3D representations of topographic surfaces. That is the reason why we tried to use photogrammetry to 3D reconstruct the brain surface. In this process, there are four main steps: (1) acquisition of specimen's photographs; (2) calculation of the camera position from some referenced points; (3) generation of a point cloud; (4) processing of the point cloud.

The model is based on photographs taken from different angles to record the total contour of the object, with a minimum overlapping (30%) of the images. The optimal lighting is a natural and indirect light, so that shaded areas are avoided. The photographs are then included in the AGISOFT Photoscan Professional Software environment 1.1 (AGISOFT PhotoScan LLC, 2014, Saint Petersburg, Russia), with the correspondent methodology [21]. After this processing, the overlapped photographs generate a point cloud. In our case, we used a total number of 32 photographs, which produced the correspondent point cloud in approximately 25 min, obtaining a mesh with 9944 vertex and 18,741 faces (Figure 1).

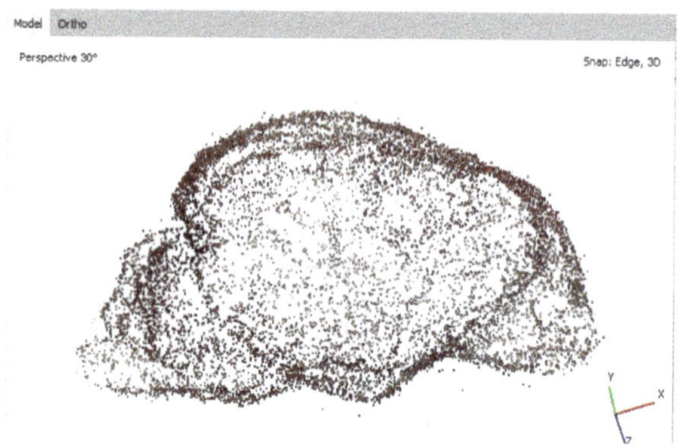

Figure 1. Example of point cloud obtained by the overlapping of a number of photographs.

An additional step is to include several control points into the model with x, y and z values to establish the model size. Further, as the points' coordinates and the different camera positions are known, it is possible to create a color texture map by projecting the original photographs onto the mesh surface. Finally, the resulting 3D model is exported as an OBJ file.

3. Results

As mentioned before, segmentations and reconstructions were possible in all cases, even in those from low resolution (0.23 T) MR images. Therefore, the quality of the results from 4.7 T, 1.5 T and 0.23 T MR images was good enough for students to recognize these structures and to understand the topographical relation they have (Figures 2–4).

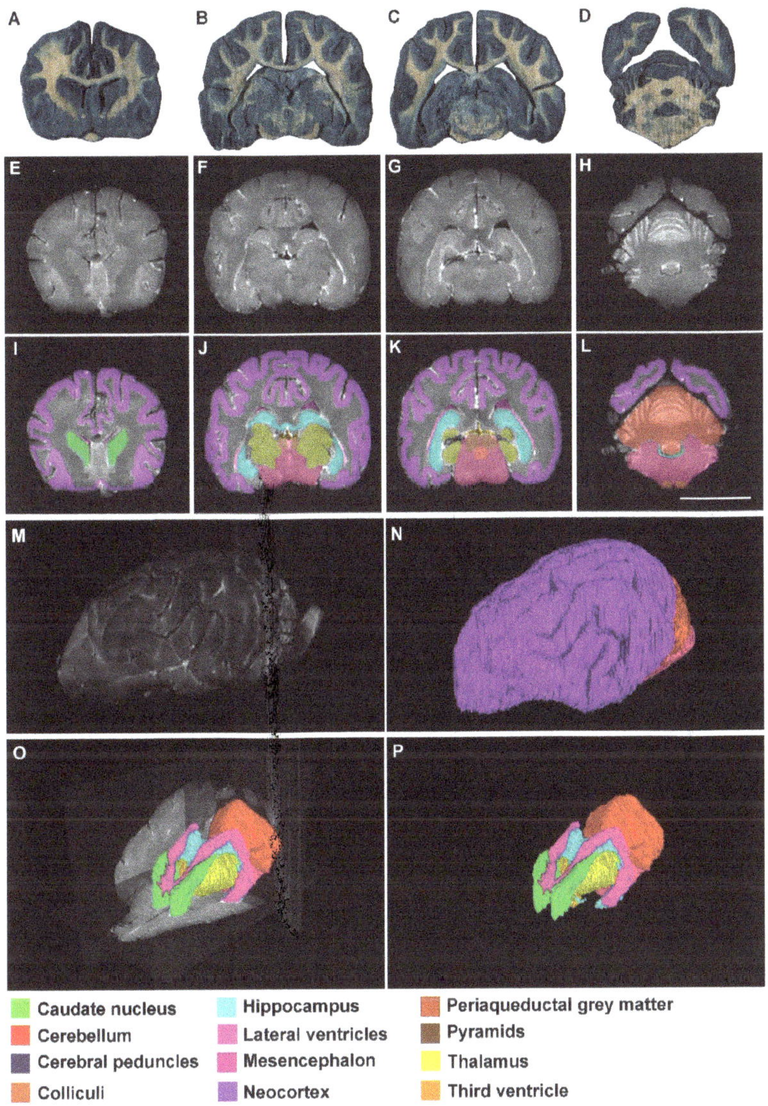

Figure 2. Images of dog brains without any signs of neural disease: (**A–D**) thick transversal sections (0.3 mm) stained with Mulligan's solution. The levels are approximately equivalent to that shown in (**E–H**) and (**I–L**); (**E–H**) Ex vivo transversal MR images (4.7 T) in the anterior–posterior axis; (**I–L**) Segmented structures with EspINA analyzer (see the color legend at the bottom of the figure); (**M**) 3D reconstructed brain with ImageJ software, taking the same stack of MR images as the basis; (**N**) 3D reconstructed brain with EspINA analyzer, taking the same stack of MR images as the basis; (**O**) 3D reconstruction of the structures of interest, using EspINA software analyzer. Observe the orthogonal planes of the MR images after removing the neocortex; (**P**) same as in (**O**) without the orthogonal planes. Scale bar in (**L**): 20 mm in (**A–L**).

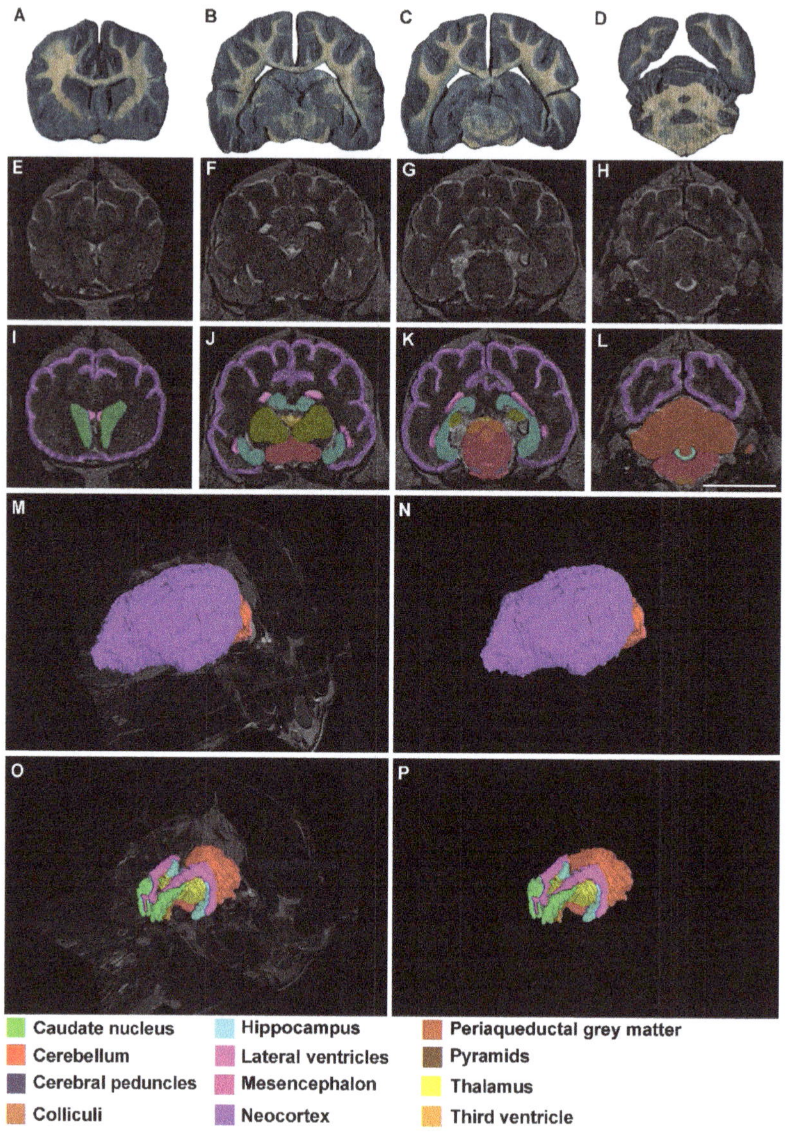

Figure 3. Images of dog brains without any signs of neural disease: (**A–D**) thick transversal sections (0.3 mm) stained with Mulligan's solution. The levels are approximately equivalent to that shown in (**E–H**) and (**I–L**); (**E–H**) dog 1 in vivo transversal MR images (1.5 T) in the anterior–posterior axis; (**I–L**) segmented structures with EspINA analyzer (see the color legend at the bottom); (**M**) 3D reconstructed brain with ImageJ software, taking the same stack of MR images as the basis; (**N**) 3D reconstructed brain with EspINA analyzer, taking the same stack of MR images as the basis; (**O**) 3D reconstruction of the structures of interest, using EspINA analyzer. Observe the orthogonal planes of the MR images after removing the neocortex; (**P**) same as in (**O**) without the orthogonal planes. Scale bar in (**L**): 20 mm in (**A–L**).

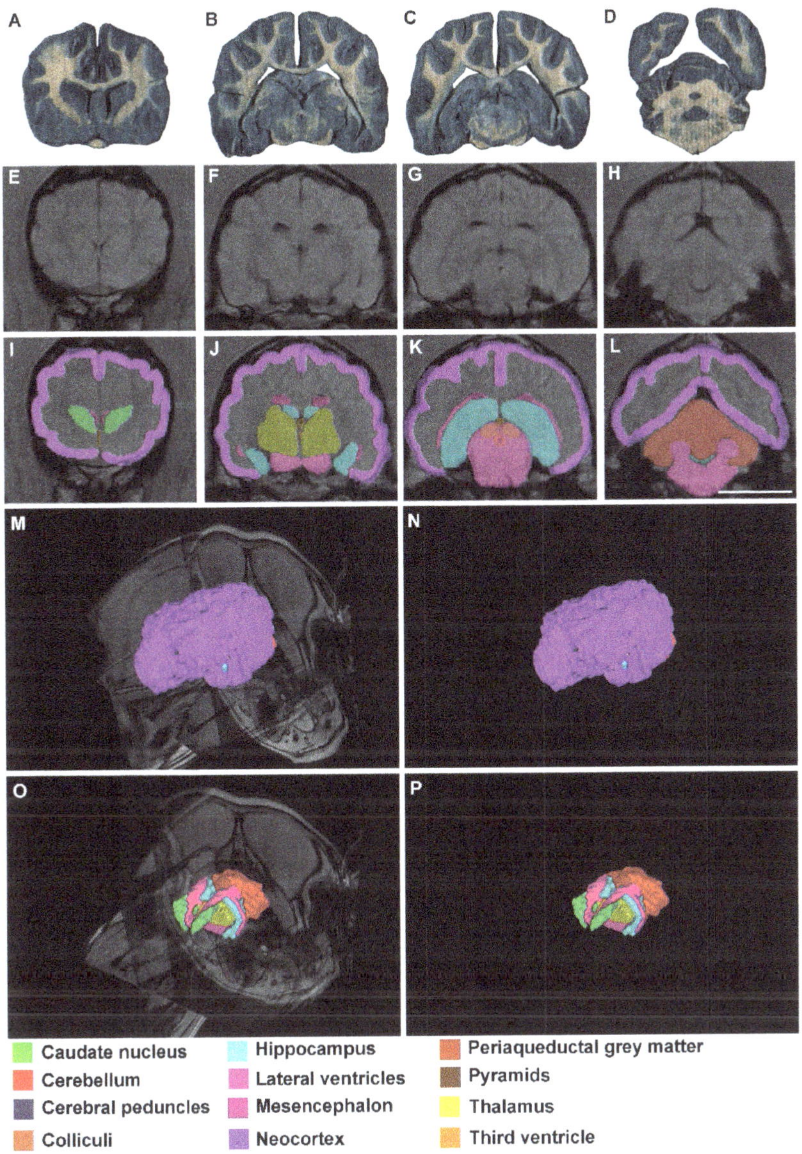

Figure 4. Images of dog brains without any sign of neural disease: (**A–D**) thick transversal sections (0.3 mm) stained with Mulligan's solution. The levels are approximately equivalent to that shown in (**E–H**) and (**I–L**); (**E–H**) dog 3 in vivo transversal MR images (0.23 T) in the anterior–posterior axis; (**I–L**) segmented structures with EspINA analyzer (see the color legend at the bottom); (**M**) 3D reconstructed brain with ImageJ, taking the same stack of MR images as the basis; (**N**) 3D reconstructed brain with EspINA analyzer, taking the same stack of MR images as the basis; (**O**) 3D reconstruction of the structures of interest, using the EspINA software. Observe the orthogonal planes of the MR images after removing the neocortex; (**P**) same as in (**O**) without the orthogonal planes. Scale bar in (**L**): 20 mm in (**A–L**).

To demonstrate the value of our teaching tool, we segmented and reconstructed in 3D 2 similar clinical cases, from different MR images 1.5 T and 0.23 T. The first case is shown in Figure 5. A French bulldog (dog 2) revealed the presence of an intra-axial and rounded mass (16 × 16 × 22 mm) localized in the left piriform lobe, by means of the 1.5 T MRI scanner. The lesion was T2W and Fluid-attenuated Inversion Recovery (FLAIR) hyperintense and T1-weighted (T1W) hypointense and showed a mild peripheral contrast enhancement that produced a mild peripheral vasogenic edema and a discrete mass effect, produced by the lesion and the edema itself. This lesion could be compatible with a neoplastic process, most likely a low-grade glioma such as an astrocytoma, due to the location, appearance and breed predisposition. The study also showed the presence of a left-sided otitis media, likely secretory, and aberrant turbinates, as an additional finding. Figure 6 shows images of another French bulldog (dog 4) that was scanned with the 0.23 T low field MRI. The encephalon presented an intra-axial oval mass (17.4 × 15.8 × 13.2 mm) located in the left-brain hemisphere. The lesion was hyperintense in T2W and FLAIR, and hypointense and mildly heterogeneous in T1W and T2*W images. No peripheral edema or cerebellar herniation were identified. In addition, a dorsolateral band of contrast enhancement was evident in post-contrast T1W images. The white matter and the corpus callosum appeared partially obliterated by the mass. On this occasion, a glioma was also considered for the main differential diagnosis, although other neoplastic or inflammatory conditions could not be ruled out. As shown in Figures 5 and 6, in both cases it was possible to segment and reconstruct the lesion as well as the surrounding structures from MR images of different resolutions. Thus, for the first time, our results reveal that EspINA is a very suitable analyzer to create and combine this type of 3D reconstructions, including pathological cases.

Concerning photogrammetry, it was possible to generate very precise 3D models from the whole brain (Figure 7). However, it was not possible to reconstruct either brain sections or MR images with enough quality to be used as a teaching tool.

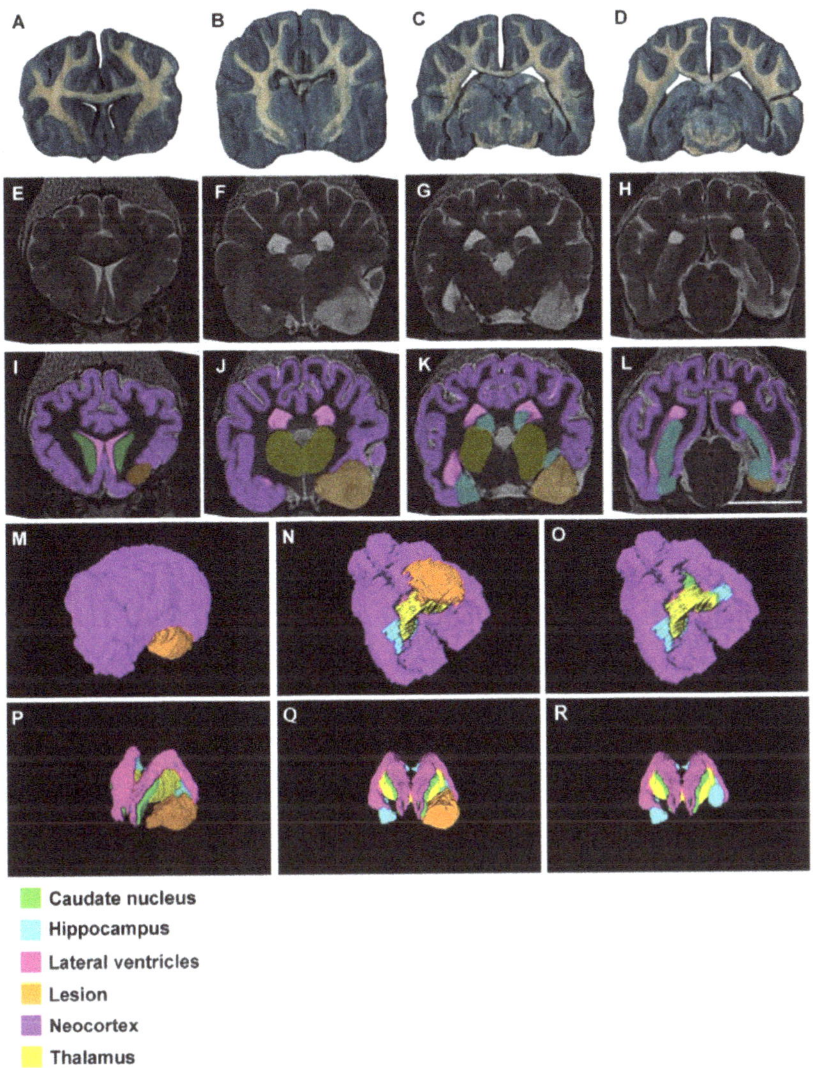

Figure 5. Images of a normal mixed-breed dog brain (**A–D**) and a 9 year old French bulldog with a tumor (dog 2) (**E–R**): (**A–D**) thick transversal sections (0.3 mm) stained with Mulligan's solution. There are no signs of neural disease. The levels are approximately equivalent to that shown in (**E–H**) and (**I–L**); (**E–H**) in vivo transversal MR images (1.5 T) in the anterior–posterior axis. Note the presence of a lesion located ventrally, extending from the caudate nucleus level rostrally to the mesencephalon caudally; (**I–L**) EspINA segmented structures of interest in relation to the lesion (in orange) location (see the color legend at the bottom); (**M**) craniolateral EspINA 3D reconstructed brain. Observe the lesion in orange; (**N**) ventral EspINA 3D reconstructed brain. Observe the lesion in orange. (**O**) has the same 3D view as in (**N**). This time, the lesion has been removed to show the possibilities of our innovative tool; (**P**,**Q**) craniolateral and cranial 3D brain reconstructions, respectively. Observe the lesion (in orange) surrounded by some of the structures of interest, after removing the neocortex; (**R**) is the same as in (**Q**), after the lesion removal to show that, among other brain regions, the lesion affects the pyriform lobe and the hippocampus and compresses the lateral ventricle of the left hemisphere. Scale bar in (**L**): 20 mm in (**A–L**).

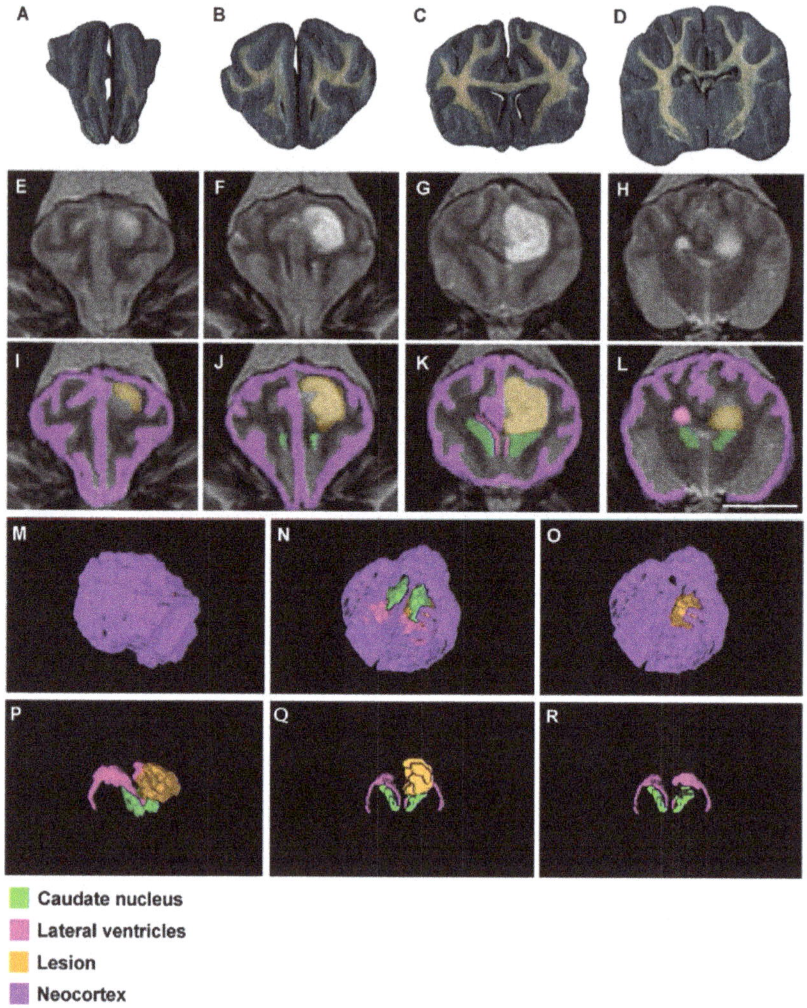

Figure 6. Images of a normal mixed-breed dog brain (**A–D**) and a 6 year old French bulldog with a tumor (dog 4) (**E–R**): (**A–D**) thick transversal sections (0.3 mm), stained with Mulligan's solution. There are no signs of neural disease. The levels are approximately equivalent to that shown in (**E–H**) and (**I–L**); (**E–H**) in vivo transversal MR images (0.23 T) in the anterior–posterior axis. Note the presence of a glioma located dorsally, extending from the rostral part of the telencephalon, dorsal to the caudate nucleus, to the diencephalon caudally; (**I–L**) EspINA segmented structures of interest, in relation to the lesion (in orange) location (see the color legend at the bottom); (**M**) dorsolateral 3D view of the EspINA reconstructed brain. Observe the lesion (barely visible) in orange; (**N**) ventral EspINA reconstructed brain. Observe the lesion in orange and its relation to different neural structures. (**O**) has the same 3D view as in (**N**). This time, the neural structures have been removed to show the possibilities of our innovative tool; (**P,Q**) lateral and cranial 3D EspINA reconstructions, respectively. Observe the lesion (in orange) surrounded by some of the structures of interest, after removing the neocortex; (**R**) is the same as in (**Q**), after the lesion removal to show that, among other brain regions, the lesion affects the sensorimotor cortex, the caudate nucleus and compressed lateral ventricle of the right hemisphere. Scale bar in (**L**): 20 mm in (**A–L**).

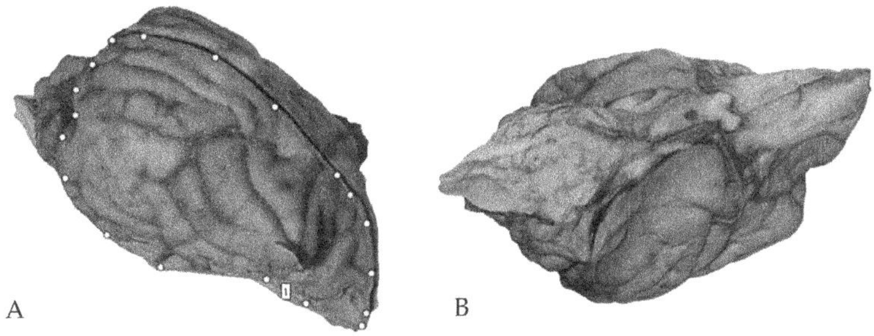

Figure 7. 3D models of the whole brain reconstructed by means of photogrammetry. (**A**) dorsolateral view; (**B**) ventral view.

4. Discussion

As mentioned before, the main goal of this present paper was to ascertain the value of EspINA to generate neural 3D reconstructions, proceeding from different quality MR images (4.7 T, 1.5 T and 0.23 T) and thus, to create a useful tool not only for anatomy students, but additionally for clinicians to understand and identify a multitude of neurological problems. An additional advantage of our educational tool is the possibility to combine neuroanatomy and clinical neurology. According to our experience, students frequently face many difficulties in their learning of anatomy and particularly of neuroanatomy. Hence, there have been continued efforts directed at incorporating new methods of teaching, learning and assessment that are aimed at logical learning and a long-term retention of anatomical knowledge. Thus, no single method for teaching anatomy, either medical or veterinary, can provide supremacy over another. On the other hand, anatomy study should not be completed in the first years of veterinary or medical school. Instead, students may continue the process of understanding anatomy (in the case of this present manuscript, neuroanatomy) in the higher years. To enhance this learning, it is normal to implement a type of "multimodal" system by combining different teaching systems: the more traditional approaches, with lectures and dissection combined with more innovative methods such as models, imaging, computer-assisted learning, peer teaching, 3D reconstructions or team-based learning [7,14,22–33].

Concerning medical neuroanatomy, different educational tools have been additionally developed over time [17,22,34–36]. In recent years, artificial intelligence (AI) has gained popularity. AI uses machine learning models to store, compute, analyze and even augment huge amounts of data to be retrieved when needed [37]. However, in our opinion, there are important limitations; for example, the cost of servers, training of students and employment of trained technical personnel to run and maintain either AI installations and apps or the development of tools. Furthermore, of course, this includes the need of adequate computers or internet connectivity to access such tools.

In summary, all these works have different approaches to the study of neuroanatomy and are, in general, useful educational tools that make the teaching–learning process much easier. However, it is noteworthy that, contrary to the method we propose with EspINA, in no case is anatomy combined with clinical neurology, which would be a further step in the integration of basic and applied disciplines, which should be one of the main goals of university education.

In respect to veterinary anatomy, the situation is very similar to that described before. The alternative methods to improve its learning, in comparison to other traditional techniques, are diverse [4,5,12,38–50]. If we focus on veterinary neuroanatomy, the use of digital teaching, 3D reconstructions and computer-assisted resources is also widespread [2,3,15,16]. Especially interesting is the use of MRI and CT scanning to create a fully interactive educational and training package for the neurovascular system of the canine brain [17]. They use a 1.5 T unit for the MR, Amira 5.6 for surface reconstruction and Mudbox to determine the aspect of the geometry. The authors combine automatic and manual segmentations, although they recognize that the poor signal from MR images 1.5 T may hinder the accurate reconstruction of anatomical structures, especially in the case of automatic segmentations. In addition, the MR dataset failed to provide an image of the entire brain. This means that the 3D reconstruction of these missing regions was by approximation, which could have impacted the anatomical accuracy of the canine brain. We consider this fact to be an important limitation, as accuracy is important when talking about neuroanatomy. In our case, it is possible to segment different quality MR images with EspINA, with high precision. Additionally, in our case, segmenting manually makes EspINA's accuracy greater, taking into consideration that details are critical in anatomy to understand morphology, topography and the relations between brain structures.

Each of the methods described before offer their own advantages and disadvantages. An ideal example of our 3D EspINA reconstructions' benefits is the possibility to focus on challenging complicated anatomical areas, or on different neural problems by segmenting the cerebral areas or structures of interest from different quality MR images (0.23, 1.5 and 4.7 T). For the first time, we have created an educational tool that combines neuroanatomy and neuropathology, contrary to what is reflected in previous publications, that are only focused on the brain anatomy. Despite all the potential benefits of this educational method, there are also a few limitations. For example, appreciating complex 3D spatial relationships requires a strong understanding of anatomy and mental 3D visualization skills, that not all students have. Another probable restriction is the use of manual segmentation tools, because to date, there are no automatic algorithms to adequately represent neural structures. Thus, using a more semi-automated or automated approach to the segmentation process could help to overcome this issue which, on the other hand, is possible when using EspINA to segment other brain structures, for example, different types of synapses [51]. In any case, we show this analyzer to be achievable in the creation of a training, educational and clinical application, using MR images of different qualities as the basis.

Although it is not the main goal of this present paper, we tried to determine if alternative methods used to make 3D reconstructions in other sciences could be applied to the study of the brain. As mentioned before, we tried to demonstrate whether photogrammetry could additionally be useful to produce 3D reconstructions of the brain, either from biological specimens, brain sections or MR images. At this point, there are no previous data in the literature on the use of photogrammetry in biology or veterinary medicine. Although our results so far are promising, we need further investigations to confirm if this is possible, as well as to discover the advantages and disadvantages in the use of this technique for the study of the encephalon.

5. Conclusions

Our contribution is important as we demonstrate, for the first time, that by using EspINA it is possible to obtain segmented structures and 3D reconstructions from 0.23, 1.5 and 4.7 T MR images. We show that this combination (imaging techniques and EspINA 3D reconstructions) is an optimal tool to help anatomists, veterinary students and clinicians have a better understanding of brain anatomy or neural lesion location. In other words, it is a step forward to facilitate the study and comprehension of neural structures for anatomy students and a new way for clinicians to accurately identify different lesions or pathologies, taking anatomy as the basis. Of course, this combination may not replace other methods to study brain anatomy; however, it can change the concept of veterinary anatomy teaching and learning. Our method provides a 3D reality that ensures the knowledge of neuroanatomy and can be a good basis for neurology practice, either medical or surgical. The lack of similar resources in this field suggests that this method introduces a new dimension into veterinary education and training. In summary, the use of EspINA 3D reconstructions is a step forward to integrate anatomy and clinical knowledge, as it has the potential to be used alongside other methodologies for the training of future veterinary practitioners.

On the other hand, we have investigated whether the use of photogrammetry could also be interesting in neuroanatomy 3D reconstructions. Our results are, so far, promising, especially when it comes to the reconstruction of the whole brain. However, it is still too early to confirm that photogrammetry is an additional interesting tool for teaching neuroanatomy.

Author Contributions: Conceptualization, J.G.-S. and L.B.-L.; methodology, R.S.-F., M.I.G.-R., M.E.F.-V. and D.C.; software, L.B.-L., L.M.d.P., P.P.-L. and I.S.-Á.; validation, R.M.-O., N.M., S.J. and M.J.H.-F.; formal analysis, L.M.d.P., P.P.-L. and I.S.-Á.; investigation, L.M.d.P., P.P-L. and I.S.-Á.; resources, R.S.-F., M.I.G.-R., M.E.F.-V. and D.C.; data curation, L.B.-L.; writing—original draft preparation, J.G.-S. and L.B.-L.; writing—review and editing, N.M. and S.J.; visualization, R.S.-F. and M.I.G.-R.; supervision, J.G.-S. and L.B.-L.; project administration, J.G.-S. and L.B.-L.; funding acquisition, J.G.-S. All authors have read and agreed to the published version of the manuscript.

Funding: This research was supported by funding from the Complutense University of Madrid, Innova Projects 88/2021-2022 and 278/2021-2022.

Institutional Review Board Statement: Not applicable.

Informed Consent Statement: Not applicable.

Data Availability Statement: The data presented in this study are available on request from the corresponding author.

Acknowledgments: The authors thank Juncal Fernández-Garayzábal for her help in translating and editing this manuscript.

Conflicts of Interest: The authors declare no conflict of interest.

References

1. Wakuri, H.; Zhang, Y.; Liu, B.; Yang, W. What is anatomy for? Considerations on the body as a whole and whole anatomy. *Okajimas Folia Anat. Jpn.* **1998**, *75*, 173–184. [CrossRef] [PubMed]
2. Schoenfeld-Tacher, R.M.; Horn, T.J.; Scheviak, T.A.; Royal, K.D.; Hudson, L.C. Evaluation of 3D additively manufactured canine brain models for teaching veterinary neuroanatomy. *J. Vet. Med. Educ.* **2017**, *44*, 612–619. [CrossRef]
3. Foss, K.D.; Seals, C.D.A.; Hague, D.W.; Mitek, A.E. Effectiveness of supplementary materials in teaching the veterinary neurologic Examination. *J. Vet. Med. Educ.* **2022**, *49*, 492–499. [CrossRef] [PubMed]
4. Khayruddeen, L.; Livingstone, D.; Ferguson, E. Creating a 3D learning tool for the growth and development of the craniofacial skeleton. *Adv. Exp. Med. Biol.* **2019**, *1138*, 57–70. [CrossRef] [PubMed]
5. Guimarães, B.; Firmino-Machado, J.; Tsisar, S.; Viana, B.; Pinto-Sousa, M.; Vieira-Marques, P.; Cruz-Correia, R.; Ferreira, M.A. The role of anatomy computer-assisted learning on spatial abilities of Medical students. *Anat. Sci. Educ.* **2019**, *12*, 138–153. [CrossRef]
6. Memon, I. Cadaver dissection is obsolete in medical training! A misinterpreted notion. *Med. Princ. Pract.* **2018**, *27*, 201–210. [CrossRef]
7. Araujo Cuauro, J.C. Aspectos históricos de la enseñanza de la anatomía humana desde la época primitiva hasta el siglo XXI en el desarrollo de las ciencias morfológicas. *Rev. Argent. Anat. Online* **2018**, *9*, 87–97.
8. Van Ginnekeng, C.J.; Vanthournout, G. Rethinking the learning and evaluation environment of a veterinary course in gross anatomy: The implementation of an assessment and development center and an E-Learning platform. *J. Vet. Med. Educ.* **2005**, *32*, 537–543. [CrossRef]
9. Guevar, J. The evolution of educational technology in veterinary anatomy education. *Adv. Exp. Med. Biol.* **2020**, *1260*, 13–25. [CrossRef]
10. Krucker, T.; Lang, A.; Meyer, E.P. New polyurethane-based material for vascular corrosion casting with improved physical and imaging characteristics. *Microsc. Res. Tech.* **2006**, *69*, 138–147. [CrossRef]
11. Riederer, B.M. Plastination and its importance in teaching anatomy. Critical points for long-term preservation of human tissue. *J. Anat.* **2014**, *224*, 309–315. [CrossRef] [PubMed]
12. Croy, B.A.; Dobson, H. Radiology as a tool for teaching veterinary anatomy. *J. Vet. Med. Educ.* **2003**, *30*, 264–269. [CrossRef] [PubMed]
13. Sandhu, G.S.; Solorio, L.; Broome, A.M.; Salem, N.; Kolthammer, J.; Shah, T.; Flask, C.; Duerk, J.L. Whole animal imaging. *Rev. Syst. Biol. Med.* **2010**, *2*, 398–421. [CrossRef] [PubMed]
14. Langlois, J.; Bellemare, C.; Toulouse, J.; Wells, G.A. Spatial abilities training in anatomy education: A systematic review. *Anat. Sci. Educ.* **2020**, *13*, 71–79. [CrossRef]

15. Christ, R.; Guevar, J.; Poyade, M.; Rea, P.M. Proof of concept of a workflow methodology for the creation of basic canine head anatomy veterinary education tool using augmented reality. *PLoS ONE* **2018**, *13*, e0195866. [CrossRef] [PubMed]
16. Hadžiomerović, N.; Hadžiomerović, A.I.; Avdić, R.; Muminović, A.; Tandir, F.; Bejdić, P.; Pandžić, A. Students' performance in teaching neuroanatomy using traditional and technology-based methods. *Anat. Histol. Embryol.* **2023**, *52*, 115–122. [CrossRef]
17. Raffan, H.; Guevar, I.; Poyade, M.; Rea, P.M. Canine neuroanatomy: Development of a 3D reconstruction and interactive ap-plication for. *PLoS ONE* **2017**, *12*, e0168911. [CrossRef]
18. Falkingham, P.L. Acquisition of high-resolution three-dimensional models using free, open-source, photogrammetric software. *Palaeontol. Electron.* **2012**, *15*, 15.1.1T. [CrossRef]
19. Herrero, M.J.; Pérez-Fortes, A.P.; Escavy, J.I.; Insua-Arévalo, J.M.; De La Horra, R.; López-Acevedo, F.; Trigos, L. 3D model generated from UAV photogrammetry and semi-automated rock mass characterization. *Comput. Geosci.* **2022**, *163*, 105121. [CrossRef]
20. Forlizzi, V.; Miranda-Solís, F.; Pérez Cruz, J.C.; Cahuantico-Choquevilca, L.A.; Morán, G.; Baldoncini, M. Tinción de Mulligan en Neuroanatomía: Protocolización de la técnica. *Rev. Argent. Anat. Online* **2020**, *11*, 31–34.
21. Bythell, J.; Pan, P.; Lee, J. Three-dimensional morphometric measurements of reef corals using underwater photogrammetry techniques. *Coral Reefs* **2001**, *20*, 193–199. [CrossRef]
22. Krontiris-Litowitz, J. Using truncated lectures, conceptual exercises, and manipulatives to improve learning in the neuroanatomy classroom. *Adv. Physiol. Educ.* **2008**, *32*, 152–156. [CrossRef] [PubMed]
23. Petersson, H.; Sinkvist, D.; Wang, C.; Smedby, O. Web-based interactive 3D visualization as a tool for improved anatomy learning. *Anat. Sci. Ed.* **2009**, *2*, 61–68. [CrossRef] [PubMed]
24. Johnson, E.O.; Charchanti, A.V.; Troupis, T.G. Modernization of an anatomy class: From conceptualization to implementation. A case for integrated multimodal–multidisciplinary teaching. *Anat. Sci. Educ.* **2012**, *5*, 354–366. [CrossRef] [PubMed]
25. Preece, D.; Williams, S.B.; Lam, R.; Weller, R. "Let's get physical": Advantages of a physical model over 3D computer models and textbooks in learning imaging anatomy. *Anat. Sci. Educ.* **2013**, *6*, 216–224. [CrossRef]
26. Ghosh, S.K. Cadaveric dissection as an educational tool for anatomical sciences in the 21st century. *Anat. Sci. Educ.* **2017**, *10*, 286–299. [CrossRef]
27. Langlois, J.; Bellemare, C.; Toulouse, J.; Wells, G.A. Spatial abilities and anatomy knowledge assessment: A systematic review. *Anat. Sci. Educ.* **2017**, *10*, 235–241. [CrossRef]
28. Joseph, M.; Singh, B. Recent advances and changing face of anatomy teaching and Learning in medical education. *Natl. J. Clin. Anat.* **2019**, *8*, 49–52. [CrossRef]
29. Yuen, J. What is the role of 3D printing in undergraduate anatomy education? A scoping review of current literature and recommendations. *Med. Sci. Educ.* **2020**, *30*, 1321–1329. [CrossRef]
30. Bernard, F.; Richard, P.; Kahn, A.; Fournier, H.D. Does 3D stereoscopy support anatomical education? *Surg. Radiol. Anat.* **2020**, *42*, 843–852. [CrossRef]
31. Bogomolova, K.; Vorstenbosch, M.A.T.M.; El Messaoudi, I.; Holla, M.; Hovius, S.E.R.; van der Hage, J.A.; Hierck, B.P. Effect of binocular disparity on learning anatomy with stereoscopic augmented reality visualization: A double center randomized controlled trial. *Anat. Sci. Educ.* **2023**, *16*, 87–98. [CrossRef] [PubMed]
32. Chytas, D.; Salmas, M.; Demesticha, T.; Noussios, G.; Paraskevas, G.; Chrysanthou, C.; Asouhidou, I.; Katsourakis, A.; Fiska, A. A review of the use of virtual reality for teaching radiology in conjunction with anatomy. *Cureus* **2021**, *13*, e20174. [CrossRef] [PubMed]
33. Asghar, A.; Naaz, S.; Patra, A.; Ravi, K.S.; Khanal, L. Effectiveness of 3D-printed models prepared from radiological data for anatomy education: A meta-analysis and trial sequential analysis of 22 randomized, controlled, crossover trials. *J. Educ. Health Promot.* **2022**, *11*, 353. [CrossRef]
34. Manson, A.; Poyade, M.; Rea, P. A recommended workflow methodology in the creation of an educational and training application incorporating a digital reconstruction of the cerebral ventricular system and cerebrospinal fluid circulation to aid anatomical understanding. *BMC Med. Imaging* **2015**, *15*, 44. [CrossRef]
35. Ocampo-Navia, M.I.; Gómez-Vega, J.C. Techniques for an anatomic approach to the study of the brain: A review. *Univ. Med.* **2021**, *62*, 22–32. [CrossRef]
36. Jacquesson, T.; Simon, E.; Dauleac, C.; Margueron, L.; Robinson, P.; Mertens, P. Stereoscopic three-dimensional visualization: Interest for neuroanatomy teaching in medical school. *Surg. Radiol. Anat.* **2020**, *42*, 719–727. [CrossRef] [PubMed]
37. Abdellatif, H.; Al Mushaiqri, M.; Albalushi, H.; Al-Zaabi, A.A.; Roychoudhury, S.; Das, S. Teaching, learning and assessing anatomy with artificial intelligence: The road to a better future. *Int. J. Environ. Res. Public Health* **2022**, *19*, 14209. [CrossRef]
38. Leandro, R.M.; Foz Filho, R.P.P.; De Silvio, M.M.; Quilici, A.P.; Sattin, M.M.; Paretsis, B.F.; Souza, V.A. Construction of the equine digestive system: A tool for teaching topographical anatomy. *J. Vet. Med. Educ.* **2019**, *46*, 108–115. [CrossRef] [PubMed]
39. Xiberta, P.; Boada, I. IVET, an interactive veterinary education tool. *J. Anim. Sci.* **2019**, *97*, 932–944. [CrossRef]
40. Suñol, A.; Aige, V.; Morales, C.; López-Beltran, M.; Feliu-Pascual, A.L.; Puig, J. Use of three-dimensional printing models for veterinary medical education: Impact on learning how to identify canine vertebral fractures. *J. Vet. Med. Educ.* **2019**, *46*, 523–532. [CrossRef]
41. Little, W.B.; Artemiou, E.; Fuentealba, C.; Conan, A.; Sparks, C. Veterinary students and faculty partner in developing a virtual three-dimensional (3D) interactive touch screen canine anatomy table. *Med. Sci. Educ.* **2019**, *29*, 223–231. [CrossRef] [PubMed]

2. Wilhite, R.; Wölfel, I. 3D Printing for veterinary anatomy: An overview. *Anat. Histol. Embryol.* **2019**, *48*, 609–620. [CrossRef] [PubMed]
3. DeBose, K. Virtual anatomy: Expanding veterinary student learning. *J. Med. Libr. Assoc.* **2020**, *108*, 647–648. [CrossRef] [PubMed]
4. Oberoi, G.; Eberspächer-Schweda, M.C.; Hatamikia, S.; Königshofer, M.; Baumgartner, D.; Kramer, A.M.; Schaffarich, P.; Agis, H.; Moscato, F.; Unger, E. 3D printed biomimetic rabbit airway simulation model for nasotracheal intubation training. *Front. Vet. Sci.* **2020**, *7*, 587524. [CrossRef] [PubMed]
5. Lee, J.S.; Park, T.H.; Ryu, J.Y.; Kim, D.K.; Oh, E.J.; Kim, H.M.; Shim, J.-H.; Yun, W.-S.; Huh, J.B.; Moon, S.H.; et al. Osteogenesis of 3D-printed PCL/TCP/bdECM scaffold using adipose-derived stem cells aggregates; an experimental study in the canine mandible. *Int. J. Mol. Sci.* **2021**, *22*, 5409. [CrossRef] [PubMed]
6. Canright, A.; Bescoby, S.; Dickson, J. Evaluation of a 3D computer model of the equine paranasal sinuses as a tool for veterinary anatomy education. *J. Vet. Med. Educ.* **2023**, *50*, 234–242. [CrossRef]
7. Plewa, B.; Skieresz-Szewczyk, K.; Jackowiak, H. Three-dimensional characteristic of fungiform papillae and its taste buds in European bison (*Bison bonasus*), cattle (*Bos taurus*), and Bison bonasus hybrid. *BMC Vet. Res.* **2022**, *18*, 21. [CrossRef] [PubMed]
8. Senos, R.; Ramos Leite, C.A.; Dos Santos Tolezano, F.; Roberto-Rodrigues, M.; Pérez, W. Using videos in active learning: An experience in veterinary anatomy. *Anat. Histol. Embryol.* **2023**, *52*, 50–54. [CrossRef]
9. Kapoor, K.; Singh, A. Veterinary anatomy teaching from real to virtual reality: An unprecedented shift during COVID-19 in socially distant era. *Anat. Histol. Embryol.* **2022**, *51*, 163–169. [CrossRef]
0. Hammerton, C.; Yip, S.W.L.; Manobharath, N.; Myers, G.; Sturrock, A. Are 3D printed models acceptable in assessment? *Clin. Teach.* **2022**, *19*, 221–228. [CrossRef]
1. Montero-Crespo, M.; Dominguez-Alvaro, M.; Rondon-Carrillo, P.; Alonso Nanclares, L.; DeFelipe, J.; Blazquez-Llorca, L. Three-dimensional synaptic organization of the human hippocampal CA1 field. *Elife* **2020**, *9*, e57013. [CrossRef] [PubMed]

animals

MDPI

Article

Flipped Classroom to Facilitate Deeper Learning in Veterinary Undergraduate Students: An Educational Change Pilot Study Limited to the Imaging Module Bones

Sibylle Maria Kneissl [1,*], Alexander Tichy [2] and Sophie Felicia Mitlacher [3]

[1] Diagnostic Imaging, Department for Companion Animals and Horses, University of Veterinary Medicine, 1210 Vienna, Austria

[2] Platform Bioinformatics and Biostatistics, Department for Biomedical Services, University of Veterinary Medicine, 1210 Vienna, Austria

[3] eLearning and New Media, Vicerectorate for Teaching Affairs and Clinical Veterinary Medicine, University of Veterinary Medicine, 1210 Vienna, Austria

* Correspondence: sibylle.kneissl@vetmeduni.ac.at

Simple Summary: All veterinary undergraduate students used an existing eLearning platform to access relevant text and selected image examples before radiology class. Only for the randomly selected students in a flipped classroom (FC) was this content amended with purposeful audio content and concrete tasks. The FC consisted of 20 students and the traditional classroom (TC) consisted of 40. The mean pre-class scores difference of students in the FC versus TC was +1.7/20 points; the mean post-class scores difference was +3/20 points. The chance of answering item 10 of the formative test (describe site of the fracture) correctly was about seven times higher for FC compared to TC learners (OR = 6.96; $p = 0.002$). The questionnaire revealed more satisfaction and greater task value in the FC compared to TC ($p = 0.048$). Higher scores, greater task value, and more positive emotions are observed in the FC compared to the TC.

Abstract: In a flipped classroom, learners study at home and do the 'homework' in class. This approach respects the limitations of memory and allows more interaction between learners. The overall vision is self-paced activities for learners with decreased boredom and greater task value, which should facilitate deeper learning. To implement a flipped classroom, a bumpy incremental change process characterized by periods of relative stillness punctuated by the acceleration of pace was planned. All veterinary undergraduate students used an existing eLearning platform to access relevant text and selected image examples before class. Only for the randomly selected students in the flipped classroom (FC) was this content amended with purposeful audio content and concrete tasks. Further, FC learners discussed their opinions in an online class forum. To measure the educational change, a pre- and post-class formative test and a standardized questionnaire for students in the FC versus in the traditional classroom (TC) were performed. To assess engagement, students were invited to measure all learning activities, categorized into attendance, or self-study. The educational change project resulted in more commitment and less resistance from teachers. The FC consisted of 20 students, while the TC had 40. The mean pre-class scores difference between FC students and TC students was +1.7/20 points, and the mean post-class scores difference was +3/20 points. The chance of answering item 10 of the formative test (describe site of the fracture) correctly was about seven times higher for FC compared to TC learners (OR = 6.96; $p = 0.002$). The questionnaire revealed more satisfaction and greater task value in the FC compared to TC ($p = 0.048$). FC students invested 21 h into the course on average, while TC students invested 16 h. The results of this pilot agree with previous reports: A transparent process was helpful to initiate mainly positive interactions between teachers and students. Higher scores, higher chance to give the correct answer, greater task value, and more positive emotions are observed in the FC compared to the TC. Higher measures of learning time are not expected to affect exam results but indicate more engagement.

Keywords: flipped classroom; veterinary medicine; education; training

1. Introduction

In a flipped classroom, learners study at home and do the 'homework' in class. In the current face-to-face radiology training system (year 3), based on the evidence in the literature [1–4], a pilot flipped classroom called bones will affect the learning of students.

Students, as with all human beings, mainly operate depending on the social positions in which they develop and live [5]. "Engagement" is a state of vigor, dedication, and absorption [6]. Too-high demands and unfair rewards are drivers against engagement [5,6]. Veterinary students are inherently motivated to help and treat animals. This intrinsic force for action is supported by learning more about diagnostic imaging and clinical reasoning [7,8]. "Autonomy" is the right to or condition of self-government, which permits learners to take more onus for their own learning. More autonomy increases vitality, creativity, well-being, and performance [5]. Autonomous support is the didactic attempt to offer students a classroom environment that supports the need for autonomy. In contrast, control orientated teaching prescribes the way to think, feel, or behave. Reeve et al. [9] describe the dialectic conjunction that students have with teachers and corresponding learning activities. In simple words, a motivating (not controlling) teaching style and dedicated learning activities result in student satisfaction. Such satisfaction, in turn, enhances the quality and extent of self-governed engagement. In practice, a motivating style means catching the learner's attitude, animating inner impetus, providing answers to requests, endorsing negative emotions, relying on instructive, non-pressuring wording, and displaying patience [9–11].

The rationale is based on the concept of the cognitive load theory [12,13], which is built upon two commonly accepted ideas. The first is that there is a limit to how much new information the human brain can process at the same time. The second is that there are no known boundaries to how much accumulated data can be passed on at the same time [14–16]. Hence, the overall aim is to increase instructional opportunities that fit within the characteristics of a working memory aiming at reducing cognitive load in class [14]. The other theory this rationale is based on is the participation metaphor [17]. The participation metaphor sees learning as a social interaction where the learner constructs content meaning, beliefs, or behaviors from active participation in a community of practice. Students have different approaches to learning: surface, deep, and strategic [18]. Deep learning follows behaviors such as the intention to understand the material. Deep learning approaches are related to higher-quality outcomes, better grades, and more satisfaction [19]. Hence, designing learning activities with concrete tasks might moderate learning from surface to deep learning [20–22], fostered by an eLearning community of practice. The third theory is based on the concept of a zone of proximal development [23], defined as the distance between the current and the potential development level of a learner. The current level matches what a learner can do without assistance, and the proximal zone of development corresponds to what a learner can do with the guidance of an expert or in collaboration with more competent peers. Therefore, another aim of this study is to create opportunities for collaborative learning, which in turn might foster the proximal zone of development.

This project is amending the current system where an online eLearning platform (Blackboard Learn, Anthology Inc., Boca Raton, FL, USA) exists and files with selected cases are stored for students in a dedicated course to prepare for pre-class and discuss the images in class. However, they are stored as stand-alone items, and students must be eager to locate them and understand what they are expected to do. The overall vision for this project is that students are active rather than silent recipients, the learning environment is flexible and intentional, and teachers are coaches rather than traditional lecturers. At the core of the new educational design is self-paced learning, decreased boredom, and greater task value so that deep learning is facilitated. The change discussed in this project is limited to one module called bones and serves as a pilot for larger changes.

2. Materials and Methods

2.1. Approval and Study Design

All students were informed about the purpose and content of the study. Students deliberately documented their study time and submitted answers to a satisfaction questionnaire; therefore, an exemption to the requirement for ethical approval was granted by the Ethics Committee of the Medical University of Vienna. Students also knew that their personal data were unidentifiable; thus, no ethical committee approval was required.

2.2. Methods for the Strategic Plan of the Educational Change Project

To implement a flipped classroom, a bumpy incremental change process characterized by periods of relative stillness and punctuated by the acceleration of pace was planned. A specific action plan using Kotter's Eight-Stage Process for Successful Organizational Transformation [24] was developed right away and streamlined repetitively with additional ideas formed while thinking about the vision, educational gap (Appendix A), stakeholders (Appendix B), and SMART goals (Appendix C). The project was conceived as a linear model of change. Similarly, it is likely to be an open-ended, ongoing process that will have to be aligned and realigned with individual opinions or periodic questionnaires. A stakeholder analysis was performed to identify all relevant parties and potential sources of resistance. SMART goals were defined by the guiding team. An empathy map served as a tangible document [25] to establish a common ground for understanding what students say, think, do, and feel. A gap analysis was performed to understand where we are now and where we want to be. The new setting was illustrated to improve understanding in the guiding team.

2.3. Methods for the Flipped Classroom

When the academic year starts, a staff member of the Vicerectorate for Teaching Affairs and Clinical Veterinary Medicine divides 200 veterinary undergraduate students randomly into 10 groups. At Diagnostic Imaging, two groups (40 students) were randomly assigned to a control group and one group (20 students) to attend the flipped classroom (FC). The grouping was triggered by best matches regarding learner and teacher (S.M.K.) time slots. Further, two control groups might balance variation in students' performance. All students used an existing eLearning platform (Blackboard Learn, Anthology Inc., Boca Raton, FL, USA) for students of the FC, this content was amended with purposeful audio content and concrete tasks. Table 1 provides an overview of the study design. Further, FC learners discussed their opinions in an online class forum. To measure the educational change, a pre- and post-class formative test and a standardized questionnaire (Appendix D) (Poll Everywhere, Poll Everywhere Inc., San Francisco, CA, USA) for students in FC versus in traditional classroom (TC) were performed. To assess engagement, students were invited to measure all learning activities (time load) [26]. Time load was individually assessed using the mobile App Studo (Studo GmbH, Graz, Austria). The time load entries consisted of the time required for attendance, self-study, and writing student papers per course. Entries could be changed retrospectively for up to 106 days (correlating to the time span of the longest course). A free-text field was also available for students to submit additional comments.

2.4. Statistical Analysis

Data were analyzed using IBM SPSS v28. Results of pre- and post-class formative tests for FC and TC were mainly reported descriptively since specific student-IDs could not be assigned to each other. However, to measure differences in the outcome of FC versus TC in the longitudinal cohort study, two relevant items of the pre- and post-class formative tests were analyzed using chi square (χ^2) test and summarized using the odds ratio (OR). The difference in satisfaction scores between the two groups was analyzed using the Mann–Whitney U-test. A p-value below 5% ($p < 0.05$) was seen as significant.

Table 1. Study design.

Chronology	Flipped (Interventional) Group	All students (or Traditional Group When Explicitly Mentioned) Participating in This Study
Before class	S.M.K. prepared a dedicated bone module using 2 PowerPoint files with embedded audio and 4 concrete activities. Further, students were provided the outline of this study. Students watched material and posted opinions in the corresponding discussion boards.	• PowerPoint files including selected images with descriptions are provided as stand-alone files. Further, students have access to a DICOM image platform to enlarge or contrast selected image examples. • Pre-class test • Access learning time
In class	Workshop (2 h): Students pose their questions in shape of formative assessment.	Traditional Group only (4 h): face-to-face learner and teacher dialogue (mainly in the shape of summative assessment)
After class		• Post-class test • Questionnaire

3. Results

3.1. Educational Change Project Strategy

The educational change project was introduced on 22 September 2022 at the end of a regular group meeting. The invitation to be part of a guiding team was accepted by six educators (S.M.K. included). One guiding group member (S.M.K.) participated actively in the FC teaching, while five supervised the pilot. The first guiding team meeting was on 28 September 2022. The guiding group produced an empathy map, and the opportunity was used to define roles as well as to describe the process and the anticipated product. The overall vision, the educational gap (Appendix A), stakeholder analysis (Appendix B), and SMART goals (Appendix C) were revised. It was obvious that the two senior members had supporting and critical voices reaching from no change needed to cultural change expected (from teacher- to learner-centered). The three younger team members behaved as supportive contributors. Additionally, the group reflected on the heterogeneity of learners, including learning attitudes, anticipated fears, and expectations, as well as the importance of good feedback from teachers. Hence, all tools used were useful to describe the project Critical voices could be felt from the first moment of the educational change project. Major resistance was not evident during the meeting. We agreed on getting written feedback on what has been said, heard, and provided after the first guiding team meeting. All were assured that this is a bottom-up change project where growth hopefully equals change, and the writer's role is providing and enabling [27].

Later, three persons gave written feedback: One opposing and two supporting. The critical arguments were that there is nothing new to be acknowledged, online material is existing, and the in-class session is interactive. S.M.K. reminded of supportive facts for the change project, such as more pre-class activities, including concrete interactive tasks, as well as pre- and post-class testing compared to providing access to reading material and imaging examples with limited guidance.

The action plan helped to understand the need to form a guiding team to design the educational change process as a bottom-up change. The writer mainly expects the guiding team to quality-assess suggestions and shape the product together into a fine-tuned local asset. This agrees with the change characterized by scale [28].

3.2. eLearning Environment and Workshop

All veterinary undergraduate students used an existing eLearning platform. The eLearning platform is an online learning application where teachers and students can interact by posting or retrieving learning material (text, images, audio, or video), lesson plans, or selected literature. The content can be organized using learning modules or simply folders to help students to navigate through the course content. However, the online material is stored in an interdisciplinary course where course work from other disciplines is stored, too, and a student must be eager to login into the correct interdisciplinary course, navigate within the course to the discipline (Diagnostic Imaging), and then identify and select relevant material before the radiology lessons.

Only for the randomly selected FC students was this content amended with a general introduction to orientate within this module, purposeful audio content to focus on the most relevant information, and concrete tasks. The purposeful audio content included two PowerPoint files with embedded audio, one with collected statements about reading fractures, and one about reading singular bone lesions. Each PowerPoint file had 4–5 slides and focused on major and minor imaging signs (i.e., reading bone fractures and osteolytic lesions) [29]. The concrete tasks consisted of four activities (i.e., understanding imaging patterns of fractures; classifying Salter-Harris fractures; describing fractures, the normal sequence of fracture healing, and abnormal fracture healing). One example is provided in Appendix E. FC learners submitted a total of 54 comments into the online class forum to share opinions and clarify questions. Peer feedback was friendly, interactive, focused, and constructive. Sometimes students reminded each other of the information not given but overseen. In other instances, not helpful classifications, such as type of osteolysis, were correctly questioned by students.

The workshop task for FC learners was to design the lesson. Students posed a total of 17 questions that demonstrated high interest, good preparation, the necessity to document new terminology with images, and problems that learners entering clinics have with clinical reasoning. Most learners were active. Roles of questioning, listening, or noting learners were well distributed. Questions mirrored prior understanding that needed minor or major reconstruction of knowledge. The educator (S.M.K.) guided learning by suited illustrations or verbal descriptions; she could build upon a solid socket of knowledge and skills. Overall, the observed readiness for understanding imaging patterns was higher among FC compared to TC learners. The questions of learners challenged the teacher and reduced boredom while teaching.

3.3. Test Results and Time Load Measures

The FC consisted of 20 students, while the TC consisted of 40. The mean pre-class scores difference between FC students and TC students was +1.7/20 points; the mean post-class scores difference was +3/20 points (Table 2).

Table 2. Results comparing the intervention to the control group.

Averaged Per Student	Flipped (Intervention) Group	Traditional (Control) Group
Pre-Test [averaged points out of 20]	13.1	11.4
Post-Test [averaged points out of 20]	15.5	12.5
Time load [averaged hours]	20.6	16.4

Odds ratios for selected test items were stated in Table 3. While the two groups did not differ in the pre-test regarding the number of correct answers to item 10 (describe site of the fracture) or 20 (describe a cortical lesion), both items show significant differences in the post-class test in favor of FC learners. The chance of answering item 10 correctly was about seven times higher compared to TC learners (OR = 6.96; $p = 0.002$). Between the pre- and post-class test results, there were no significant improvements for item 20; but a significant effect regarding item 10 was demonstrated for FC learners (OR = 12; $p < 0.001$).

Table 3. Odds ratios of item 10 and 20 comparing FC to TC test results.

Odds Ratio	Pre-Class Test	Post-Class Test
FC versus TC result (item 10)	1.14	6.96 *
FC versus TC result (item 20)	2.7	4.5 *

* significant improvement in favor of FC learners.

FC students invested 21 h into the course on average, while TC students invested 16 h. No student has used the available free-text field for additional comments within the App Studo (Studo GmbH).

3.4. Questionnaire

The questionnaire revealed more satisfaction and greater task value in the FC compared to TC ($p = 0.048$). Further, students´ perspectives were collected using an open-end question as the last item (Appendix D). Three responses from TC learners concentrated on the need to get normal image examples or improved labelling of abnormal images in their respective figure legends. Twelve responses from the FC learners focused on the improved learning environment supporting deeper learning by (a) dedicated activities, (b) online discussions among peers, and (c) teacher feedback in a non-threatening environment (formative assessment) in the workshop. No student commented about having spent more time or feeling time pressure.

4. Discussion

The results of this pilot agree with previous reports: Higher scores [30], higher chance to give the correct answer [30], greater task value [31], and more positive emotions [31,32] were observed in the FC compared to the TC. A similar concept has been applied before by O'Connor et al. [1]; the authors observed 10.5% higher scores, greater task value, and more positive emotions in the flipped learning class compared to the traditional learning class. Higher measures of learning time are not expected to affect exam results but indicate more engagement [33–35]. Further, a transparent process was helpful to initiate mainly positive interaction between teachers and students [36,37].

Regarding the overwhelming positive emotions and extra time efforts of FC learners, it is likely that FC meets the adapted values of the new generation better [38]: The learners have high expectations and ask for transparent learning conditions [39,40]. They know how to deal with educational online resources and enjoy interacting as peers. The physical campus does not disappear, but it has a different function, such as individual feedback versus traditional classroom teaching. It is advisable that teachers from different universities interact and share online learning material to manage the new faculty workload as a collaborative community.

In the following section, selected elements for autonomous supportive teaching related to the FC project are discussed through the lens of the teacher.

4.1. Create an Online Working Space That Includes the Formal Framework

The online space includes the latest information about the formal framework, including good examples of various radiologic bone conditions. The framework supports the "Teach Less, Learn More" idea, which aims to engage students, prepare them for this specific task, and make learning meaningful for them [8]. Likewise, responsibility for learning is given to the student, increasing autonomy and fostering the idea of running one's own learning journey [41].

4.2. Create Specific Agendas with Concrete Tasks

Meaningful tasks that address multiple goals allow for control over the learning process and engage students in evaluating their own work and progress [42]. In that setting, learners are supposed to assemble outside of class and cooperate with their team affiliates to figure out authentic issues [43,44].

Especially weak students need more time to manage learning objectives appropriately [45–47]. To ensure enough study time, exposure to more learning opportunities is especially useful. Students may pace their learning time to their individual needs and master the needed competencies more effectively and efficiently [48].

4.3. Emphasize Intragroup Cooperation and Foster Positive Peer Interaction

Cooperative learning enhances motivation and learning [49–53]. Conditions that support cooperation are positive interdependence [50] and individual accountability [51], which promote interaction, trust, and conflict resolution. One reason for the enhanced learning is the elaborated explanations given to peers by peers. Peer-to-peer support is a promising format that can alleviate teaching pressure for faculty and offer education to students at their own cognitive level in a safe educational environment [54,55].

By creating a peer group, learning opportunities are multiplied, and social support is increased, thus enhancing social competence, self-confidence, self-esteem, and resilience [50]. Peer coaching is also an encouraging format for social development when established within a non-evaluative environment. The overall result can be more resilience to deal with unexpected occurrences during a learning task [56].

4.4. Improved Feedback to Learners

Traditionally, an undergraduate veterinary student can be physically present and hardly active and will pass the radiology course when having attempted to read three to four radiologic cases under supporting teacher guidance. Hence, there is an active and individual dialogue between student and teacher in the TC, but students feel as though they are in a constant (threatening) summative assessment. The discussion boards on the eLearning platform and the face-to-face workshop implemented in the FC improved the overall feedback loop between learners and teachers by providing meaningful and good quality oral or written feedback in a non-threatening formative assessment. The power of dedicated and meaningful feedback has been demonstrated to raise self-esteem, clarify goals, and empower students for self-directed learning [57–61].

As stated above, one limitation of this study was the resistance of an individual teacher to change. Possibly, this educator is worried about losing resources, which is supported by the conservation of resources theory [62], or she could not grasp the chance of change as a learning opportunity [63]. Future studies may explore reasons for resistance to change and consider conditions needed for better cooperation, such as positive interdependence [49], appropriate social skills [64], resilience [65], or improved appreciative inquiry [66]. In the present case, the planned changes are meant mainly to enrich a program through interactive tasks, peer mentoring, and improved feedback that will increase and eventually ignite self-determined motivation and autonomy. Although this changing process is within the institutional logic [67] that describes itself as learner-centered [68], opinions about teaching methods or teachers being explicitly learner-centered vary. Hence, this educational change project is a further step in the same direction and guides team members to have different opinions about the necessity of change.

Another limitation of this study was that the default settings of the test software used are limited to group observations and do not allow individual tracking. It is likely that an FC depends on student performance, meaning that higher-level learners students outperform compared to lower-level learners [69]. In future studies, we will observe students as individuals.

5. Conclusions

The key-project aims are less cognitive load and deeper learning by implementing an FC for veterinary undergraduate students in veterinary radiology. The project was successful in observing engagement and better grades for FC students. The bottom-up bumpy incremental change resulted in more commitment and less resistance from teachers. The transparent process was helpful to initiate mainly positive interaction. This agrees with the idea of distributional leadership [70], where transparent rules and roles are an effective start [20,36,37,71].

In a subsequent project, the module bones will be amended with the module joints and thorax. This will allow the team of teachers to agree on learning outcomes, select relevant teaching material, and design corresponding tasks. In this phase, it will be essential to allow tracking of individual learners to get longitudinal information of and measure anticipated differences between learners attending TC and FC or different students' levels. Further, it will be necessary to learn more about the veterinary students' and educators' perspectives regarding their needs. Debatably, these studies are needed to explore if all undergraduate veterinary students study before class and master the shift in the learning responsibility.

Author Contributions: Conceptualization, S.M.K. and S.F.M.; methodology, S.M.K., A.T. and S.F.M.; validation, S.M.K., A.T. and S.F.M.; formal analysis, S.M.K., A.T. and S.F.M.; investigation, S.M.K.; data curation, S.M.K., A.T. and S.F.M.; writing—original draft preparation, S.M.K.; writing—review and editing, S.M.K., A.T. and S.F.M.; visualization, S.M.K., A.T. and S.F.M.; supervision, S.M.K.; project administration, S.M.K. All authors have read and agreed to the published version of the manuscript.

Funding: Open Access Funding by the University of Veterinary Medicine Vienna.

Institutional Review Board Statement: Ethical review and approval do not require the formal vote of the Ethics Committee, Medical University of Vienna. An exemption to the requirement for ethical approval was granted by the Ethics Committee of the Medical University of Vienna.

Informed Consent Statement: All students were informed about the purpose and content of the study. Students also knew that their personal data were unidentifiable.

Data Availability Statement: The datasets used and analysed during the current study are available from the corresponding author on reasonable request.

Acknowledgments: We would like to acknowledge the work of the guiding group for dedicated feedback during this educational change project.

Conflicts of Interest: The authors declare no conflict of interest.

Appendix A. Educational Gap

Departure point: Where are we now?

- Summative oral assignment with varying levels
- Students with surface learning
- Teachers with repetitive tasks
- eLearning environment with hardly defined tasks

Goal: Where do we want to be?

- Summative written assignment with standardized levels
- Students with deep learning
- Teachers with challenging new tasks
- eLearning environment with clearly defined roles and tasks

Appendix B. Stakeholder Analysis

Stakeholder	Opposed	Neutral	Supportive
Learner		x	x
Teacher *	x	x	x
eLearning Team			x
Head of Division			x
Vice-Rector for Teaching Affairs and Clinical Veterinary Medicine			x

* Senior teachers who are not willing to invest extra efforts in eLearning content will need a special focus to be converted from opposed to neutral, or even better, from neutral to supportive. A motivator could be off-clinic time to implement eLearning content or outsourcing work to student employees.

Appendix C. SMART Goals

Criterion	Description
Specific	To develop a pre-class formative test. To develop a clearly defined marking grid. To develop at least four concrete pre-class eLearning activities. To design a workshop. To develop a post-class summative test.
Measurable	Using time load measurements to measure engagement. Using assessment to drive learning (and measure understanding). Using a questionnaire to measure student´s satisfaction.
Attainable	Developing and agreeing on learning activities and questions for summative assessment will need several discussion rounds. Time load measurements and course questionnaires are well established at this site.
Realistic	Twelve weeks is a reasonable period to implement a pilot that serves for larger changes depending on its outcome.
Time bound	The academic year starts Oct 1st in Austria. An eLearning Pilot will be performed using a student cohort in January 2023.

Appendix D. Satisfaction and Task Value Questionnaire according to O'Connor, Fried (1)

Item Number	Question
1	I was very interested in the content of the eLearning environment.
2	I am happy I understood the material taught in the eLearning environment.
3	I worry whether I am sufficiently prepared for the on-site training.
4	My enjoyment of the eLearning environment made me want to learn the material.
5	I often think about what else I would rather be doing during the on-site training.
6	I felt intimidated during the question-and-answer segments in the on-site training.
7	Is there anything else you want to share?

Appendix E. Activity Classifying Singular Bone Lesions

This table shows assessment criteria and imaging features of bone lesions. Study it carefully. Then classify the femoral and ulnar bone lesions (Figure A1) using the listed imaging criteria. Post your opinion into the discussion board or react to opinions posted.

Criterion	Aggressive Bone Lesion	Non-Aggressive Bone Lesion
Example	Osteomyelitis, Osteosarcoma	Bone cyst, Osteoma
Osteolysis type	Moth-eaten or permeative	geographic
Transition zone	Long and poorly demarcated	Well demarcated, eventually showing a sclerotic rim
Compact bone	Interrupted	Preserved
Periosteal reaction	Interrupted, irregular	Solid, smooth

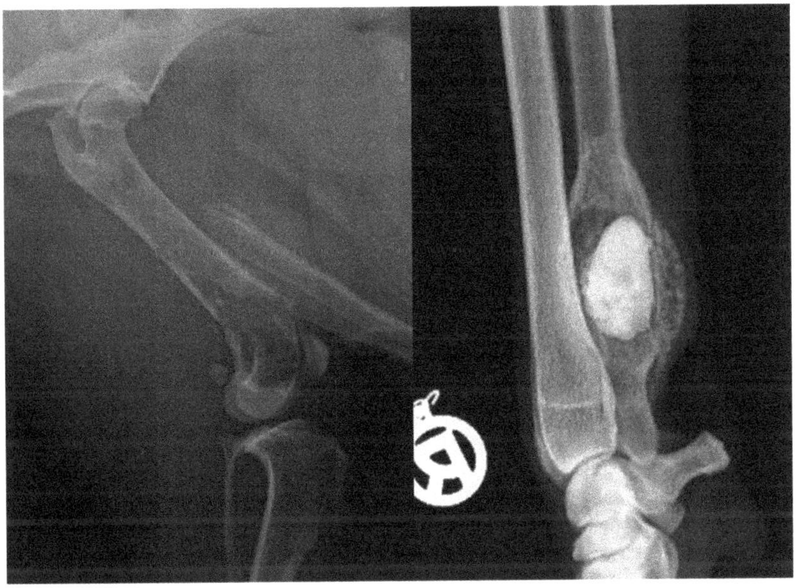

Figure A1. Mediolateral view of the left upper leg (**left side**) and the right distal lower arm (**right side**).

References

1. O'Connor, E.E.; Fried, J.; McNulty, N.; Shah, P.; Hogg, J.P.; Lewis, P.; Zeffiro, T.; Agarwal, V.; Reddy, S. Flipping radiology education right side up. *Acad. Radiol.* **2016**, *23*, 810–822. [CrossRef]
2. Ge, L.; Chen, Y.; Yan, C.; Chen, Z.; Liu, J. Effectiveness of flipped classroom vs traditional lectures in radiology education: A meta-analysis. *Medicine* **2020**, *99*, e22430. [CrossRef]
3. Evans, L.; Vanden Bosch, M.L.; Harrington, S.; Schoofs, N.; Coviak, C. Flipping the Classroom in Health Care Higher Education: A Systematic Review. *Nurse Educ.* **2019**, *44*, 74–78. [CrossRef]
4. Vavasseur, A.; Muscari, F.; Meyrignac, O.; Nodot, M.; Dedouit, F.; Revel-Mouroz, P.; Dercle, L.; Rozenblum, L.; Wang, L.; Maulat, C.; et al. Blended learning of radiology improves medical students' performance, satisfaction, and engagement. *Insights Into Imaging* **2020**, *11*, 61. [CrossRef] [PubMed]
5. Ryan, R.M.; Deci, E.L. Self-determination theory and the facilitation of intrinsic motivation, social development, and well-being. *Am. Psychol.* **2000**, *55*, 68–78. [CrossRef]
6. Bakker, A.; Demerouti, E. Towards a model of work engagement. *Career Dev. Int.* **2008**, *13*, 209–223. [CrossRef]
7. Linn, A.; Khaw, C.; Kildea, H.; Tonkin, A. Clinical reasoning—A guide to improving teaching and practice. *Aust. Fam. Physician* **2012**, *41*, 18–20.
8. Klevin, T.; Jude, C.; Tan, C. Engaging our learners: Teach less, learn more. In *Innovation in Education*; Larkley, J., Maynhard, V., Eds.; National Library Board: Singapore, 2013; pp. 153–177.
9. Reeve, J.; Deci, E.; Ryan, R. Self-determination theory: A dialectical framework for understanding the sociocultural influences on student motivation. In *Research on Sociocultural Influences on Motivation and Learning: Big Theories Revisited*; McInerney, D., Van Etten, S., Eds.; Information Age Press: Greenwich, CT, USA, 2004; Volume 4, pp. 31–59.
10. Reeve, J. Autonomy-Supportive Teaching: What It Is, How to Do It. In *Building Autonomous Learners*; Woon Chia, L., Keng, J., Ryan, R., Eds.; Springer Science+Business Media: Singapore, 2016.

11. Reeve, J. Why teachers adopt a controlling motivating style toward students and how they can become more autonomy supportive. *Educ. Psychol.* **2009**, *44*, 159–178. [CrossRef]
12. Sweller, J.; Ayres, P.; Kalyuga, S. *Cognitive Load Theory*; Springer Science+Business Media: New York, NY, USA, 2011.
13. Sweller, J.; Chandler, P. Why some material is difficult to learn. *Cogn. Instr.* **1994**, *12*, 185–233. [CrossRef]
14. Paas, F.; van Gog, T.; Sweller, J. Cognitive Load Theory: New conceptualizations, specifications, and integrated research perspectives. *Educ. Psychol. Rev.* **2010**, *22*, 115–121. [CrossRef]
15. Plass, J.L.; Moreno, R.; Brünken, R. *Cognitive Load Theory: Theory and Applications*; Cambridge University Press: Cambridge, UK, 2010.
16. Reedy, G. Using cognitive load theory to inform simulation design and practice. *Clin. Simul. Nurs.* **2013**, *11*, 350–360. [CrossRef]
17. Sfard, A. On two metaphors for learning and the dangers of choosing just one. *Educ. Res.* **1998**, *27*, 4–13. [CrossRef]
18. Entwistle, N.; Tait, H. Approaches to studying and perceptions of the learning environment across disciplines. *New Dir. Teach. Learn.* **1995**, *64*, 93–103. [CrossRef]
19. Ramsden, P. *Approaches to Learning*; Routledge Falmer: Oxford, UK, 2003.
20. Butcher, D.; Davies, C.; Highton, M. *Designing Learning: From Module Outline to Effective Teaching*; Routledge: Oxon, UK, 2019.
21. Plant, E.; Ericsson, K.; Hill, L.; Asberg, K. Why study time does not predict grade point average across college students: Implications of deliberate practice for academic performance. *Contemp. Educ. Psychol.* **2005**, *30*, 96–116. [CrossRef]
22. Walker, M. *Higher Education Pedagogies*; SRHE and Open University Press: Berkshire, UK, 2005.
23. Vygotsky, L.S. *Mind in Society: The Development of Higher Psychological Processes*; Harvard University Press: Cambridge, MA, USA, 1978.
24. Kotter, J.P.; Wyman, O. *Leading Change*; Harvard Business School Press: Boston, MA, USA, 2013.
25. Yee, J.; White, H.; Lennon, L. Valuing Design. 2015. Available online: https://valuingdesign.org/ValuingDesign_Report_2015.pdf (accessed on 2 March 2023).
26. Kneissl, S.; Tomiska, T.; Rehage, J. Measuring Time Load Using a Mobile Application to Monitor Curriculum Workload. *J. Vet. Med. Educ.* **2022**, *50*, e20210127. [CrossRef]
27. Uhl-Bien, M.; Arena, M. Leadership for organizational adaptability: A theoretical synthesis and integrative framework. *Leadersh. Q.* **2018**, *29*, 89–104. [CrossRef]
28. Todnem By, R. Organisational change management: A critical review. *J. Chang. Manag.* **2005**, *5*, 369–380. [CrossRef]
29. Lamb, C.R. Applying the concept of major and minor findings: Guidance for trainees and exam candidates. *Vet. Radiol. Ultrasound* **2022**, *63*, 649–652. [CrossRef]
30. Sukut, S.L.; Mayer, M.N.; D'Eon, M.F.; Burbridge, B.E.; Waldner, C.L. Comparing Two Resources Used to Teach Pulmonary Patterns for a Flipped Veterinary Radiology Course. *J. Vet. Med. Educ.* **2021**, *48*, 211–216. [CrossRef]
31. Yang, C.; Yang, X.; Yang, H.; Fan, Y. Flipped classroom combined with human anatomy web-based learning system shows promising effects in anatomy education. *Medicine* **2020**, *99*, e23096. [CrossRef] [PubMed]
32. Decloedt, A.; Franco, D.; Martlé, V.; Baert, A.; Verwulgen, A.; Valcke, M. Development of Surgical Competence in Veterinary Students Using a Flipped Classroom Approach. *J. Vet. Med. Educ.* **2021**, *48*, 281–288. [CrossRef] [PubMed]
33. Brint, S.; Cantwell, A. Undergraduate time use and academic outcomes: Results from the University of California undergraduate experience survey 2006. *Teach. Coll. Rec.* **2010**, *112*, 2441–2470. [CrossRef]
34. Gleason, J.; Walstad, W. An empirical test of an inventory model of student study time. *J. Econ. Educ.* **1988**, *19*, 315–321. [CrossRef]
35. Kuhlee, D. Brauchen wir eine Workload-Diskussion? Zur Rolle formaler Studienworkloads für das Lern- und Studierhandeln. Eine empirische Studie bei Lehramts-Studierenden des Master of Education. *Das. Hochschulwesen* **2012**, *60*, 79–87.
36. Gordon, L.J.; Rees, C.E.; Ker, J.S.; Cleland, J. Leadership and followership in the healthcare workplace: Exploring medical trainees' experiences through narrative inquiry. *BMJ Open* **2015**, *5*, e008898. [CrossRef] [PubMed]
37. Storey, J.; Holti, R. *Towards a New Model of Leadership for the NHS*; NHS Leadership Academy: London, UK, 2013.
38. Gillispie, V. Using the Flipped Classroom to Bridge the Gap to Generation Y. *Ochsner J.* **2016**, *16*, 32–36.
39. Ng, E.; Schweitzer, L.; Lyons, S. New Generation, Great Expectations: A Field Study of the Millennial Generation. *J. Bus. Psychol.* **2010**, *25*, 281–292. [CrossRef]
40. Seemiller, C.; Megan, G. Generation Z: Educating and Engaging the Next Generation of Students. *SAGE J.* **2017**, *22*, 21–26. [CrossRef]
41. Reeves, S.; Fletcher, S.; Barr, H.; Birch, I.; Boet, S.; Davies, N.; McFadyen, A.; Rivera, J.; Kitto, S. A BEME systematic review of the effects of interprofessional education: BEME Guide No. 39. *Med. Teach.* **2016**, *38*, 656–668. [CrossRef]
42. Perry, N.E.; Hutchinson, L.; Thauberger, C. Mentoring Student Teachers to Design and Implement Literacy Tasks that Support Self-Regulated Reading and Writing. *Read. Writ. Q.* **2007**, *23*, 27–50. [CrossRef]
43. Parmelee, D.; Michaelsen, L.K.; Cook, S.; Hudes, P.D. Team-based learning: A practical guide: AMEE Guide No. 65. *Med. Teach.* **2012**, *34*, e275–e287. [CrossRef]
44. Parmelee, D.X.; Michaelsen, L.K. Twelve tips for doing effective Team-Based Learning (TBL). *Med. Teach.* **2010**, *32*, 118–122. [CrossRef]
45. Kyndt, E.; Berghmans, I.; Dochy, F.; Bulckens, L. Time is not enough. Workload in higher education: A student perspective. *High. Educ. Res. Dev.* **2014**, *33*, 684–698. [CrossRef]
46. Stinebrickner, R.; Stinebrickner, T. Time-use and college outcomes. *J. Econ.* **2004**, *121*, 243–269. [CrossRef]

7. Molloy, E. Time to Pause: Feedback in Clinical Education. In *Clinical Education in the Health Professions*; Molloy, E., Delaney, C., Eds.; Elsevier: Sydney, NSW, Australia, 2009; pp. 128–146.
8. Oudbier, J.; Spaai, G.; Timmermans, K.; Boerboom, T. Enhancing the effectiveness of flipped classroom in health science education: A state-of-the-art review. *BMC Med. Educ.* **2022**, *22*, 34. [CrossRef] [PubMed]
9. Johnson, D.; Johnson, R.; Smith, K. Cooperative Learning: Improving University Instruction by Basing Practice on Validated Theory. *J. Excell. Coll. Teach.* **2013**, *25*, 85–118.
0. Johnson, D.; Johnson, R.; Smith, K. The state of cooperative learning in postsecondary and professional settings. *Educ. Psychol. Rev.* **2007**, *19*, 15–29. [CrossRef]
1. Slavin, R. *Cooperative Learning: Theory, Research, and Practice*, 2nd ed.; Allyn & Bacon: Boston, MA, USA, 1995.
2. Slavin, R. Introduction based on cooperative learning. In *Handbook of Research on Learning and Instruction*; Mayer, P., Alexander, P., Eds.; Routledge: Oxon, UK, 2011.
3. Thomas, L. *Building Student Engagement and Belonging in Higher Education at a Time of Change*; Paul Hamlyn Foundation: London, UK, 2012.
4. Yiend, J.; Weller, S.; Kinchin, I. Peer observation of teaching: The interaction between peer review and developmental models of practice. *J. Furth. High. Educ.* **2014**, *38*, 465–484. [CrossRef]
5. Ten Cate, O.; Durning, S. Peer teaching in medical education: Twelve reasons to move from theory to practice. *Med. Teach.* **2007**, *29*, 591–599. [CrossRef]
6. Schwellnus, H.; Carnahan, H. Peer-coaching with health care professionals: What is the current status of the literature and what are the key components necessary in peer-coaching? A scoping review. *Med. Teach.* **2014**, *36*, 38–46. [CrossRef]
7. McKimm, J. Giving effective feedback. *Br. J. Hosp. Med.* **2009**, *70*, 158–161. [CrossRef] [PubMed]
8. Barton, K.L.; Schofield, S.J.; McAleer, S.; Ajjawi, R. Translating evidence-based guidelines to improve feedback practices: The interACT case study. *BMC Med. Educ.* **2016**, *16*, 53. [CrossRef] [PubMed]
9. Boud, D.; Walker, D. Making the most of experience. *Stud. Contin. Educ.* **1990**, *12*, 61–80. [CrossRef]
0. Orsmond, P.; Merry, S. The importance of self-assessment in students' use of tutors' feedback: A qualitative study of high and non-high achieving biology undergraduates. *Assess. Eval. High. Educ.* **2013**, *38*, 737–753. [CrossRef]
1. Plymouth University. 7 Steps to Effective Feedback. 2011. Available online: https://www.plymouth.ac.uk/uploads/production/document/path/2/2394/7_steps_effective_feedback_2011__3_pdf (accessed on 2 March 2023).
2. Hobfoll, S.E. Conservation of resources. A new attempt at conceptualizing stress. *Am. Psychol.* **1989**, *44*, 513–524. [CrossRef]
3. Sundberg, K.; Josephson, A.; Reeves, S.; Nordquist, J. Power and resistance: Leading change in medical education. *Stud. High. Educ.* **2017**, *42*, 445–462. [CrossRef]
4. Lewin, K. Group decision and social change. In *Readings in Social Psychology*; Maccoby, E., Newcomb, T., Hartley, E., Eds.; Holt, Rinehart and Winston: New York, NY, USA, 1958.
5. King, D.D.; Newman, A.; Luthans, F. Not if, but when we need resilience in the workplace. *J. Organ. Behav.* **2016**, *37*, 782–786. [CrossRef]
6. Bushe, G.R.; Kassam, A.F. When Is Appreciative Inquiry Transformational?: A Meta-Case Analysis. *J. Appl. Behav. Sci.* **2005**, *41*, 161–181. [CrossRef]
7. Gordon, L.; Cleland, J.A. Change is never easy: How management theories can help operationalise change in medical education. *Med. Educ.* **2021**, *55*, 55–64. [CrossRef] [PubMed]
8. Curriculum Committee. Curriculum Veterinärmedizin 2019. Available online: https://www.vetmeduni.ac.at/fileadmin/v/z/mitteilungsblatt/curricula/2019-06_Curriculum_Diplomstudium_Veterinarrmedizin.pdf (accessed on 2 March 2023).
9. Zhou, X. A conceptual review of the effectiveness of flipped learning in vocational learners' cognitive skills and emotional states. *Front. Psychol.* **2023**, *13*, 1039025. [CrossRef] [PubMed]
70. Yukl, G.A. *Leadership in Organizations*, 7th ed.; Prentice-Hall: Upper Saddle River, NJ, USA, 2013.
71. Academy, N.L. *The Healthcare Leadership Model: The Nine Dimensions of Leadership Behaviour*; NHS Leadership Academy: Leeds, UK, 2013.

animals

MDPI

Project Report

Evaluation of an Interprofessional Blended Learning Course Focusing on Communication within Veterinary Teams

Sylva Agnete Charlotte Heise [1,*], Sandra Wissing [2], Verena Nerschbach [3], Ellen Preussing [4], Andrea Tipold [2] and Christin Kleinsorgen [1,*]

1 E-Learning-Consulting, Centre for E-Learning, Didactics and Educational Research, University of Veterinary Medicine Hannover, 30559 Hannover, Germany
2 Centre for E-Learning, Didactics and Educational Research, Clinical Skills Lab, University of Veterinary Medicine, 30173 Hannover, Germany; andrea.tipold@tiho-hannover.de (A.T.)
3 Clinic for Small Animals, University of Veterinary Medicine Hannover, 30559 Hannover, Germany
4 Lightwings Preussing, VetAcademy, 8134 Adliswil, Switzerland
* Correspondence: sylva.heise@tiho-hannover.de (S.A.C.H.); christin.kleinsorgen@tiho-hannover.de (C.K.)

Simple Summary: This study explores the impact of a blended learning course on enhancing interprofessional communication skills among veterinary students and apprentices training to become veterinary assistants. The course, which was first implemented during the COVID-19 pandemic, utilizes a blended learning design with online modules, synchronous seminars and simulation training. The results show an increase in knowledge and improved self-assessment of communication skills, with positive feedback on the course structure. Challenges such as limited resources are noted, emphasizing the need for ongoing data collection to refine the teaching methods and maximize the benefits for participants in future runs of the course.

Abstract: Based on the importance of communication and teamwork in veterinary practice, we explored the impact of a blended learning course designed to enhance interprofessional communication skills among veterinary students and apprentice assistants. The blended learning course design included online modules, synchronous (online) seminars, and simulation training sessions. The asynchronous online elements should complement the varied schedules of different professions and meet the individual needs of participants, especially considering the challenges posed by the COVID-19 pandemic. The course structure, evaluations, and outcomes were documented, showing a positive impact on knowledge gain concerning communication and self-assessment in communication skills. In the pretest, the participants scored 43.18% correct answers to a knowledge test, whereas 71.50% correct answers were given in the posttest. Some participants indicated an improvement in the self-assessment of their skills. For example, before the training only 13.64% answered the question "How prepared do you feel regarding your communication skills for entering the profession?" with "Very good" or "Good", versus 50.00% in the posttest. There were also only 22.73% of participants who agreed to having sufficient understanding of the roles of other professional groups, while in the posttest, 81.82% agreed. The evaluations highlighted positive feedback on the organization, learning environment, and overall course structure. However, challenges such as limited resources, especially time and financial constraints, influenced the implementation and ongoing development of the course. Subsequent runs of the course could gather more data to further improve the teaching of veterinary interprofessional communication. This ongoing data collection would allow continuous insights into and adjustments to the teaching methods, ensuring maximum benefit for veterinary students and apprentice assistants.

Keywords: interprofessional; team communication; teamwork; communication course; interprofessional course; blended learning; flipped classroom

1. Introduction

Communication and establishment of personal relationships between veterinarians and pet owners influence the quality and outcomes of medical treatments [1,2]. The veterinarian must actively obtain information from and provide information to the pet owner, and not just during the anamnesis. Especially after starting a treatment schedule, it is essential to maintain good communication with the owner to determine whether the animal's health has improved or deteriorated. In the meantime, not only veterinarians and owners are often involved in the care of the animal but also other professions and groups [3]. Especially in larger practices or clinics, communication within the team is crucial to ensure the treatment is implemented and pursued efficiently and without errors. A recent study from the UK shows that not only communication with owners is important but also good team communication is crucial [4]. In this study, communication problems were identified as a contributing factor in about 80% of cases of alleged professional negligence, with about half of these including communication problems within the team or between different teams.

The successful treatment of animals often involves several specialized veterinarians, veterinary assistants, animal physiotherapists, nutrition specialists, and others [3]. This is the reason why interprofessional teamwork is gaining significance, as the success of treatments depends not only on expertise but also on effective collaboration among the professions. It is also proven that interprofessional education can positively influence the organizational climate and job satisfaction, which is shown by a scoping review based on the literature of professionals in different medical fields (except veterinary medicine), where the effect of the IPE (Interprofessional Education) of post-graduates is shown [5].

Communication skills are currently mostly taught as an elective in the veterinary curriculum in Germany [6–10]. A competence model including a list of communication competences has been established [11]; however, longitudinal integration and implementation are still in progress. The SOFTVETS-Competence Model [11] also includes interprofessional team communication. At the University of Veterinary Medicine Hannover (TiHo Hannover), Germany, training of communication competences for veterinary students is explicitly provided in the subject of Veterinary Professional Studies and Propaedeutics. Additional content is offered in elective courses as well as intramural practical training at the Small Animal Clinic [8]. However, the emphasis is primarily on communication with pet owners, not on team communication. In Germany's training catalog for veterinary assistants, communication with pet owners is emphasized, but there is no explicit mention of interprofessional communication skills either [12]. Furthermore, the training of veterinary assistants differs markedly from that of veterinary students. Most of the three year training period is workplace-based, with only short periods of vocational school blocks, while veterinary students spend 8 of 11 terms at the university and mainly gain practical experience in internships in the 9th and 10th terms. It is important to recognize that professional roles, qualifications and academic standards vary internationally. Due to differences in training structures and naming conventions across countries, there may be potential for misunderstanding [13]. In Germany, veterinary assistants undergo a three-year vocational training program organized by the regional veterinary chamber [12]. This comprehensive program includes theoretical modules alongside practical work at veterinary practices. Veterinary assistants support veterinarians in various tasks, such as animal treatment and examination, pre- and post-operative care, X-rays, client guidance and administrative duties.

A promising interprofessional pilot project was already carried out in the UK several years ago [14], but no similar educational projects have been reported in Germany, nor does the national ordinance include any adjustments toward communication or interprofessional competences in Germany yet [10]. Thus, we aim that this pilot project will lead to further curriculum development. In Germany, communication competences as well as interprofessional competences are already anchored in the national catalog of learning objectives in the study programs of human medicine [15] and dentistry [8,16]. This indicates that other healthcare sectors have already recognized the relevance, and we in veterinary medicine should also take this step.

Since the two professions of veterinarians and veterinary assistants are both trained at the TiHo, but only alongside each other and not together, a pilot project should improve this situation and close this gap in veterinary education. It should also address the lack of communication training within the team, which has not been covered in the academic curriculum and has only been thought between owner and veterinary assistant during training. In order to make a joint learning intervention accessible for both professions, a blended learning course was designed, i.e., a mixture of online learning and face-to-face learning [17]. At the time of the implementation of the course, there were still contact restrictions due to COVID-19, so face-to-face teaching was mainly reserved for the clinical–practical subjects and the elective courses mostly took place online. Therefore, the external circumstances influenced the course planning toward a blended learning concept. The course structure also simplified the organization with different professions. In order to take advantage of the benefits of the flipped classroom design, the theoretical content was initially elaborated independently in order to use the later attendance time more effectively for application and transfer tasks [18–20]. An elective interprofessional communication course was created and evaluated with the aim of exploring knowledge, attitudes and self-assessment of communication skills.

The research questions were as follows:

- How do participants score on a knowledge test before and after an interprofessional communication course?
- How do participants rate their self-assessment of communication skills before and after an interprofessional communication course?
- How do participants evaluate a blended learning interprofessional communication course?

2. Materials and Methods

2.1. Creation of the Course

In the winter term of 2022/2023, the course "Interprofessional communication for veterinary practice" was offered for the first time to students of veterinary medicine and apprentices training to become veterinary assistants, in the following referred to as apprentice assistants. An overview of the course design is illustrated in Figure 1. We chose the concept of a flipped classroom to enable asynchronous learning of the theory to be able to use the in-person meetings more effectively to apply what has been learned [19,21,22]. This format enables personalized learning according to one's own learning style [23]. There were no significant differences in the evaluation of the teaching approach between students of different performance levels, which indicates that all students can benefit from this concept. The basic structure of an asynchronous online course was already proven suitable for imparting communication skills [24]. It was created and provided by the TiHo Moodle platform. The course comprised nine interactive modules in which theoretical content was delivered by means of texts, videos, and interactive tasks. The tools of the Moodle platform as well as the H5P software (Versions 1.17.2) were used for this purpose. A blended learning event was chosen because online delivery of theoretical content was easily achievable and, for both professions, flexible in terms of time [25,26]. The module topics were created in accordance with the core competencies of the WHO and the recommendations of the IpEC [27,28]. Each module was available for completion for 1–3 weeks, with an average estimated processing time of 2 h. At the end of each module, tasks had to be completed to verify successful participation. These tasks included quizzes, interactive videos, audio recordings, or text composition. For the course design, thematically relevant videos were created with professional actors as best-practice or worst-case examples, focusing on typical situations and conflicts within veterinary practice.

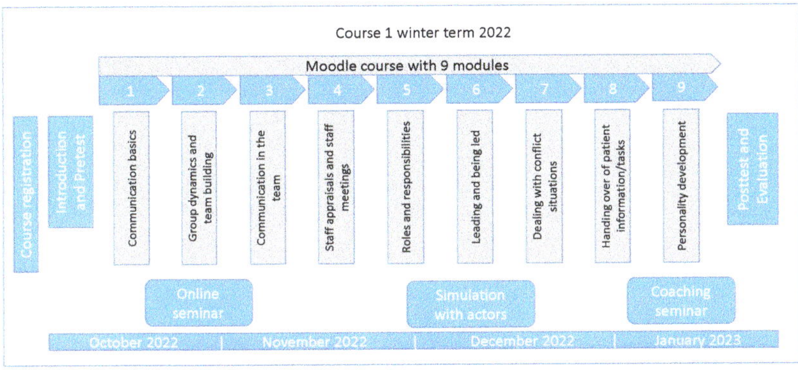

Figure 1. Overview of the blended learning course design from the winter term 2022/2023.

In addition to the online course, a synchronous online seminar was conducted to delve deeper into the learning content and explore topics related to biases, potential prejudices, and professional roles. Furthermore, simulation training sessions with professional actors were offered (two hours per participant) to apply the learned theoretical content in a practical context. This training took place in the communication facility at the Clinical Skills Lab at TiHo Hannover, which is a consultation room with cameras and microphones and a one-way mirror [29]. For this purpose, six scenarios were developed, each with three versions, to encompass all the possible combinations (actor, veterinary assistant, veterinary assistant; actor, veterinary assistant, veterinarian; actor, veterinarian, veterinarian). The simulation training was designed to provide an opportunity to practice communication strategies in a safe learning environment without putting the well-being of animals or people at risk. The scenarios were debriefed through multi-source feedback (360-degree feedback) immediately following the training. The feedback was provided by participating and observing participants (veterinary student, apprentice assistant) as well as by the actors and course facilitators. Finally, one professional communication coaching event was provided, focusing on topics such as stress management and resilience.

2.2. Creation of the Questionnaire

To assess knowledge and attitudes regarding communication skills before and after the course, a pretest and posttest as well as an evaluation to rate the course design were developed. The individual components of the tests are listed in Table 1. To allow for a pseudonymous comparison of the results of the two tests, participants were asked to provide a unique code and some personal data. Participation was anonymized, with only the IP address allowing inferences about the identity of the participants.

Table 1. Overview of the pre- and posttest questions.

	Number of Questions	
Question Type	**Pretest**	**Posttest**
Demographic data	8	3
Knowledge test	26	26
Needs assessment (RIPLS) [30]	19	19
Self-assessment	16	16
Previous experience	1	0
Course expectations	4	0
Evaluation questions	0	69

The questions for the needs assessment were the original 19 items of the validated German version of the Readiness for Interprofessional Learning Scale [30]; however, the results of this analysis are not included in this paper, as these are described in more detail in another report [31]. The rating questions were designed with a five-point response scale (1 = strongly agree to 5 = strongly disagree; 1 = yes, definitely to 5 = no, not at all, 1 = very good to 5 = very poor). Self-assessment questions were also created with a five-point response scale (1 = very good to 5 = very poor, 1 = yes, definitely to 5 = no, not at all). In addition to these scales, the option "no answer" was enabled for all the questions.

The self-assessment questions and statements were based on the CSAS (Communication Skills Attitude Scale) [32] and were supplemented and validated within the working group. Similar statements have already been used in a previous study exploring veterinary students' and apprentice assistants' need for communication training [33].

The knowledge test section comprised 26 single-choice questions aligned with the course modules. Each single-best answer question comprised one attractor and two to four distractors. For the knowledge questions, the response "Don't know" was also provided. An example question from this section is the following: "In which order are the teambuilding phases by Tuckman described?".

The posttest was created similarly to the pretest. It included the collection of gender, year of birth, profession, and the unique code. The knowledge test, self-assessment, and needs assessment were repeated. In addition, a final evaluation of the event was conducted, where aspects like organization and technology, learning environment and support, sustainability and the structure of individual components were rated. The evaluation was divided into 10 different sections, consisting of a total of 66 single-choice or rating questions. Participants always had the option to select "No response", leading to varying dataset sizes in some cases. Within these categories, 32 statements were provided for respondents to answer as rating questions. The scaling of the responses was five-point (1 = strongly agree to 5 = strongly disagree). The clarity of the nine modules was also assessed (1 = very clear to 5 = not clear) as well as the content depth (1 = too detailed to 5 = too superficial). Lastly, participants were asked to rate the helpfulness of the course modules and components (asynchronous Moodle course, synchronous online seminar, communication coaching, simulation session) for their learning success (1 = very helpful to 5 = not helpful). Finally, a filter question was asked to ascertain whether the respondent was a veterinary student or an apprentice assistant to determine the most appropriate placement of the course in their academic or training year (veterinary students: 1st to 6th academic year; apprentice assistants: 1st to 3rd training year).

For the data analysis, Microsoft Office Excel 2010 (Microsoft Corporation, Redmond, WA, USA) was used, and for the statistical analyses, SAS Enterprise Guide 7.1 (SAS Institute Inc., Cary, NC, USA) was employed.

The conducted surveys adhered to the regulations stipulated concerning general data protection. Prior to answering the questionnaires, written consent was obtained from all the participants. Additionally, a unique code was assigned to each questionnaire to ensure the collection of anonymized, matched samples. Participation was voluntary and anonymous. Apart from the raw IP addresses, no identifiable data were gathered, ensuring respondent anonymity. Participants had the option to skip any question or select "No answer". This research adhered to the ethical standards of the University of Veterinary Medicine Hannover, Foundation. Approval for the entire project was granted by the university's Data Protection Officer. Students who participated voluntarily provided consent for their data to be processed in line with the EU General Data Protection Regulation of 2018 (General Data Protection Regulation Art. 6 I 1 lit. e i.V.m. 89 and Lower Saxony Data Protection Act § 3 I 1 No. 1 NHG, § 13). All the collected data were analyzed and handled anonymously in accordance with the university's data protection regulations. The university's doctoral thesis committee, acting as the ethics committee, reviewed and sanctioned the project in line with ethical guidelines governing research involving human participants.

Upon request, the corresponding author can provide the data used in this study. However, these data are not publicly accessible due to ethical considerations and privacy restrictions.

3. Results

The course was offered for the first time in the winter term 22/23. Apprentice assistants (veterinary assistants in training) were informed via email, while veterinary students could enroll in the course as an elective course via online registration. In the pilot course, 18 veterinary students and 13 prospective veterinary assistants registered for the elective course. Of the latter, only 11 actually started the course and 6 of them successfully completed the entire course and additionally participated in the posttest as well. All the veterinary students completed the course in full, including assignments and tests. Altogether, 22 paired samples were collected using individual codes. All the subsequent analyses refer to n = 22, compromising 6 paired tests from apprentice assistants and 16 from veterinary students.

In the following, we will summarize the evaluations, considering "Strongly agree" and "Agree" as positive and "Disagree" and "Strongly disagree" as negative responses.

3.1. Demographic Data

Most of the participants were female (n = 21, 95.45%) and were born between 1984 and 2003. Less than half of them had already participated in previous communication training (n = 8, 36.36%). Almost all the participants had experience of teamwork at work (n = 21, 95.45%). Almost an equal number had already gained experience in teamwork related to sports or hobbies (n = 20, 90.91%).

3.2. Knowledge Test

In the pretest, 190 correct answers were identified in the knowledge test, while in the posttest, the number increased to 291, resulting in a knowledge gain of 53.16%. The number of incorrect answers also increased from 45 to 72, representing an increase of 60%. In the pretest, the "Don't know" option was selected 180 times, whereas in the posttest, it was only chosen 38 times, indicating a reduction of −78.89%. Since the knowledge test questions were not set as mandatory, there was the option to continue the questionnaire without providing an answer. This was observed more frequently in the posttest than in the pretest. The differences in answering the entire knowledge test are depicted in Figure 2.

3.3. Communication Skills Assessment

All three questions regarding the self-assessment of one's communications skills showed a positive trend between the pretest and the posttest. The ratings of the three questions are shown in Figure 3. The most obvious change was observed in question three. The response "Very good" was chosen more than three times as often in the posttest (n = 4, 18.18%) compared to the pretest (n = 1, 4.55%), and the same applied to "good" (Pretest: n = 2, 9.09%, Posttest: n = 7, 31.82%). In the posttest "Very bad" was no longer selected and the selection of "Bad" decreased to approximately one-sixth of its previous frequency (Pretest: n = 7, 31.82%, Posttest: n = 1, 4.55%).

Self-assessment questions 1–3:

1. How do you rate your communication skills with pet owners?
2. How do you rate your communication skills within a team?
3. How prepared do you feel regarding your communication skills for entering the profession?

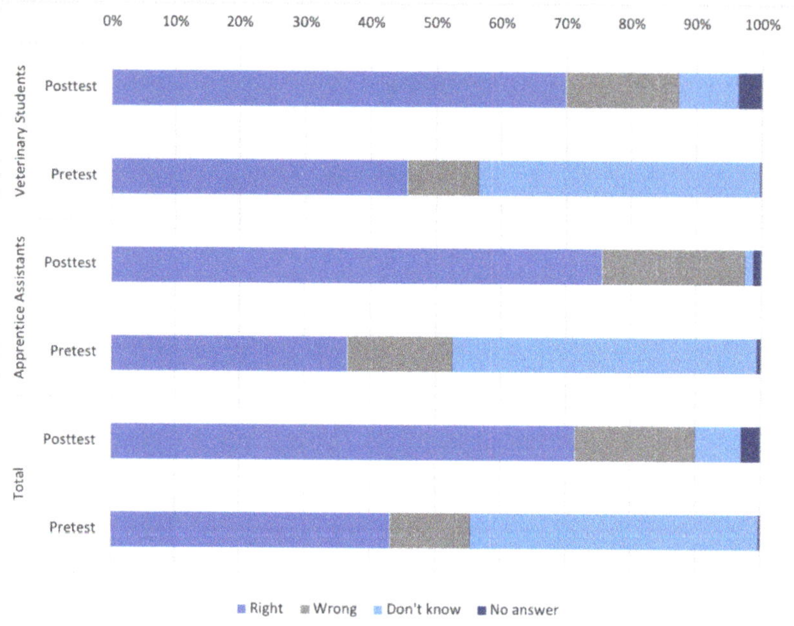

Figure 2. The 26 knowledge-based questions summarized and sorted by professions, presented as an overview, comparing the pre- and posttest.

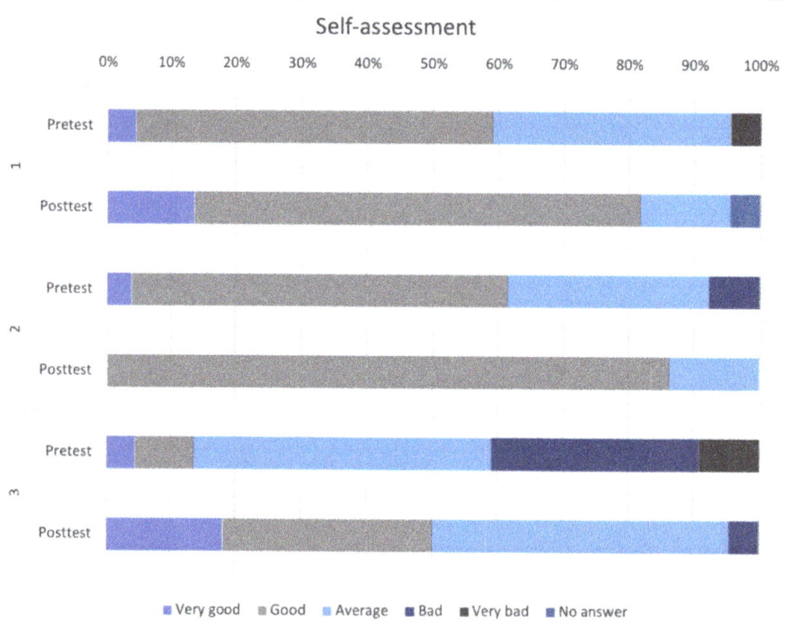

Figure 3. Comparative representation of self-assessment questions 1–3 between the pre- and posttest.

The additional questions regarding one's communication skills and their assessment are shown in Figure 4. The majority of the participants saw room for improvement in their communication skills in the pretest and chose "Yes, definitely" or "Yes, rather" (n = 13, 59.09%). In the posttest, this value decreased by about half (n = 7, 31.82%). In the pretest, a huge number of participants rated themselves as not prepared for potential conflicts within the team (n = 7, 31.82%) and two participants even chose "No, not at all". In the posttest, these selection options were almost not chosen at all.

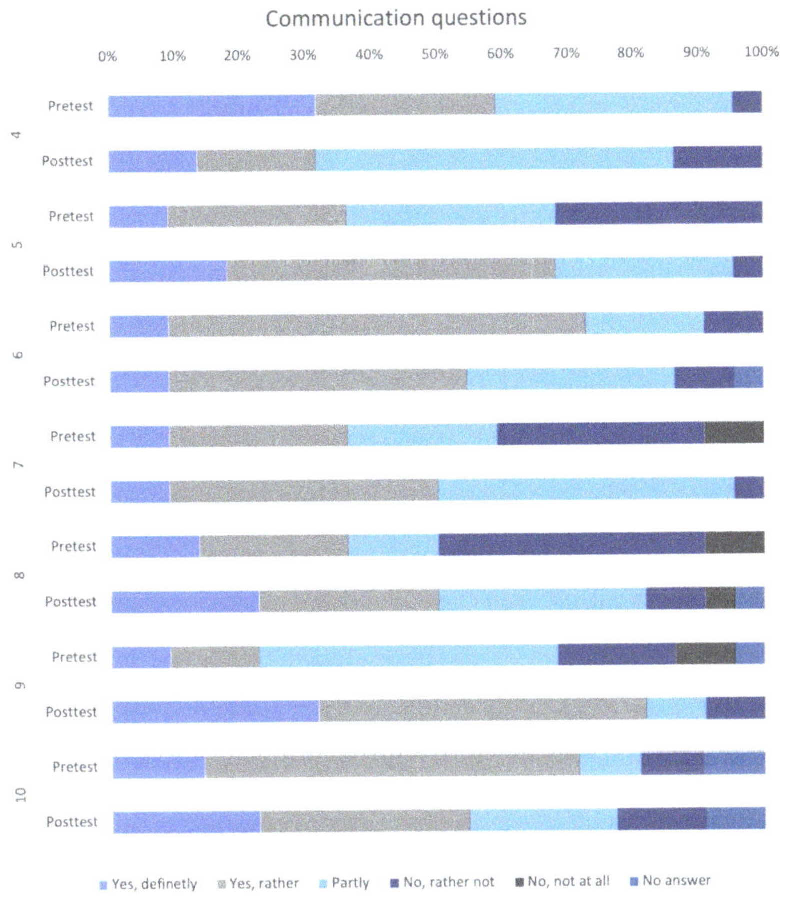

Figure 4. Comparative representation of self-assessment questions 4–10 between the pre- and posttest.

Self-assessment questions 4–10:

4. Do you see room for improvement in your communication skills?
5. Do you feel well-prepared for employee discussions?
6. Can you delegate tasks effectively to others?
7. Do you feel well-prepared for potential conflict situations within a team?
8. Has your study/training helped you acquire communications skills?
9. Do you feel you have sufficient understanding of the roles of other professional groups?
10. Do you wish for interprofessional events in the timetable?

Communication statements 11–16 are depicted in Figure 5. With the exception of statement 16, these were all rated very positively. Statements 11 to 15 were not rated differently in the pre- and in the posttest. The statement "I don't have time in my educations/studies to learn communication skills". received higher ratings of "Rather not true" and "Not true" in the posttest (n = 14, 63.63%) than in the pretest (n = 11, 50%).

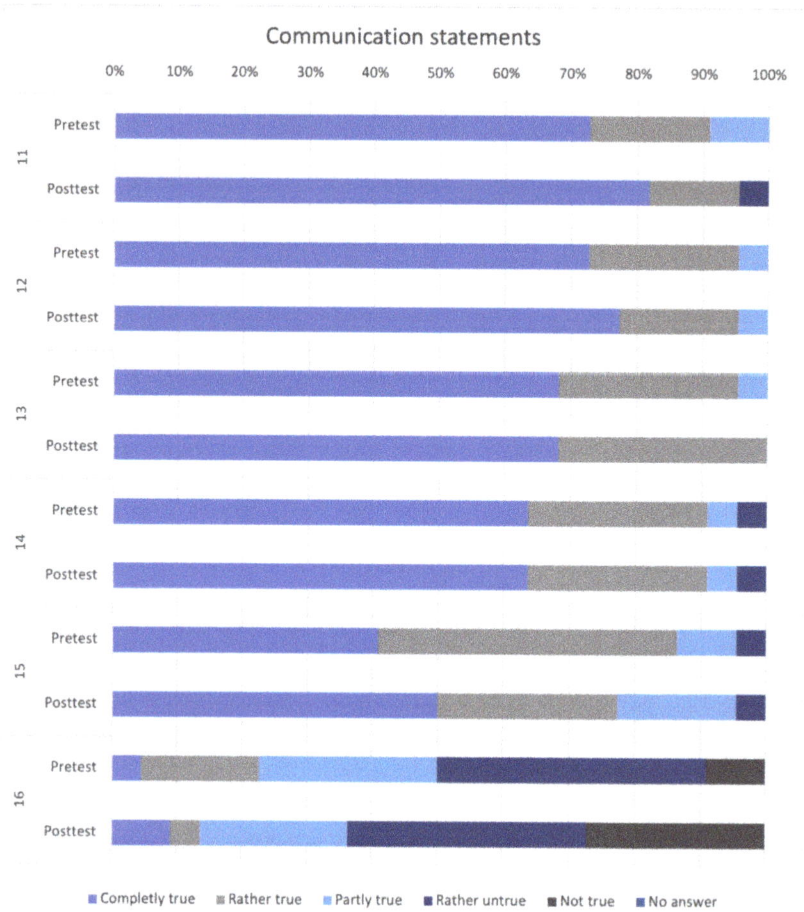

Figure 5. Comparative representation of self-assessment statements 11–16 between the pre- and posttest.

Communication statements 11–16:

11. Communication skills are important for my everyday life.
12. Learning communicative skills enhances my ability to conduct customer/patient conversations.
13. Learning communicative skills improves my ability to communicate within a team.
14. Through communication training in education/studies, I can learn to better handle conflict situations in my future professional life.
15. I believe that communication skills can be learned.
16. I don't have time in my education/studies to learn communication skills.

3.4. Evaluation

The evaluation of the course was filled out 25 times; in the following, we only focus on 22 of the paired samples.

3.4.1. Organization and Technology

The majority of the respondents found the organization of the event to be well-executed (n = 21, 95.45%). Participation in the Moodle course also went smoothly for the majority
(n = 19, 86.36%). The overall course concept, which included an asynchronous online course, (online) seminars, and in-person meetings, received positive ratings (n = 20, 90.91%).

3.4.2. Learning Atmosphere and Support

The results of the evaluation part "Learning atmosphere and support" are shown in Figure 6.

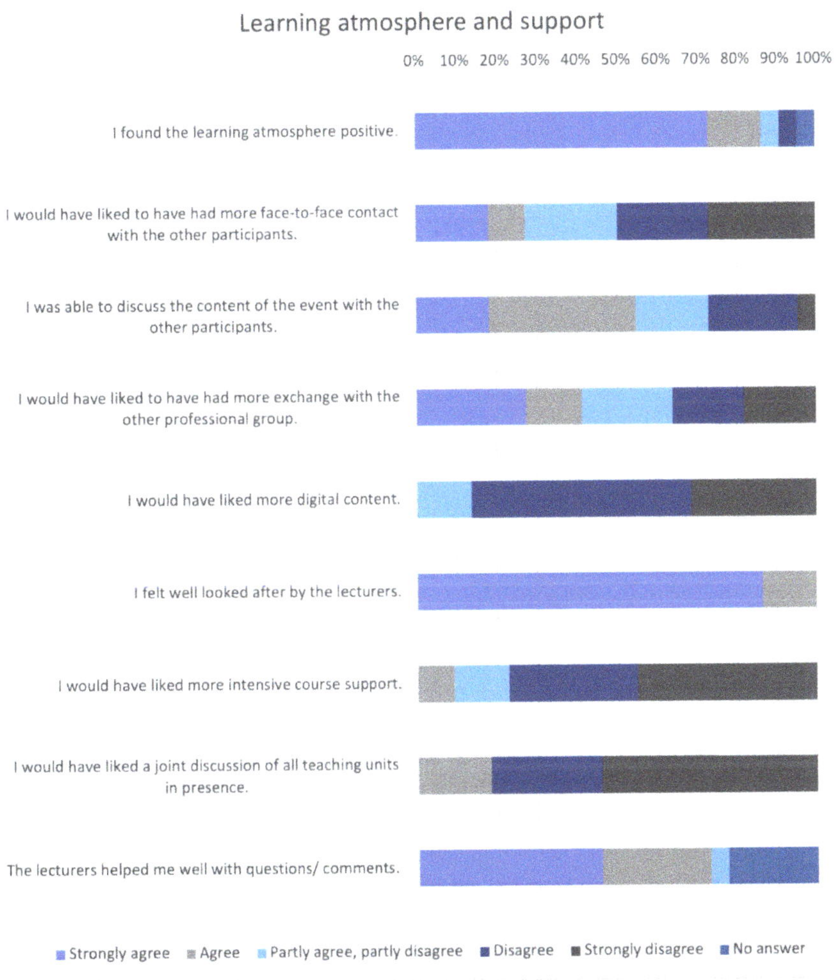

Figure 6. Evaluation of the learning atmosphere and the support.

Most participants evaluated the learning environment positively (n = 16, 72.73%, "Strongly agree"; n = 3, 13.64%, Agree"). In response to the statement "I would have liked more face-to-face contact with other participants", varied responses arose. Nonetheless, more participants disagreed with this statement (n = 5, 22.73% "Disagree", n = 6, 27.27% "Strongly disagree").

Participants indicated that they had sufficiently compared notes with other participants about the course content (n = 18.18%, n = 4 "Strongly agree"; n = 8, 36.36% "Agree"). No participant chose to agree with the item "I would have liked more digital content". All the participants felt well looked after by the lecturers. Five participants chose not to select an answer for the item "The lecturers helped me well with questions/comments".

3.4.3. Sustainability

The results from the section "Sustainability" of the evaluation are shown in Figure 7.

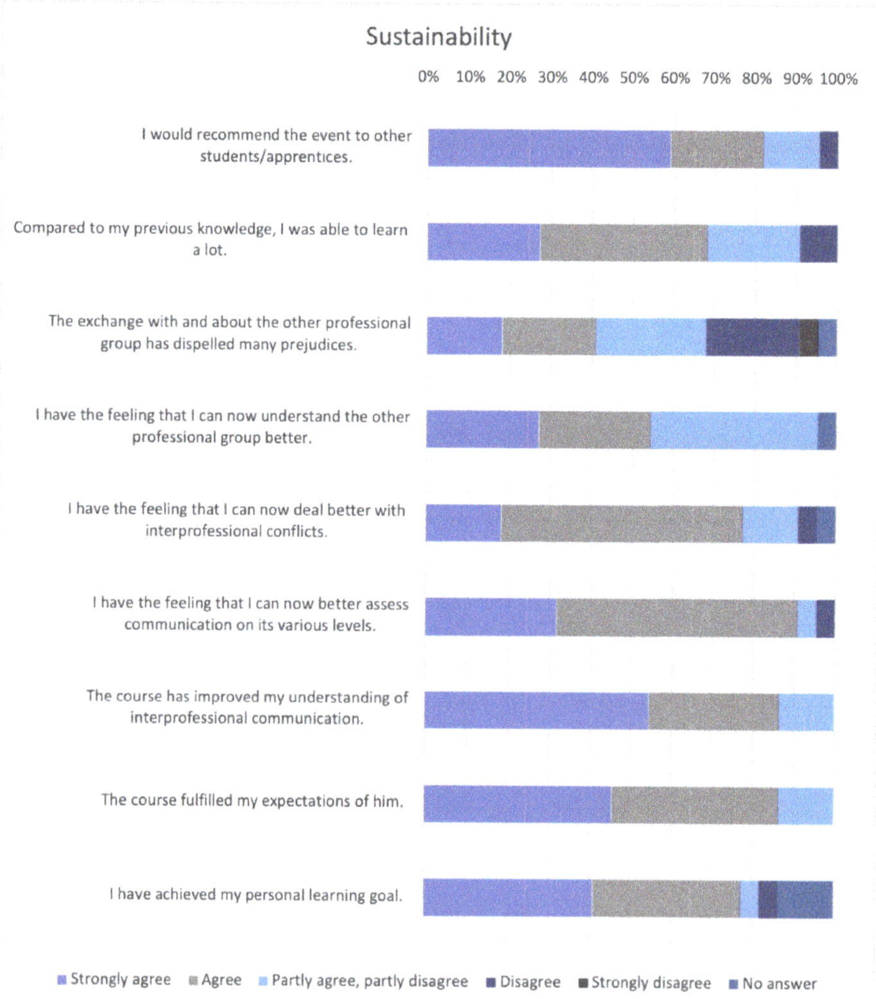

Figure 7. Evaluation of the sustainability.

Most participants stated that they would recommend the event to other veterinary students/apprentice assistants (n = 18, 82.81%). Regarding the extent of the learning achieved, most participants agreed that they had learned a lot (n = 15, 68.18%). The respondents stated that their understanding of the other respective professional group had improved (n = 12, 54.55%). The course mostly fulfilled the expectations of the participants (n = 19, 86.36%).

3.4.4. Structure

All the results of the section "structure" of the evaluation are displayed in Figure 8.

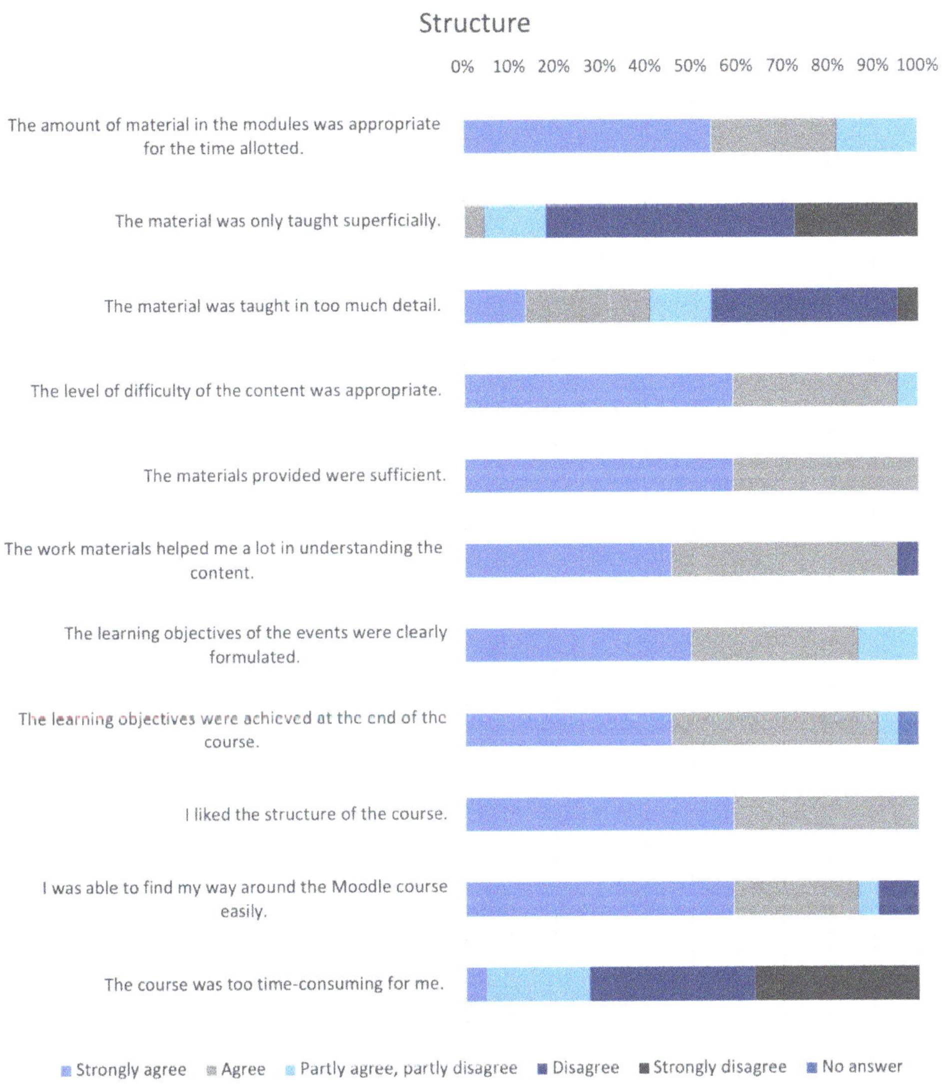

Figure 8. Structure evaluation.

The majority of participants rated the amount of content as appropriate for the scheduled period (n = 18, 81.82%). Most respondents disagreed that the content had been covered too superficially (n = 18, 81.82%). The level of difficulty was mostly rated appropriate (n = 21, 95.45%). All the provided learning materials were rated as sufficient (n = 22, 100%). All the participants liked the structure of the course (n = 22, 100%).

3.4.5. Comprehensibility

Six of the nine modules were exclusively rated as "Very understandable" and "Rather understandable". In the modules "Communication basics" and "Leading and being led" and "Personal development", one person each gave "Partly" as an answer for these modules. Additionally, in the "Leading and being led" module, one person also marked it as "Rather incomprehensible".

3.4.6. Professional Depth

The professional depth of all the online course modules was rated by the participants on a scale from "Much too detailed" to "Much too superficial". All the modules were mostly rated as "Exactly right".

All the results of the evaluation of the helpfulness of the modules are shown in Figure 9. The module "Staff appraisals and staff meeting" was the best rated module (n = 20, 90.91%). The module "Communication basics" was the lowest rated module (n = 12, 54.55%).

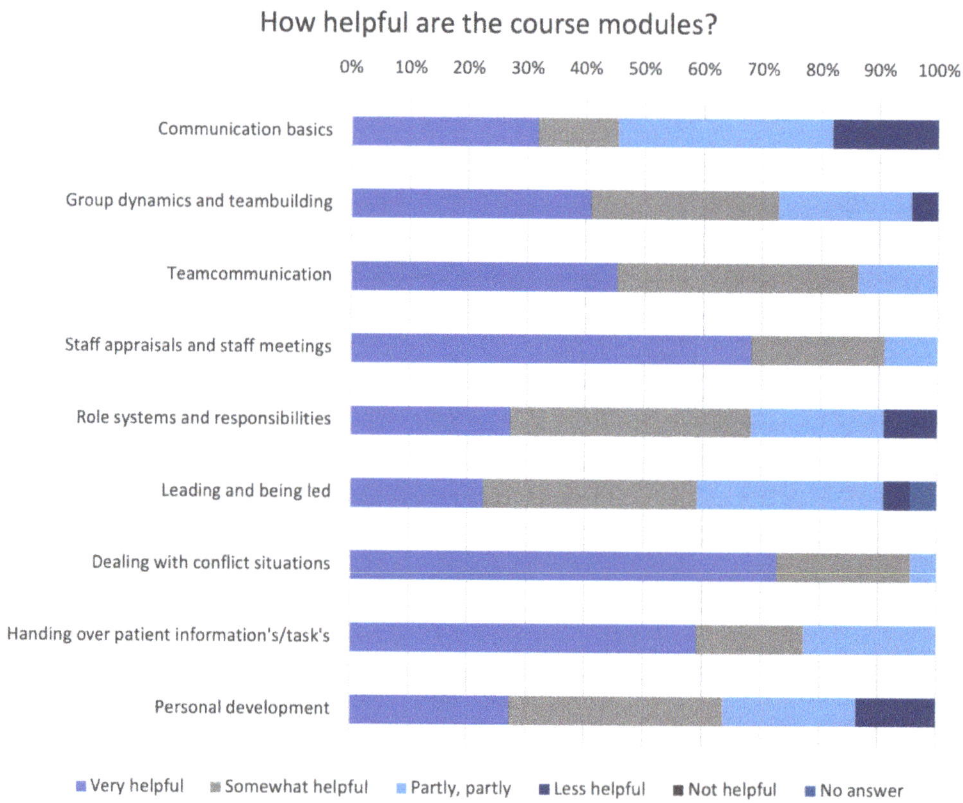

Figure 9. Presentation of the evaluation of the rating of the helpfulness of the modules.

Figure 10 presents all the results of the rating of the components' helpfulness. The simulation training was the best rated part of the course (n = 17, 77.27%), whereas the lowest rated component was the online seminar (n = 5, 22.73%).

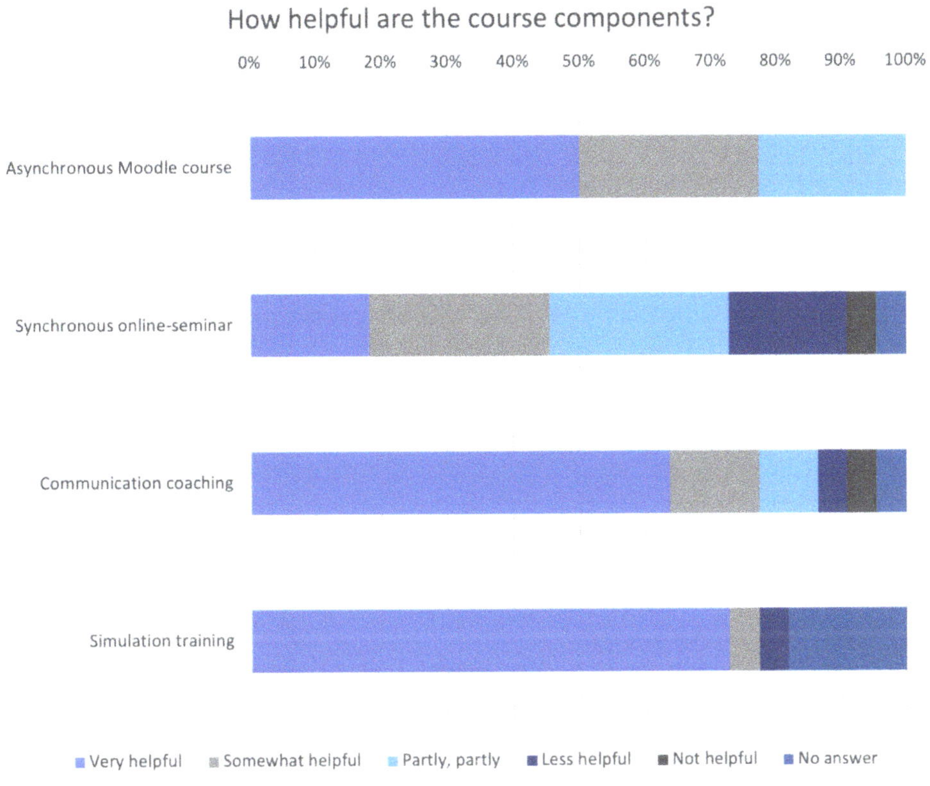

Figure 10. Evaluation of the rating regarding how helpful the components of the course are.

The veterinary students and apprentice assistants were asked in which academic or trainee year they would find an interprofessional communication course appropriate. The veterinary students were in strong agreement, particularly recommending the third academic year (n = 11, 68.75%). The apprentice assistants' responses were less conclusive, with half of the respondents favoring the first year of training (n = 3, 50%).

4. Discussion

Communication is unanimously recognized as a core competency in the medical and veterinary health professions [34,35]. Although this competency has not yet been mandatorily incorporated into veterinary medicine, it is taught to varying extents at German universities [8,10]. As part of the interprofessional communication course in the winter term 22/23, a positive effect on the knowledge and self-assessment of the communication skills of veterinary students and apprentice assistants was observed. Furthermore, the evaluation confirmed that both professional groups positively evaluated the blended learning course, particularly the simulation training. The implementation and reporting of any course evaluation on interprofessional courses in the veterinary field are relatively rare [14]. Even if there are papers about communication courses in this field [36–38] and about interprofessional courses in other healthcare sectors [39–41], the gap in veterinary medicine is huge.

The pilot project "Interprofessional Team Communication for Veterinary Practice" enjoyed a positive response, which is an indication to us that veterinary students and apprentice assistants appreciate the relevance of the subject matter. Several studies also show that the attitude toward interprofessional education is mostly positive, even if a lot of students do not have much knowledge about it [42,43]. Our aim was to demonstrate the potential of an interprofessional learning intervention in veterinary medicine. After the initial veterinary interprofessional intervention in England in 2011 yielded positive results [14], the anticipated curriculum adjustments did not materialize. Therefore, more than 10 years later, with this project in Germany, we aimed to take the next step in this direction and focus on the course structure to help to close the research gap. With this project, we also sent a response to the various calls for action from overarching organizations [28,44]. The alternative to interprofessional learning is uniprofessional education, which is the current format being used mostly in veterinary medicine, especially for veterinary students.

Implementing the course went smoothly for the veterinary students, whereas the apprentice assistants encountered greater difficulty in completing the course, as measured by the number of apprentice assistants who did not complete the course entirely. That could be due to the fact that veterinary students are required to fulfill a specific number of elective hours, whereas the apprentice assistants voluntarily took the course alongside their regular workload in the clinics and received only a certificate of attendance for it. Improvement is needed in this regard. Time resources need to be provided to potential participants to successfully engage in interprofessional courses with similar prerequisites and motivations. Previous studies also indicate that it is not only the apprentice assistants who may have encountered difficulties in completing the course, even students seemed to prefer the blended learning approach; they also mentioned lack of discipline and problems with their time management as being obstacles preventing them from completing blended learning courses [45]. These might also be reasons especially contributing to the issues faced by the apprentice assistants.

The improved self-assessment of the participants' communication skills post-course provides an indication of the effectiveness of the multi-week training, even if studies show that the self-assessment is not always an accurate tool to measure clinical competencies, especially for low-performing students [46]. A study indicated that also shorter durations resulted in fewer measurable differences among participants but showed positive changes on the part of the pet owners [47]. As already assessed by Bahramsoltani et al. [37], especially the practical training is useful for an improvement in communications skills. This was also obvious in our evaluation when comparing the online course with the practical learning sessions. The blended learning concept also facilitated the organization of the course with the different professions and different daily routines. Nevertheless, the evaluation indicated a desire for more interaction. In particular, the simulation training was resource-intensive. In addition to preparing the scenarios and training and paying the actors, time and space capacities were also limitations.

An extensive evaluation was administered as a posttest, directly after completing the course. The course structure proved suitable for the event, although some participants wished for more in-person interaction during the course. As aforementioned, asynchronous online courses were already proven suitable for imparting communication skills in veterinary education [24]. The asynchronous elements combined several advantages, like flexibility, repeatability, and better understanding through multimedia use [48]. Combined with the practical training, we used the already established flipped classroom concept [22,49]. Blended learning is an already approved learning method for veterinary medicine, especially for clinical skills like communication [50]. Furthermore, there are also hints that the learning outcome after blended learning compared to traditional learning is higher [21,26]. However, every teaching and learning model's natural has its advantages and disadvantages. This format allows students to tailor their learning to their individual needs. The course design was chosen because unnecessary contacts should still be avoided at TiHo Hannover due to COVID-19 infection numbers [51]. The use of videos to reflect on simulated situations is particularly suitable for training the ability to perceive and reflect [52]. After completing the pilot course, our aim was to continue and to make the content available and accessible for further persons and professions. Due to the limited resources, the course was exclusively conducted online, with two synchronous online seminars covering the topics prejudices and conflict potentials and resilience and stress management. Also, in the next winter term, the course was offered again. This time complemented by two additional online modules covering the topics of the seminars, as synchronous online seminars posed a challenge in finding an available time slot for all the professions. There is particular scope here to create opportunities for online collaboration and teamwork in asynchronous settings. More feedback and especially peer-centered activities were reported by students who studied mostly in synchronous settings in comparison with mostly asynchronous settings [53]. Furthermore, it must be highlighted how virtual collaboration is defined and to what extent virtual collaboration is achievable within asynchronous settings [54]. Also, the need for technical and facilitating support for online group processes and tasks with shared purposes must be considered in course design and, in particular, during the implementation.

The long-term aim of this pilot project is the implementation of an interprofessional communication course, or ideally, the longitudinal integration of this content into the curriculum. In this context, the major hurdles in the medical field have already been explored regarding implementation, with organizational challenges being prominent and highly qualified instructors playing a crucial role in the execution [55]. There was previously also a study that measured the benefit of team communication training, the results of which showed an improvement in productive teamwork after such training [56]. It is shown that especially with the longitudinal implementation, further challenges arise in logically embedding individual content into various sessions [57]. However, resources are also described as a limiting factor. Faculties that have not yet offered integrated interprofessional teaching mainly cite funding limitations and limited participation from other disciplines as reasons [58]. Both arguments we can understand well after piloting the course and running a second and third adapted learning intervention with limited financial resources.

It should be emphasized that although the apprentice assistants performed slightly lower on average in the pretest regarding the knowledge-based questions (36.54% correct answers) compared to the veterinary students (45.67%), they performed even better in the posttest (75.64% correct answers by apprentice assistants, 69.95% correct answers by veterinary students). Regarding the knowledge test, as was to be expected, an increase in knowledge from 53,16% could be demonstrated by the increase in the number of correct answers after completion of the course. However, there is still room for improvements as not all participants were able to answer all the questions correctly. Therefore, improvements could either be made in the knowledge test or also in teaching and learning material to achieve better outcomes. The chosen answer "Don't know" decreased, which also speaks in favor of the increase in competence. Nevertheless, we also observed an increase in incorrect answers in the posttest. This observation shows an increase in self-confidence in choosing a wrong answer rather than selecting "Don't know" and can be described as a supposed increase in competence. The guessing of answers, instead of choosing "Don't know", could be observed in the Progress Test of Veterinary Medicine as well [59]. This is a phenomenon that has not yet been fully explained by studies, but also in the Progress Test of Veterinary Medicine and a study about self-regulated learning the amount of both correct and incorrect answers increased with growing knowledge, while the "Don't know" response decreased [59,60]. These findings suggest a notable boost in self-assurance, implying that the uptick in incorrect responses can also be construed as a positive advancement. However, it has been already shown that veterinary medical students do not always assess their own abilities realistically [46].

Due to the small sample size resulting from a small number of participants, particularly the even smaller number of paired samples, the study's statements are limited. We had a relatively small sample size, further skewed by the disproportional distribution of the two surveyed professions. While the sample size of this study may not initially appear particularly large, the response rate of the apprentice assistants was very high. Out of a total of 21 apprentice assistants working at the University of Veterinary Medicine, 13 enrolled in the course. Furthermore, generating connected samples proved to be challenging, as some codes could not be assigned to the participants. Similar issues have been observed in other studies at the TiHo [61]. Because of the sample number, we focused on descriptive analysis in this paper.

The pretest was conducted immediately before the course began, and the posttest was administered immediately afterwards. To assess the sustainable learning outcomes and long-term changes in attitude and self-assessment, it would be beneficial to conduct additional tests at intervals of several weeks to months after the completion of the course, as in a previous study [62]. We used the same questions in the pre- and posttest, but the test bias is likely to be minimal in our study, as several months elapsed between the two tests and neither the questions nor the correct answers were disclosed. As a further outlook, we anticipate running additional iterations of the course after the pilot phase. These iterations can provide us with comparative insights into which teaching format is most effective. By attaining a larger sample size, this would enable us to explore differences among various professions.

5. Conclusions

Overall, the blended learning approach received positive feedback, proving to be organizationally beneficial and suitable for our event. Looking ahead to the continuation of the course, we anticipate further evaluations that will likely yield additional insights. Bearing in mind that communication teaching in veterinary medicine still receives little attention, with this positive example of an interprofessional course, we hope to influence curriculum adjustments and demonstrate the relevance and benefits of interprofessional education.

Additional investigation is warranted to explore the relationship between learning, shifts in performance or attitudes and the resulting impact on healthcare outcomes. This area of inquiry remains open for further exploration, with the potential to deepen our understanding of the mechanisms underlying educational interventions in healthcare settings and their ultimate effect on patient care and job satisfaction. Based on our findings, we can encourage other institutions to incorporate interprofessional education. Furthermore, there is a need for communication training, which is currently not adequately offered to all. Incorporating simulation training in various contexts, including interprofessional settings, could help improve communication in future workplaces. Collaboration among different educational institutions is necessary to provide access to such courses for various professions. To mitigate organizational challenges, the blended learning concept appears to be a promising approach for the implementation of interprofessional training in veterinary and veterinary associated professions.

Author Contributions: S.A.C.H. and C.K.: Study design, data collection, data analysis, results interpretation, and writing and review of the manuscript. A.T.: Study design, results interpretation and review of the manuscript. E.P.: Course design. S.W.: Study design, data collection. V.N.: Study design. All authors have read and agreed to the published version of the manuscript.

Funding: This study was supported by the project Innovation Plus 2022/2023, No. T0049 of the Ministry of Science and Culture of Lower Saxony. This Open Access publication was funded by the Deutsche Forschungsgemeinschaft (DFG, German Research Foundation) 491094227 "Open Access Publication Funding" and the University of Veterinary Medicine Hannover, Foundation.

Institutional Review Board Statement: This study was conducted in accordance with the ethical standards of the University of Veterinary Medicine Hannover Foundation. The entire project was approved by the university's data protection officer. The voluntarily participating students consented to the processing of their data in accordance with the EU General Data Protection Regulation of 2018 (General Data Protection Regulation Art. 6 I 1 lit. e i.V.m. 89 and Lower Saxony Data Protection Act § 3 I 1 No. 1 NHG, § 13). All the collected data were evaluated and processed anonymously in accordance with the data protection regulation of the university. Due to the lack of an ethics approval code, the doctoral thesis committee of the university, which acts as the university's ethics committee, validated the project in accordance with ethical guidelines regarding research with human participants and approved this study. Written consent to participate in the study was obtained from all the participants. The data protection officer reviewed the proposed project regarding observance of the Data Protection Law and gave permission to perform this study. All of the data obtained were processed and evaluated anonymously and in compliance with EU's General Data Protection Regulation. All the data presented in this study are available on request from the corresponding author. The data are not publicly available due to ethical and privacy restrictions.

Informed Consent Statement: Informed consent was obtained from all the subjects involved in this study. Consent forms were approved by the data protection officer and the doctoral thesis committee of the university.

Data Availability Statement: All the data presented in this study are available on request from the corresponding author. The data are not publicly available due to ethical and privacy restrictions.

Acknowledgments: We wish to thank all the enrolled participants in the courses and evaluations. Furthermore, we appreciate the work of our actors, who professionally performed and improvised during the simulation sessions, providing thoughtful feedback to students and course facilitators.

Conflicts of Interest: The authors declare that this research was conducted in the absence of any commercial or financial relationships that could be construed as a potential conflicts of interest.

References

1. Hamood, W.J.; Chur-Hansen, A.; McArthur, M.L. A qualitative study to explore communication skills in veterinary medical education. *Int. J. Med. Educ.* **2014**, *5*, 193–198. [CrossRef]
2. Pun, J.K.H. An integrated review of the role of communication in veterinary clinical practice. *BMC Vet. Res.* **2020**, *16*, 394. [CrossRef]
3. Kinnison, T.; May, S.A.; Guile, D. Inter-professional practice: From veterinarian to the veterinary team. *J. Vet. Med. Educ.* **2014**, *41*, 172–178. [CrossRef] [PubMed]
4. Russell, E.; Mossop, L.; Forbes, E.; Oxtoby, C. Uncovering the 'messy details' of veterinary communication: An analysis of communication problems in cases of alleged professional negligence. *Vet. Rec.* **2022**, *190*, e1068. [CrossRef]
5. Medina-Cordoba, M.; Cadavid, S.; Espinosa-Aranzales, A.F.; Aguia-Rojas, K.; Bermudez-Hernandez, P.A.; Quiroga-Torres, D.A.; Rodriguez-Duenas, W.R. The effect of interprofessional education on the work environment of health professionals: A scoping review. *Adv. Health Sci. Educ. Theory Pract.* **2023**, 1–18. [CrossRef] [PubMed]
6. Gruber, C.; Dilly, M.; Bahramsoltani, M.; Kleinsorgen, C.; Engelskirchen, S.; Ramspott, S.; Ehlers, J.P. Communication as teaching content of veterinary studies—A joint position paper from the DVG specialist group "communication and didactics" and the GMA veterinary medicine committee. *GMS J. Med. Educ.* **2021**, *38*, Doc84. [CrossRef] [PubMed]
7. Kleinsorgen, C.; Ramspott, S.; Ehlers, J.P.; Gruber, C.; Dilly, M.; Engelskirchen, S.; Bernigau, D.; Bahramsoltani, M. Kommunikative Kompetenzen im Studium der Veterinärmedizin in Deutschland—Ansätze für die Entwicklung eines Mustercurriculums. *Berl. Münchener Tierärztliche Wochenschr.* **2020**, *133*, 12–21. [CrossRef]
8. Pohl, A.; Klass, L.G.; Kleinsorgen, C.; Bernigau, D.; Pfeiffer-Morhenn, B.; Arnhold, S.; Dilly, M.; Beitz-Radzio, C.; Wissing, S.; Vogt, L.; et al. Integration and potential of teaching communication skills in the study of veterinary medicine in Germany. *GMS J. Med. Educ.* **2021**, *38*, Doc53. [CrossRef] [PubMed]
9. Ramspott, S.; Beitz-Radzio, C.; Stucki, P.; Eule, J.C. Ergebnisse "Lernziele im Bereich Kommunikation". In Proceedings of the 61. Jahreskongress der Dt. Gesellschaft für Kleintiermedizin, Berlin, Germany, 12–15 November 2015.
10. Ordinance concerning the Certification of Veterinary Surgeons (Verordnung zur Approbation von Tierärztinnen und Tierärzten—TAppV). 2006. Available online: https://www.gesetze-im-internet.de/tiermedfangausbv/BJNR252200005.html (accessed on 9 January 2024).
11. Kleinsorgen, C.; Steinberg, E.; Domotor, R.; Piano, J.Z.; Rugelj, J.; Mandoki, M.; Radin, L. "The SOFTVETS Competence Model"—A preliminary project report. *GMS J. Med. Educ.* **2021**, *38*, Doc50. [CrossRef] [PubMed]
12. Niedersachsen, T. Verordnung über die Berufsausbildung zum Tiermedizinischen Fachangestellten/zur Tiermedizinischen Fachangestellten. 2005. Available online: https://www.gesetze-im-internet.de/tiermedfangausbv/BJNR252200005.html (accessed on 9 January 2024).
13. Harvey, L.; Ladyman, R.; Farnworth, M. International differences in the journey toward compulsory veterinary nurse registration. *Vet. Nurse* **2014**, *5*, 538–542. [CrossRef]

14. Kinnison, T.; Lumbis, R.; Orpet, H.; Welsh, P.; Gregory, S.; Baillie, S. Piloting interprofessional education interventions with veterinary and veterinary nursing students. *J. Vet. Med. Educ.* **2011**, *38*, 311–318. [CrossRef]
15. Wissing, F. National Competency-Based Learning Objective Catalogue for Dental and Human Medicine. *Bundesgesundheitsblatt Gesundheitsforschung Gesundheitsschutz* **2018**, *61*, 170. [CrossRef]
16. Ruttermann, S.; Sobotta, A.; Hahn, P.; Kiessling, C.; Hartl, A. Teaching and assessment of communication skills in undergraduate dental education—A survey in German-speaking countries. *Eur. J. Dent. Educ.* **2017**, *21*, 151–158. [CrossRef]
17. Hrastinski, S. What Do We Mean by Blended Learning? *TechTrends* **2019**, *63*, 564–569. [CrossRef]
18. Harris, B.F.; Harris, J.; Reed, L.; Zelihic, M. Flipped Classroom: Another Tool for Your Pedagogy Tool Box. *Dev. Bus. Simul. Exp. Learn.* **2016**, *43*, 325–333.
19. Matthew, S.M.; Schoenfeld-Tacher, R.M.; Danielson, J.A.; Warman, S.M. Flipped Classroom Use in Veterinary Education: A Multinational Survey of Faculty Experiences. *J. Vet. Med. Educ.* **2019**, *46*, 97–107. [CrossRef] [PubMed]
20. Tolks, D.; Schäfer, C.; Raupach, T.; Kruse, L.; Sarikas, A.; Gerhardt-Szép, S.; Kllauer, G.; Lemos, M.; Fischer, M.R.; Eichner, B.; et al. An introduction to the Inverted/Flipped Classroom Model in Education and Advanced Training in Medicine and in the Healthcare Professions. *GMS J. Med. Educ.* **2016**, *33*, Doc46. [CrossRef]
21. Dooley, L.M.; Frankland, S.; Boller, E.; Tudor, E. Implementing the Flipped Classroom in a Veterinary Pre-clinical Science Course: Student Engagement, Performance, and Satisfaction. *J. Vet. Med. Educ.* **2018**, *45*, 195–203. [CrossRef]
22. González-Montaña, J.R.G.; Alonso- Diez, A.J.; Domínguez, J.C.; Martínez-Pastor, F.; Alonso de la Verga, M.E. Adapted model of flipped classroom in Veterinary Medical Pathology teaching: Students' perception. In Proceedings of the 8th International Conference on Higher Education Advances (HEAd'22), Valencia, Spain, 15–17 June 2022.
23. Muca, E.; Cavallini, D.; Raspa, F.; Bordin, C.; Bergero, D.; Valle, E. Integrating New Learning Methods into Equine Nutrition Classrooms: The Importance of Students' Perceptions. *J. Equine Vet. Sci.* **2023**, *126*, 104537. [CrossRef]
24. Artemiou, E.; Adams, C.L.; Toews, L.; Violato, C.; Coe, J.B. Informing web-based communication curricula in veterinary education: A systematic review of web-based methods used for teaching and assessing clinical communication in medical education. *J. Vet. Med. Educ.* **2014**, *41*, 44–54. [CrossRef] [PubMed]
25. Tayebinik, M.; Puteh, M. Blended Learning or E-Learning? *Int. Mag. Adv. Comput. Sci. Telecommun.* **2012**, *3*, 103–110.
26. Vallee, A.; Blacher, J.; Cariou, A.; Sorbets, E. Blended Learning Compared to Traditional Learning in Medical Education: Systematic Review and Meta-Analysis. *J. Med. Internet Res.* **2020**, *22*, e16504. [CrossRef]
27. Interprofessional Education Collaborative IPEC. Core Competencies for Interprofessional Collaborative Practice: 2016 Update. 2016. Available online: https://ipec.memberclicks.net/assets/2016-Update.pdf; https://www.ipecollaborative.org/ipec-core-competencies (accessed on 9 January 2024).
28. WHO. *Framework for Action on Interprofessional Education & Collaborative Practice*; No. WHO/HRH/HPN/10.3; World Health Organisation: Geneva, Switzerland, 2010.
29. Rauch, M.; Bettermann, V.; Tipold, A.; Wissing, S.; Kleinsorgen, C. Use of Actors or Peers as Simulated Clients in Veterinary Communication Training. *J. Vet. Med. Educ.* **2022**, *50*, e20210055. [CrossRef]
30. Luderer, C.; Donat, M.; Baum, U.; Kirsten, A.; Jahn, P.; Stoevesandt, D. Measuring attitudes towards interprofessional learning. Testing two German versions of the tool "Readiness for Interprofessional Learning Scale" on interprofessional students of health and nursing sciences and of human medicine. *GMS J. Med. Educ.* **2017**, *34*, Doc33. [CrossRef]
31. Heise, S.A.C.; Tipold, A.; Rohn, K.; Kleinsorgen, C. Measuring Veterinarian Professions' Readiness for Interprofessional Learning in a Pre- and Post-Intervention Study. *Animals* **2024**, *14*, 229. [CrossRef]
32. Rees, C.; Sheard, C.; Davies, S. The development of a scale to measure medical students' attitudes towards communication skills learning: The Communication Skills Attitude Scale (CSAS). *Med. Educ.* **2002**, *36*, 141–147. [CrossRef]
33. Rauch, M. Interprofessionelle Bedarfsermittlung von Kommunikationsfaähigkeiten und Evaluation von Schauspielereinsatz im Kommunikationstraining in der Tiermedizin. Doctoral Thesis, Stiftung Tierärztliche Hochschule Hannover, Hannover, Germany, 2021.
34. Gaida, S.; Hartl, A.; Tipold, A.; Dilly, M. Communication identity in veterinary medicine: A grounded theory approach. *Vet. Rec. Open* **2018**, *5*, e000310. [CrossRef]
35. McDermott, M.P. Veterinary communication skills and training in the United Kingdom and the United States of America. 2018.
36. Radford, A.D.; Stockley, P.; Taylor, I.R.; Turner, R.; Gaskell, C.J.; Kaney, S.; Humphris, G.; Magrath, C. Use of simulated clients in training veterinary undergraduates in communication skills. *Vet. Rec.* **2003**, *152*, 422–427. [CrossRef]
37. Bahramsoltani, M.; Broer, S.; Langforth, S.; Eule, C.; Prior, A.; Vogt, L.; Li, T.T.; Schirone, R.; Pohl, A.; Jensen, K.C. Outcome of Communication Training in Veterinary Studies: Influence on the Perception of the Relevance of Veterinary Competencies and Self-Assessment of Communication Skills. *Animals* **2023**, *13*, 1516. [CrossRef] [PubMed]
38. Mossop, L.; Gray, C.; Blaxter, A.; Gardiner, A.; MacEachern, K.; Watson, P.; Whittlestone, K.; Robbe, I. Communication skills training: What the vet schools are doing. *Vet. Rec.* **2015**, *176*, 114–117. [CrossRef]
39. Dreier-Wolfgramm; Homeyer, S.; Oppermann, R.F.; Hoffmann, W. A model of interprofessional problem-based learning for medical and nursing students: Implementation, evaluation and implications for future implementation. *GMS J. Med. Educ.* **2018**, *35*, Doc13. [CrossRef]
40. van Diggele, C.; Roberts, C.; Burgess, A.; Mellis, C. Interprofessional education: Tips for design and implementation. *BMC Med. Educ.* **2020**, *20*, 455. [CrossRef]

41. Baldwin, D.C., Jr. Some historical notes on interdisciplinary and interprofessional education and practice in health care in the USA. 1996. *J. Interprof Care* **2007**, *21* (Suppl. S1), 23–37. [CrossRef] [PubMed]
42. Almalki, A.; Park, Y.S.; Tekian, A. Needs Assessment for Interprofessional Education: Implications for Integration and Readiness for Practice. *Healthcare* **2021**, *9*, 411. [CrossRef]
43. Singh, J.; Matthees, B. Facilitating Interprofessional Education in an Online Environment during the COVID-19 Pandemic: A Mixed Method Study. *Healthcare* **2021**, *9*, 567. [CrossRef]
44. Blackwell, M.J. Beyond philosophical differences: The future training of veterinarians. *J. Vet. Med. Educ.* **2001**, *28*, 148–152. [CrossRef]
45. Washburn, S.E.; Cook, A.K.; Tayce, J.D. Replacing a Veterinary Physiology Endocrinology Lecture with a Blended Learning Approach Using an Everyday Analogy. *J. Vet. Med. Educ.* **2022**, *49*, 61–70. [CrossRef]
46. Root Kustritz, M.V.; Molgaard, L.K.; Rendahl, A. Comparison of student self-assessment with faculty assessment of clinical competence. *J. Vet. Med. Educ.* **2011**, *38*, 163–170. [CrossRef]
47. McArthur, M.; Fitzgerald, J. Evaluation of a Communication Skills Training Program for Companion-Animal Veterinarians: A Pilot Study Using RIAS Coding. *J. Vet. Med. Educ.* **2016**, *43*, 111–125. [CrossRef]
48. Ruf, D.; Berner, M.M.; Kriston, L.; Harter, M. E-Learning—An important contribution to general medical training and continuing education? *Bundesgesundheitsblatt Gesundheitsforschung Gesundheitsschutz* **2008**, *51*, 1061–1069. [CrossRef] [PubMed]
49. Decloedt, A.; Franco, D.; Martle, V.; Baert, A.; Verwulgen, A.; Valcke, M. Development of Surgical Competence in Veterinary Students Using a Flipped Classroom Approach. *J. Vet. Med. Educ.* **2021**, *48*, 281–288. [CrossRef] [PubMed]
50. Kelly, R.F.; Mihm-Carmichael, M.; Hammond, J.A. Students' Engagement in and Perceptions of Blended Learning in a Clinical Module in a Veterinary Degree Program. *J. Vet. Med. Educ.* **2021**, *48*, 181–195. [CrossRef] [PubMed]
51. Tolks, D.; Kuhn, S.; Kaap-Fröhlich, S. Teaching in times of COVID-19. Challenges and opportunities for digital teaching. *GMS J. Med. Educ.* **2020**, *37*, Doc103. [CrossRef] [PubMed]
52. Schick, K.; Reiser, S.; Schacht, L.; Janssen, L.; Thomm, E.; Dinkel, A.; Fleischmann, A.; Berberat, P.O.; Bauer, J.; Gartmeier, M. How can communicative competence instruction inmedical studies be improved through digitalization? *GMS J. Med. Educ.* **2020**, *37*, Doc57.
53. Fabriz, S.; Mendzheritskaya, J.; Stehle, S. Impact of Synchronous and Asynchronous Settings of Online Teaching and Learning in Higher Education on Students' Learning Experience During COVID-19. *Front. Psychol.* **2021**, *12*, 733554. [CrossRef]
54. Breen, H. Virtual collaboration in the online educational setting: A concept analysis. *Nurs. Forum* **2013**, *48*, 262–270. [CrossRef]
55. Hinding, B.; Brunahl, C.A.; Buggenhagen, H.; Gronewold, N.; Hollinderbaumer, A.; Reschke, K.; Schultz, J.H.; Junger, J. Pilot implementation of the national longitudinal communication curriculum: Experiences from four German faculties. *GMS J. Med. Educ.* **2021**, *38*, Doc52. [CrossRef]
56. Hanley, A.; Kedrowicz, A.A.; Hammond, S.; Hardie, E.M. Impact of Team Communication Training on Performance and Self-Assessment of Team Functioning during Sophomore Surgery. *J. Vet. Med. Educ.* **2019**, *46*, 45–55. [CrossRef]
57. Nestel, D.; Robbe, I.J.; Jones, K.V. Personal and professional development in undergraduate health sciences education. *J. Vet. Med. Educ.* **2005**, *32*, 228–236. [CrossRef]
58. Estrada, A.H.; Samper, J.; Stefanou, C.; Blue, A. Contemporary Challenges for Veterinary Medical Education: Examining the State of Inter-Professional Education in Veterinary Medicine. *J. Vet. Med. Educ.* **2022**, *49*, 71–79. [CrossRef]
59. Herrmann, L.; Freise, F.; Tipold, A.; Schaper, E. Ergebnisse des Progress Test Tiermedizin an der Stiftung Tierärztliche Hochschule Hannover. *Berl. Münch Tierärztl Wochenschr.* **2021**, *134*, 1–11. [CrossRef]
60. Zintl, J. Untersuchungen zum Selbstregulierten Lernen in der Studieneingangsphase der Veterinärmedizin an der Tierärztlichen Hochschule Hannover. Doctoral Thesis, Tierärztliche Hochschule Hannover, Hannover, Germany, 2022.
61. Zintl, J.; Kleinsorgen, C.; Tipold, A.; Schaper, E. Die Studieneingangsphase in der Tiermedizin—Herausforderungen, Chancen und Bedarfe. *Berl. Und Münchener Tierärztliche Wochenschr.* **2023**, *135*, 1–16. [CrossRef]
62. Rhind, S.M.; Baillie, S.; Kinnison, T.; Shaw, D.J.; Bell, C.E.; Mellanby, R.J.; Hammond, J.; Hudson, N.P.; Whittington, R.E.; Donnelly, R. The transition into veterinary practice: Opinions of recent graduates and final year students. *BMC Med. Educ.* **2011**, *11*, 64. [CrossRef] [PubMed]

MDPI AG
Grosspeteranlage 5
4052 Basel
Switzerland
Tel.: +41 61 683 77 34

Animals Editorial Office
E-mail: animals@mdpi.com
www.mdpi.com/journal/animals

www.ingramcontent.com/pod-product-compliance
Lightning Source LLC
Chambersburg PA
CBHW061437210926
51850CB00008B/1538